SKIN DISEASE

Diagnosis and Treatment

SKIN DISEASE
Diagnosis and Treatment

THOMAS P. HABIF, M.D.
Adjunct Professor of Medicine
    (Dermatology)
Dartmouth Medical School
Hanover, New Hampshire

MARK J. QUITADAMO, M.D.
Assistant Professor of Medicine
    (Dermatology)
Dartmouth Medical School
Hanover, New Hampshire

JAMES L. CAMPBELL, JR., M.D., M.S.
Assistant Professor of Dermatology
    (Medicine)
University of Massachusetts
    Medical School
Worcester, Massachusetts

KATHRYN A. ZUG, M.D.
Associate Professor of Medicine
    (Dermatology)
Dartmouth Medical School
Hanover, New Hampshire

Editor: **Elizabeth M. Fathman**
Developmental Editor: **Ellen Baker Geisel**
Project Manager: **Carol Sullivan Weis**
Project Specialist: **Pat Joiner**
Designer: **Mark Oberkrom**

Illustrator: **Jeanne Robertson**
Layout Design: **Jeanne E. Genz**
Digital Color Scanning: **William P. James**
Project Organization: **Laura A. McCann**

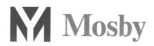

An Affiliate of Elsevier

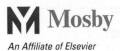

An Affiliate of Elsevier

NOTICE

Pharmacology is an ever-changing field. Standard safety precautions must be followed, but as new research and clinical experience broaden our knowledge, changes in treatment and drug therapy may become necessary or appropriate. Readers are advised to check the most current product information provided by the manufacturer of each drug to be administered to verify the recommended dose, the method and duration of administration, and contraindications. It is the responsibility of the licensed prescriber, relying on experience and knowledge of the patient, to determine dosages and the best treatment for each individual patient. Neither the publisher nor the editor assumes any liability for any injury and/or damage to persons or property arising from this publication.

Permissions may be sought directly from Elsevier's Health Sciences Rights Department in Philadelphia, USA: phone: (+1)215-238-7869, fax: (+1)215-238-2239, email: healthpermissions@elsevier.com. You may also complete your request on-line via the Elsevier Science homepage (http://www.elsevier.com), by selecting 'Customer Support' and then 'Obtaining Permissions'.

Mosby, Inc.
An Affiliate of Elsevier
11830 Westline Industrial Drive
St. Louis, Missouri 63146

Printed in the United States of America

International Standard Book Number 0-8151-3762-1

03 04 TG/KP 9 8 7 6 5

Preface

Changes in health care delivery require an increasing level of sophistication among primary care providers in all medical disciplines. Dermatology is no exception, since 10% of all out-patient medical visits to primary care physicians are for dermatologic problems.

This book was designed as a field guide for the diagnosis and management of common dermatologic conditions. Content is meant to be current, concise, and consistent rather than all-inclusive. Photographs were chosen to illustrate key diagnostic features of specific conditions. Color-coded figures represent statistical maps showing the likely distribution of skin lesions.

It is our sincere hope that this book becomes a valued and often used resource in your medical library.

Thomas P. Habif
James L. Campbell, Jr.
Mark J. Quitadamo
Kathryn A. Zug

Contents

SKIN DISEASE

Diagnosis and Treatment

1 | Topical Therapy

■ BASIC PRINCIPLES OF TREATMENT

A wide variety of medications are available for treating skin disease. Specific medications are covered in detail in the appropriate sections. Basic principles of topical treatment are discussed here.

PRESERVING THE INTEGRITY OF NORMAL SKIN

- The skin is an important barrier that must be maintained to function properly.
- Any insult that removes water, lipids, or protein from the epidermis alters the integrity of this barrier and compromises its function.
- Restoration of the normal epidermal barrier is accomplished with the use of mild soaps and emollient creams and lotions.

CREAMS AND LOTIONS

- Creams and lotions restore water and lipids to the epidermis.
- Numerous brands are available.
- Creams are thicker and more lubricating than lotions.
- The best time to apply lubricants is after washing, when the skin has been hydrated. The skin should be patted dry and the cream or lotion applied. Lubricants should not be applied to wet skin.
- Lubricants should be applied as frequently as necessary to keep the skin soft.
- It is not necessary to buy special moisturizers for the face, body, eyelids, and hands. Any moisturizer can be used in any region.
- Patients should be advised not to spend large sums on moisturizers produced by cosmetic companies. These preparations have no special properties and are sometimes extremely expensive.
- They should check with their physician for specific recommendations.

Abbreviated List of Lubricating Creams and Lotions

(There are many other effective products.)

Thicker creams and ointments

(Thicker creams and ointments are greasy but substantial and long lasting; many patients prefer evening or bedtime application.)
Vaseline petroleum jelly
Aquaphor ointment
Eucerin cream

Lighter creams

Acid Mantle
Cetaphil cream
DML cream
Moisturel cream
Nutraplus cream

Lighter lotions

Cetaphil lotion
DML lotion
Nutraderm lotion
Moisturel lotion

Special preparations

- Sarna lotion contains camphor and menthol and controls pruritus.
- Lac-Hydrin contains ammonium lactate and is highly effective for treating very dry skin. It is available by prescription and is expensive.
- Amlactin is similar to Lac-Hydrin but is less expensive and available without prescription.
- Alpha hydroxy acid moisturizers may be slightly more effective than other creams, but they usually are not worth the extra cost.

WASHING AND SOAPS

- Several mild bar and liquid soaps are suitable for treating inflammatory skin disease.
- Patients should be advised not to wash excessively. It is not necessary to bathe daily in the winter in the Northern states. Patients should wash in the axilla and groin and avoid rubbing soap daily over the entire body. They should also avoid the overaggressive use of washcloths that can exfoliate and remove the stratum corneum. Exfoliating skin may be effective for treating acne, but it interferes with the care of inflamed, sensitive skin.
- Examples of mild bar soaps include Cetaphil, Dove, Keri, Basis, Oil of Olay, and many others. Pure Ivory soap is possibly the most drying and irritating.

DRY SKIN

- The tendency to have dry skin is an inherited trait and is common in atopic patients (those with a family or personal history of hay fever, asthma, dry skin, or eczema).
- Dry skin is more severe in the winter months, when the humidity is low.
- Dry skin is most commonly seen on the hands and lower legs. Initially the skin is rough and covered with fine white scales. Thicker tan or brown scales may appear.

WET DRESSINGS

- Wet dressings, or compresses, are a valuable aid in the treatment of exudative (wet) skin diseases.
  1. Obtain a clean, soft cloth such as bed sheeting or shirt material. The cloth need not be new or sterilized.
  2. Fold the cloth and cut to fit an area slightly larger than the area to be treated.
  3. Wet the folded dressings by immersing them in the solution, and wring them out to the point of sopping wet (neither running nor just damp).
  4. Place the wet compresses on the affected area. Do not pour solution on a wet dressing to keep it wet because this practice increases the concentration of the solution and may cause irritation. Remove the compress and replace it with a new one.
  5. Leave the dressings in place for 30 minutes to 1 hour. Dressings may be used two to four times a day or continuously. Discontinue the use of wet compresses when the skin becomes dry. Excessive drying causes cracking and fissures.
- The temperature of the compress solution should be cool when an antiinflammatory effect is desired and tepid when the purpose is to debride an infected, crusted lesion.
- A wet compress should not be covered with a towel or plastic. These items inhibit evaporation, promote maceration, and increase skin temperature, which facilitates bacterial growth.

Benefits of Wet Compresses

- Inflammation suppression: The evaporative cooling causes the constriction of superficial vessels, thereby decreasing erythema and the production of serum. Wet compresses soothe acute inflammatory processes such as acute poison ivy.
- Wound debridement: The compress macerates vesicles and crust, helping debride these materials when the compress is removed.
- Drying: Repeated cycles of wetting and drying promote drying of weeping wet lesions.

■ TOPICAL CORTICOSTEROIDS

Topical corticosteroids are the most effective medications for treating inflammatory skin disease. They are very safe when used properly. They all have similar properties and differ only in strength, base, and price.

GENERIC VS. BRAND NAMES

- Many generic topical steroid formulations are available. Triamcinolone acetonide is probably the most widely used.
- Vasoconstrictor assays have shown large differences in the activity of generic formulations compared with that of brand-name equivalents: many are inferior, a few are equivalent, and a few are more potent than brand-name equivalents.
- Many generic topical steroids have vehicles with different ingredients (e.g., preservatives) than brand-name equivalents.

STRENGTH

Potency: Groups I Through VII

- The antiinflammatory properties of topical corticosteroids result in part from their ability to induce vasoconstriction of the small blood vessels in the upper dermis.
- This property is used in an assay procedure to determine the strength of each new product.
- These products are subsequently tabulated in seven groups, with group I the strongest and group VII the weakest (see Appendix D).
- The treatment sections of this book recommend topical steroids by group number rather than by generic or brand name because the agents in each group are essentially equivalent in strength.

Choosing the Appropriate Strength

- The best results are obtained when preparations of adequate strength are used for a specified length of time.
- Weaker, "safer" strengths often fail to provide adequate control. Patients whose conditions do not respond after 1 to 4 weeks of treatment should be reevaluated.

Superpotent Topical Steroids (Group I)

- Clobetasol propionate (Cormax), betamethasone dipropionate (Diprolene), and diflorasone diacetate (Psorcon) are examples of the most potent topical steroids available.

- In general, no more than 45 to 60 gm of cream or ointment should be used each week.
- Side effects are minimized and efficacy increased when medication is applied once or twice daily for 2 weeks followed by 1 week of rest.
- This cyclic schedule (pulse dosing) is continued until resolution occurs.
- A weaker topical steroid can be used intermittently for maintenance.
- Psorcon can be used with plastic dressing occlusion. The other superpotent topical steroids should not be used with occlusive dressings.
- Patients must be monitored carefully. Refills should be strictly limited.

Concentration

- The concentration of steroid listed on the tube cannot be used to compare its strength with other steroids.
- Some steroids are much more powerful than others and need be present only in small concentrations to produce the maximal effect.
- Most of the topical steroids are fluorinated. That is, a fluorine atom has been added to the hydrocortisone molecule. Fluorination increases potency.
- Products such as Westcort cream increase potency without fluorination. However, the same side effects occur with these nonfluorinated steroids.

VEHICLE

The base determines the rate at which the active ingredient is absorbed through the skin.

Creams

Creams are complex mixtures and usually contain preservatives. They have the following characteristics:

- White color and somewhat greasy texture
- Components that may cause irritation, stinging, and allergy
- High versatility (i.e., may be used in nearly any area) (Therefore creams are the base most often prescribed.)
- Best treatment for acute exudative inflammation
- Most useful vehicle for intertriginous areas (skin touches skin [e.g., groin, rectal area, axilla])

Ointments

The ointment base contains a limited number of organic compounds consisting primarily of greases, such as petroleum jelly, with little or no water. Many ointments are preservative free. Ointments have the following characteristics:

- Translucence (They look like petroleum jelly.)
- Greasy feeling that persists on skin surface
- More lubrication (Thus they are desirable for drier lesions.)
- Greater penetration of medicine than with creams and therefore enhanced potency
- Too occlusive for acute (exudative) eczematous inflammation or intertriginous areas such as the groin

Gels

Gels are greaseless mixtures. They have the following characteristics:

- A clear base, sometimes with a jellylike consistency
- Use for acute exudative inflammation, such as poison ivy, and for scalp areas where other vehicles mat the hair

Solutions and Lotions

Solutions may contain water and alcohol as well as other chemicals. They have the following characteristics:

- Clear or milky appearance
- Most useful application for the scalp because they penetrate easily through hair, leaving no residue
- Possible stinging and drying when applied to intertriginous areas such as the groin

STEROID-ANTIBIOTIC MIXTURES

- Some products contain a combination of antibiotics and corticosteroids.
- The majority of steroid-responsive skin diseases can be managed successfully without topical antibiotics.
- Neomycin is a sensitizer and may complicate an already prolonged and difficult-to-control problem such as stasis dermatitis.

Lotrisone Cream

- Lotrisone cream contains a combination of the antifungal agent clotrimazole and the corticosteroid betamethasone dipropionate. It is expensive.
- It is indicated for the topical treatment of tinea pedis, tinea cruris, and tinea corporis.
- This product is used by many physicians as the topical antiinflammatory agent of first choice.

- Most inflammatory skin diseases are not infected or contaminated by fungus.
- Lotrisone is a marginal drug for cutaneous fungal infections.

AMOUNT OF CREAM TO DISPENSE

- The amount of cream dispensed is very important.
- A sufficient amount of cream should be prescribed, and limits on duration and frequency of application should be set.
- The fingertip unit (FTU) provides the means to assess how much cream to dispense and apply.
- An FTU is the amount of ointment expressed from a tube with a 5-mm-diameter nozzle and applied from the distal skin crease to the tip of the index finger.
- One FTU weighs approximately 0.5 gm. The number of FTUs required to cover specific body areas is illustrated in Appendix C.

APPLICATION
Frequency: Intermittent dosing

These are general guidelines; specific instructions and limitations must be established for each case.

Group I topical steroids

- Difficult-to-treat inflammatory diseases such as plaque psoriasis and hand eczema respond most effectively when a group I topical steroid is applied twice a day for 2 weeks, followed by 1 week of rest.
- The schedule of 2 weeks of treatment followed by 1 week of rest is repeated until the lesions have cleared.

Group II through VII topical steroids

- Group II through VI topical steroids should be applied twice each day.
- The duration of application should be limited to 2 to 6 weeks.
- If adequate control is not achieved, treatment should be stopped for 4 to 7 days, and then another course of treatment is begun.

Methods
Simple application

- Creams and ointments should be applied in thin layers and slowly massaged into the site one to four times a day.
- It is unnecessary to wash before each application.

- Different skin surfaces vary in the ability to absorb topical medicine.
- The thin eyelid skin heals quickly with group VI or VII steroids. Higher-potency steroids should be avoided.
- The palms and soles offer a greater barrier to the penetration of topical medicine and require more potent therapy.
- Intertriginous areas (e.g., axilla, groin, rectal area, area under the breasts) respond more quickly with weaker-strength creams. The apposition of two skin surfaces performs the same function as an occlusive dressing, which greatly enhances penetration.
- The skin of infants and young children is more receptive to topical medicine and responds quickly to weaker creams. A baby's diaper has the same occlusive effect as covering with a plastic dress-

ing. The penetration of steroid creams is greatly enhanced; therefore only group VI and VII preparations should be used under a diaper.
- Inflamed skin absorbs topical medicines much more efficiently. This explains why red inflamed areas generally have such a rapid initial response when treated with weaker topical steroids.

Occlusion
- Occlusion with a plastic dressing (e.g., Saran Wrap) is an effective method for enhancing the absorption of topical steroids.
- The plastic dressing holds perspiration against the skin surface, which hydrates the top layer of the epidermis (stratum corneum).
- Topical medication penetrates a moist stratum corneum much more effectively than it penetrates dry skin.

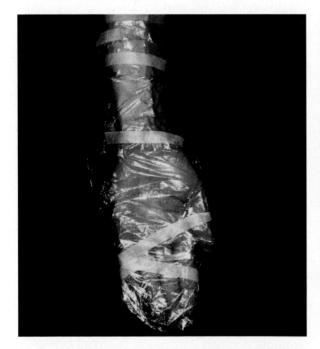

Occlusion of the hand. A plastic bag is pulled on and pressed against the skin to expel air. Tape is wound snugly around the bag.

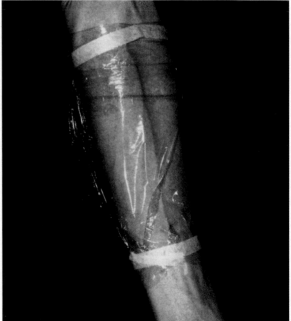

Occlusion of the arm. A plastic sheet (e.g., Saran Wrap) is wound around the extremity and secured at both ends with tape. A plastic bag with the bottom cut out may be used as a sleeve and held in place with tape or an Ace bandage.

- Eruptions that are resistant to simple application may heal quickly with the introduction of a plastic dressing.
- Nearly any area can be occluded; the entire body may be occluded with a vinyl exercise suit, which is available at most sporting goods stores.
- Occlusive dressings are used more often with creams than with ointments, but ointments may be covered if the lesions are particularly dry.
- Weaker, less expensive products (e.g., triamcinolone cream 0.1%) provide excellent results. Large quantities of this medicine may be purchased at a substantial savings.
- Occlusion of moist areas may encourage the rapid development of infection.
- Dressings should not remain on the area continuously because infection or follicular occlusion may result. If an occluded area suddenly becomes worse or if pustules develop, infection, usually with staphylococci, should be suspected. Oral antistaphylococcal antibiotics (e.g., cephalexin [Keflex] 500 mg twice a day) should be given.
- A reasonable occlusion schedule is twice daily for a 2-hour period or 8 hours at bedtime, with simple application once or twice during the day.
- Occluded areas often become dry, and the use of lubricating cream or lotion should be encouraged. A cream or lotion may be applied shortly after the medicine is applied, when the plastic dressing is removed, or at other convenient times.

Method of occlusion

- The area should be cleaned with mild soap and water. Antibacterial soaps are unnecessary.
- The medicine is gently rubbed into the lesions, and the entire area is covered with plastic (e.g., Saran Wrap, Handi-Wrap, plastic bags, or gloves).
- The dressing is secured with tape so that it is close to the skin and the ends are sealed. An airtight dressing is unnecessary. The plastic may be held in place with an Ace bandage or a sock.
- The best results are obtained if the dressing remains in place for at least 2 hours. Many patients find that bedtime is the most convenient time to wear a plastic dressing and therefore wear it for 8 hours.
- More medicine is applied shortly after the dressing is removed and while the skin is still moist.

Systemic Absorption

- The possibility of producing systemic side effects from the absorption of topical steroids is unlikely when medications are used as previously described.
- Persistent, unsupervised use of group I topical steroids over wide areas can result in significant systemic absorption and side effects.
- The number of refills of all topical steroids should be limited.

Avoid weaker, "safe" preparations

- In an attempt to avoid complications, physicians often choose a weaker steroid preparation than that indicated; the weaker preparations all too frequently fall short of expectations and fail to give the desired antiinflammatory effect. The disease does not improve but rather becomes worse because of the time wasted using the ineffective cream.
- The treatment of intense inflammation with hydrocortisone cream 0.5% is a waste of time and money. Generally, a topical steroid of adequate strength (see treatment recommendations for each disease) should be used two to four times daily for a specific length of time, such as 7 to 21 days, to obtain rapid control.

Children

- The relative safety of moderately strong topical steroids and their relative freedom from serious systemic toxicity despite widespread use in the very young has been clearly demonstrated.
- Patients should be treated for a specific length of time with a medication of appropriate strength.
- Steroid creams should not be used continually for many weeks, and patients whose conditions do not respond in a predictable fashion should be reevaluated.
- Group I topical steroids should be avoided in prepubertal children.
- Only group VI or VII agents should be used in the diaper area and for only 3 to 10 days. Growth parameters should be monitored in children on chronic topical glucocorticoid therapy.

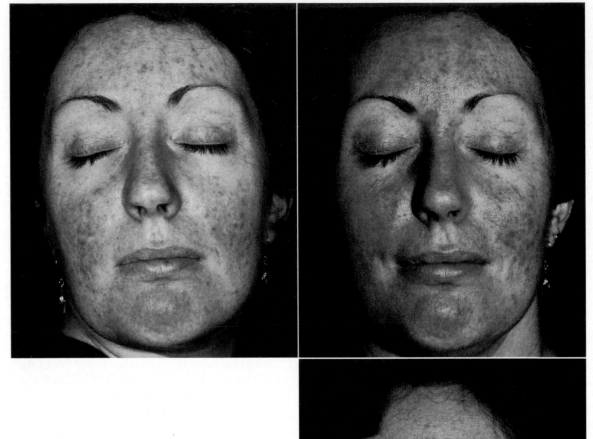

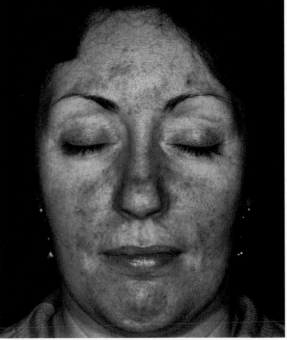

Steroid rosacea. **A,** Numerous red papules formed on the cheeks and forehead with constant daily use of a group V topical steroid for more than 5 years. **B,** Ten days after discontinuing use of the group V topical steroid. **C,** Two months after the use of topical steroids was discontinued. Telangiectasia has persisted; rosacea has improved with oral antibiotics.

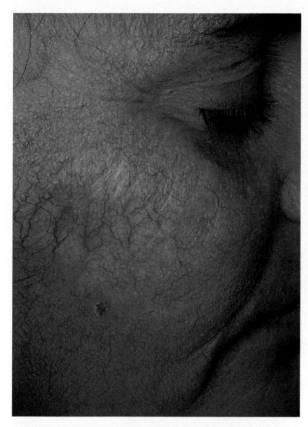

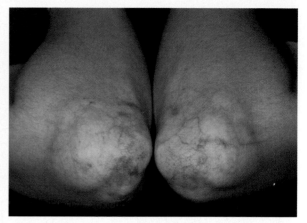

Steroid atrophy. Atrophy with prominence of the underlying veins and hypopigmentation after the use of a superpotent steroid applied daily for 3 months to treat psoriasis. Note that small plaques of psoriasis persist. Atrophy improves after topical steroids are discontinued, but some hypopigmentation may persist.

Atrophy and telangiectasia after continual use of a group IV topical steroid for 6 months. The atrophy may improve after the topical steroid is discontinued, but the telangiectasia often persists.

ADVERSE REACTIONS

Topical steroids have an excellent safety record. They can produce a number of adverse reactions, however. Once these are understood, the most appropriate strength can be prescribed confidently. The reported adverse reactions to topical steroids follow:

- Allergic contact dermatitis
- Burning, itching, irritation, dryness caused by the vehicle
- Hypertrichosis of face
- Hypopigmentation
- Miliaria and folliculitis after occlusion with plastic
- Nonhealing leg ulcers (Steroids applied to any leg ulcer retard the healing process.)
- Ocular hypertension, glaucoma, cataracts
- Rebound phenomenon (i.e., psoriasis becomes worse after treatment is stopped)
- Rosacea, perioral dermatitis, acne
- Skin atrophy with telangiectasia, stellate pseudoscars (arms), purpura, striae (from anatomic occlusion [e.g., groin, axillae])
- Skin blanching from acute vasoconstriction
- Systemic absorption
- Tinea incognito, impetigo incognito, scabies incognito

Steroid Rosacea and Perioral Dermatitis

- Steroid rosacea is a side effect observed when topical steroids are applied to the face for weeks or months.
- Erythema and pustulation occur each time attempts are made to discontinue topical treatment.

Atrophy

- Long-term use of strong topical steroids in the same area may result in thinning of the epidermis and regressive changes in the connective tissue in the dermis.

- The affected areas are often depressed slightly below normal skin and usually reveal telangiectasia, prominence of underlying veins, and hypopigmentation.
- Purpura and ecchymosis result from minor trauma.
- The face, dorsa of the hands, extensor surfaces of the forearms and legs, and intertriginous areas are particularly susceptible.
- In most cases, atrophy is reversible and may be expected to disappear in the course of several months.

Striae

- Long-term use (over months) of even weak topical steroids on the upper inner thighs or in the axillae results in striae similar to those on the abdomens of pregnant women.
- These changes are irreversible.
- Pruritus in the groin area is common, and patients are considerably relieved by the less potent steroids. Symptoms often recur after treatment is terminated. It is a great temptation to continue topical treatment on an as-needed basis. Every attempt must be made to determine the underlying process and discourage long-term use.

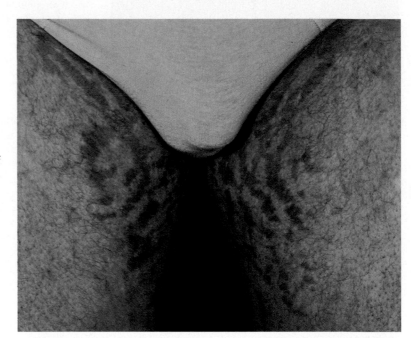

Striae of the groin after long-term use of group V topical steroids for pruritus. These changes are irreversible.

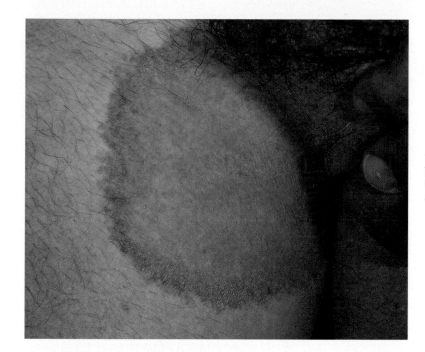

Typical presentation of tinea of the groin before treatment. A fungal infection of this type typically has a sharp, scaly border and shows little tendency to spread.

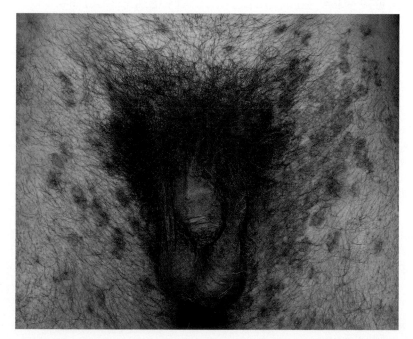

Tinea incognito. Bizarre pattern of widespread inflammation created by applying a group II topical steroid twice daily for 3 weeks to an eruption similar to that in the previous photograph. A potassium hydroxide preparation showed numerous fungi.

2 Eczema

■ ACUTE ECZEMATOUS INFLAMMATION

DESCRIPTION
- Acute eczematous inflammation is characterized by erythema, edema, and vesiculation. Weeping or oozing of acute lesions is typical. Pruritus is often severe.

HISTORY
- Causes of acute eczema include allergic contact hypersensitivity to specific allergens such as poison ivy, oak, or sumac and other allergens (such as nickel, topical medicaments, fragrance, and rubber additives). In an id reaction, vesicular reactions occur at a distant site from a fungal infection.
- Stasis dermatitis, scabies, irritant reactions, and dyshidrotic and atopic eczema may present as an acute eczematous inflammation.

SKIN FINDINGS
- Findings include erythema, edema, vesiculation, and weeping. Inflammation can be moderate to intense. Tiny, clear, fluid-filled vesicles are seen on the skin surface. Bullae may develop.

LABORATORY
- Patch testing should be considered if the distribution suggests, the problem is recurrent, or there is known occupational or other exposure to cutaneous allergens.

COURSE AND PROGNOSIS
- If the provoking factors can be avoided, the eruption improves over 7 to 10 days, with clearing usual by 3 weeks.

- Excoriation predisposes to infection and causes serum, crust, and purulent material to accumulate.

MANAGEMENT
- Cool, wet compresses and topical steroid creams allow vasoconstriction and suppress inflammation and itching. A clean cloth is soaked in Burow's cool solution and then placed on affected areas for 30 minutes. Then an appropriate topical steroid cream is applied and rubbed in.

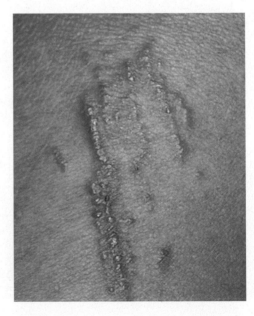

Vesicles are present in a linear distributions.

- Oral corticosteroids are reserved for severe or generalized acute eczema. The dosage is approximately 1mg/kg/day initially, tapering over 3 weeks.
- Oral antihistamines (i.e., diphenhydramine [Benadryl] and hydroxyzine [Atarax]) can relieve itching, and their sedative effect may promote sleep.
- If secondary infection is suspected, an anti–*Staphylococcus aureus* antibiotic (e.g., cephalexin, dicloxacillin) is administered for 10 to 14 days.

CAVEAT

- Causes of acute eczematous inflammation are diverse and include atopic dermatitis, id reactions, stasis dermatitis, irritant and allergic contact dermatitis, and dermatophyte infections. The clinician should look for telltale distributions and ask about prior history and exposures to help with making the diagnosis.

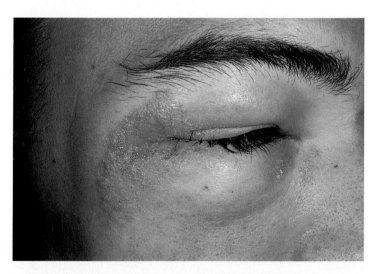

Acute inflammation causes swelling, oozing, and crusting.

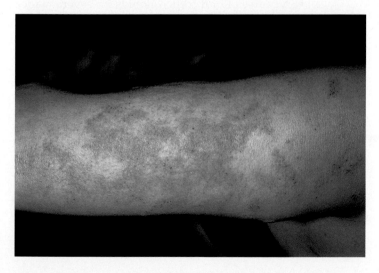

Vesicles are characteristic of the acute phase of eczematous inflammation. Itching is often intense.

■ RHUS DERMATITIS (POISON IVY)

DESCRIPTION

- Poison ivy, oak, and sumac are the most common causes of allergic contact dermatitis in the United States.
- Oleoresin (lipid-soluble portion) contains a mixture of highly allergenic catechol chemicals called *urushiols*.

HISTORY

- Contact with the plant leaf, stem, or root, even in autumn and winter, results in a pruritic bullous eruption within 8 to 72 hours of exposure in a previously sensitized individual and 12 to 21 days for an individual who has not yet been sensitized (primary sensitization).
- About half of American adults develop the rash if they are exposed; 30% to 40% require prolonged exposure to produce the dermatitis.
- About 10% to 15% of Americans cannot be sensitized.

SKIN FINDINGS

- Clinical findings vary with the quantity of oleoresin that contacts the skin, pattern of contact, individual susceptibility, and regional variations in skin reactivity.
- Findings include pruritic, edematous, linear erythematous streaks, usually with vesicles and large bullae on exposed skin.
- Airborne particulate matter from burning results in intense, pruritic facial erythema and edema; the eyelids can be dramatically swollen.

COURSE AND PROGNOSIS

- Eruption lasts 10 days to as long as 3 weeks.
- Short courses of oral corticosteroids (such as dose packs) may result in rebound phenomenon with prompt blistering when corticosteroids are discontinued.
- The rash resolves completely without scarring.
- Impetigo or cellulitis may occur from scratching and bacterial secondary infection.

DISCUSSION

- Poison ivy is not spread by blister fluid.
- The allergenic oleoresin can be spread by contaminated clothing, garden tools, or animals.
- Cross-reacting allergens include mango peel, oil of raw cashew nut shells, Japanese lacquer, and ginkgo fruit pulp.

MANAGEMENT

- The skin should be washed with soap to inactivate and remove allergic oleoresin, thereby preventing further skin penetration and contamination. Washing is most effective if done within 15 minutes of exposure.
- Exposed clothing and tools should be cleansed with soapy water.
- Short, cool tub baths with or without colloidal oatmeal (Aveeno) are soothing for itching and swelling.
- Calamine lotion controls itching, but prolonged use causes excessive drying.
- Hydroxyzine and diphenhydramine control itching and encourage sleep.
- Cold, wet compresses with tap water or Burow's solution are highly effective during the acute blistering stage. They are applied for 15 to 30 minutes several times a day for 1 to 4 days until blistering and severe itching are controlled. Tap-water cool compresses are very useful for severe facial or eyelid edema.
- A medium-potency topical steroid should be generously applied after the wet compress.
- A course of oral corticosteroids for severe, widespread inflammation is started at 0.75 to 1mg/kg/day every morning and is slowly tapered over 3 weeks.
- Poison ivy oleoresin in capsules and injectable syringes for hyposensitization has been removed from the market as a result of side effects and incomplete efficacy.

CAVEAT

- A black spot within a vesicular or bullous eruption suggests poison ivy. Oxidized urushiol leaves a black, inklike mark on the skin.

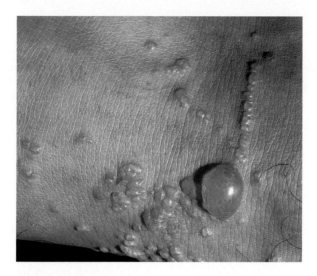

Classic presentation of poison ivy. Vesicles appear in a linear distribution and vary in size.

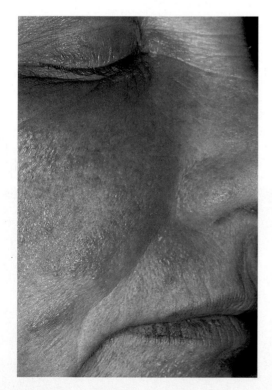

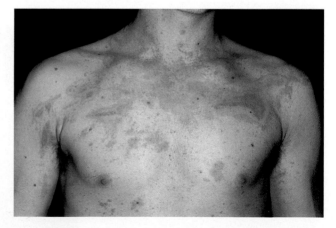

Vesicles disappear, and erythema and scaling appear as the acute phase ends. Itching is less intense.

Poison ivy can involve wide areas. The decision to use oral or topical steroids depends on the severity of the symptoms.

■ SUBACUTE ECZEMATOUS INFLAMMATION

DESCRIPTION

- The inflammation consists of itchy, red, scaling plaques in various configurations.

HISTORY

- This condition may evolve from acute (vesicular) eczema.
- Patients complain of dermatitis that has been present over a week.
- Itching is variable.
- The condition resolves spontaneously without scarring.
- Excoriation converts this condition to a chronic process.

SKIN FINDINGS

- Erythema and scaling occur in various patterns.
- Often, there are indistinct borders.
- Redness may be faint or intense.

ETIOLOGY AND CLINICAL PRESENTATION

- Contact allergy, irritation, atopic dermatitis, stasis dermatitis, nummular eczema, fingertip eczema, fungal infections are possible etiologies.

TREATMENT

Steroids

- Group II to V steroid creams two to four times a day with or without plastic occlusion are administered. Occlusion hastens resolution.
- Steroid ointments can be applied two to four times a day without occlusion.
- Tar ointments and creams (many over-the-counter preparations) provide an alternative for steroid-resistant lesions and are moderately effective in some patients.
- Wet dressing should be avoided because they cause excessive dryness.

Moisturizers

- Moisturizers are an essential part of therapy.
- They work best when applied a few hours after topical steroids.
- Application should continue for days or weeks after the inflammation has cleared.
- Frequent application is encouraged.
- Moisturizers are most effective when applied directly after the skin is patted dry after a shower.
- Creams (e.g., Eucerin, Cetaphil, DML, Acid Mantle) are better than lotions.
- Infrequent washing with mild soap (e.g., Dove, Cetaphil, Keri, Purpose, Basis) is also helpful.

Antibiotics

- Antibiotics (e.g., cephalexin, dicloxacillin) are used for secondary infection.

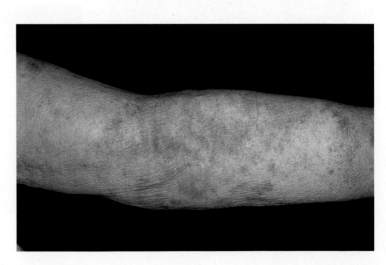

Erythema and scaling with indistinct borders are characteristic. Vesicles may never appear. This is often the initial presentation in the winter in atopic patients.

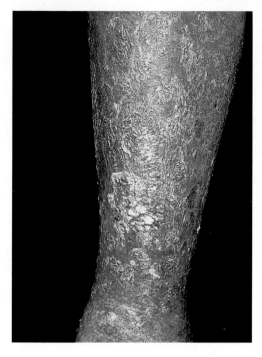

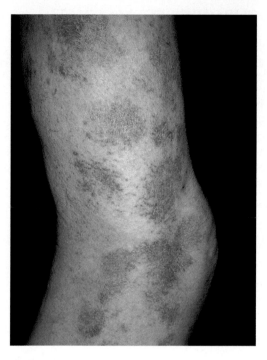

Erythema and scale can be extensive and suggest a diagnosis of psoriasis. Psoriatic plaques often have distinct borders.

The configuration of subacute inflammation varies. Plaques may be patchy or confluent.

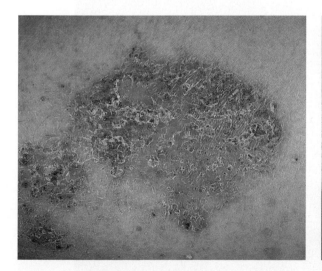

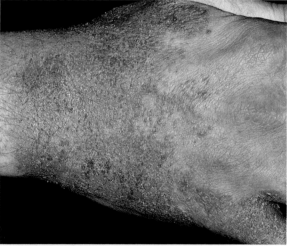

This plaque is dense and covered with scale. The borders are somewhat distinct. Differentiation from psoriasis in this case would be difficult. The history and types of plaques in other areas may be needed to confirm a diagnosis.

Atopic dermatitis. The back of the hands is a common site to find subacute irritant dermatitis.

◼ CHRONIC ECZEMATOUS INFLAMMATION

DESCRIPTION

- The skin is red, scaling, and thickened (lichenified).

HISTORY

- There is moderate to intense itching.
- Scratching and rubbing become habitual and are done unconsciously.
- The disease becomes self-perpetuating.
- Scratching leads to thick skin, which itches even more.

SKIN FINDINGS

- Intense itching can lead to excoriations.
- Inflamed, itchy skin thickens, and surface skin markings become more prominent.
- Thick plaques with deep parallel skin markings appear (lichenification).
- Sites commonly involved are those easily reached or creased areas.
- Hyperpigmentation or hypopigmentation appears.

ETIOLOGY AND CLINICAL PRESENTATION

- Atopic dermatitis, habitual scratching, lichen simplex chronicus, chapped and fissured feet, nummular eczema, asteatotic eczema, fingertip eczema, hyperkeratotic eczema are possible etiologies.

TREATMENT

- Chronic eczematous inflammation is often resistant to treatment; the key to success is breaking the itch-scratch cycle.

Topical Steroids

- Group I or II creams or ointments applied two to four times a day can be effective.
- Groups II through V steroids are used with plastic occlusion for 2 to 8 hours.
- Intralesional injections (e.g., Kenalog, 10 mg/ml) are very effective; resistant plaques are reinjected at 3- to 4-week intervals.
- Steroid-impregnated tape (e.g., Cordran tape) should be left on for 12 hours.
- Liquid nitrogen therapy or excision is performed if multiple therapies fail or if the lesion is very thick.

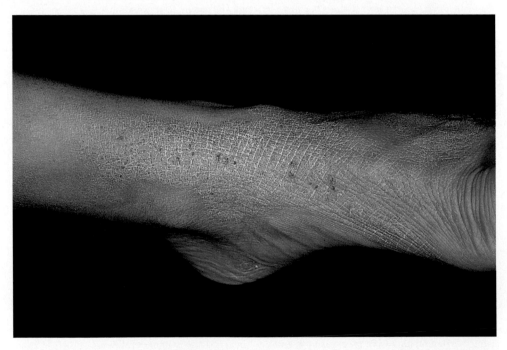

Marked accentuation of skin lines, indistinct borders, and minimal scale are all characteristics of chronic eczema.

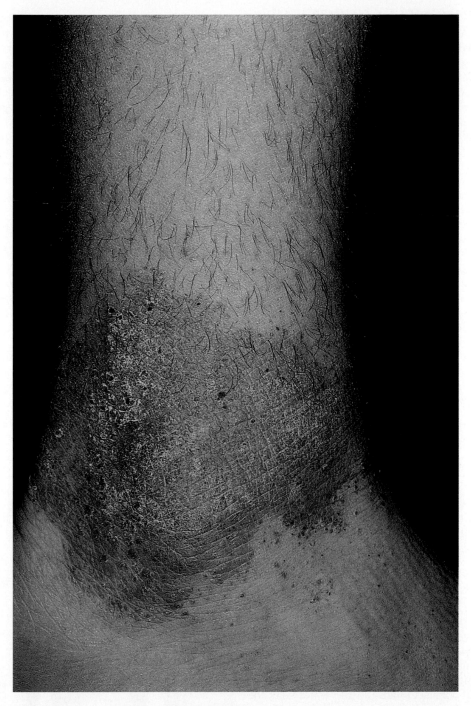

The isolated plaque is thick with accentuation of skin lines. Scratching for weeks produces this picture.

■ LICHEN SIMPLEX CHRONICUS

DESCRIPTION

- A localized plaque of chronic eczematous inflammation is created by habitual scratching. This plaque is frequently located on the wrists, ankles, and nape of the neck.

HISTORY

- This condition is more common in adults but may be seen in atopic children.

SKIN FINDINGS

- Findings include a sharply demarcated, red, scaly plaque with prominent skin lines (lichenification).
- Although this is a chronic eczematous disease, acute changes of vesiculation and weeping may result from sudden allergy to topical treatments.
- Moist scaling, serum, crust, and pustules signal secondary infection.
- Nodules, usually smaller than 1 cm and scattered randomly in the scalp, occur in patients who frequently pick at the scalp.
- The areas most commonly affected are conveniently reached; these areas include the outer portion of the lower legs, wrists and ankles, posterior neck, scalp, upper eyelids, fold behind the ear, scrotum, vulva, and anal skin.

LABORATORY

- A potassium hydroxide scraping should be considered. Tinea infection can mimic lichen simplex chronicus.

COURSE AND PROGNOSIS

- A typical plaque stays localized and shows little tendency to enlarge with time. Once established, the plaque does not usually increase in size.

TREATMENT

- Stress may play a role in some individuals and should be acknowledged and addressed.
- The patient should understand that the rash does not resolve until even minor scratching and rubbing are stopped.
- Scratching frequently takes place during sleep, and the affected area may have to be covered.
- Treatment consists of a 5-minute water soak followed by the application of a medium- to high-potency topical steroid in an ointment base.
- The treatment of the anal area, genitalia, or fold behind the ear does not require the administration of potent topical steroids; rather, these areas should be treated with group V or VI topical steroids in an ointment base.
- For scalp lesions, a group I or II steroid gel such as fluocinonide (Lidex) or solution such as clobetasol (Cormax scalp solution) is applied twice each day.
- Moist, secondarily infected areas respond to oral antibiotics and a topical steroid lotion.
- Nodules caused by picking at the scalp may be very resistant to treatment, requiring monthly intralesional injections with triamcinolone acetonide (Kenalog, 5 to 10 mg/ml).

DISCUSSION

- This condition was once referred to as *localized neurodermatitis*.
- The patient derives great pleasure from scratching to relieve the inflamed site. Loss of pleasurable sensation or continued subconscious habitual scratching may explain why this eruption frequently recurs.
- Lichen simplex chronicus affecting the genitalia or anus can be a very chronic, difficult problem causing considerable distress and frustration.

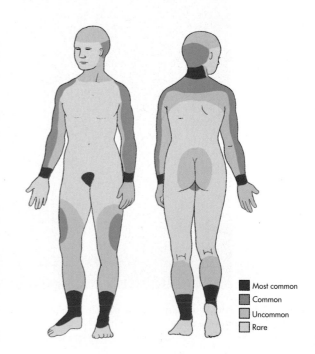

Most common
Common
Uncommon
Rare

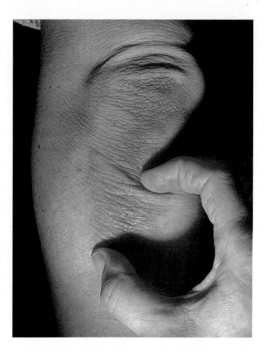

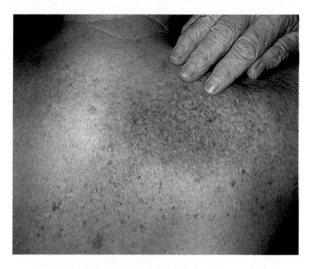

The classic presentation. Skin lines are markedly accentuated. Itching becomes more intense as the plaque thickens and a vicious cycle continues.

The upper back is another target for repetitive scratching and excoriation. Linear white scars that are evidence of a habit that has existed for months or years should be sought.

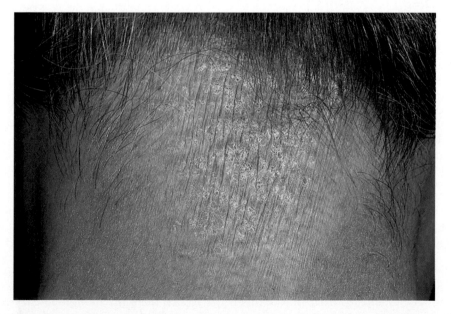

The occipital lower scalp is possibly the most common target for anxiety-induced scratching. Very thick, difficult-to-manage plaques may form and sometimes become infected. Psoriasis can present with similar features. Short courses of oral antibiotics are sometimes the appropriate initial treatment before potent topical steroids are started.

■ HAND ECZEMA

DESCRIPTION

- A common, often chronic problem with multiple causative and contributing factors, hand eczema can be categorized as follows:

<table>
<tr><td>Irritant, p. 35</td><td>Keratolysis exfoliativa, p. 38</td></tr>
<tr><td>Atopic, p. 50</td><td>Fingertip, p. 36</td></tr>
<tr><td>Allergic, p. 30</td><td>Hyperkeratotic, p. 21</td></tr>
<tr><td>Nummular, p. 40</td><td>Pompholyx (dyshidrosis),</td></tr>
<tr><td>Lichen simplex</td><td>   p. 42</td></tr>
<tr><td> chronicus, p. 18</td><td>Id reaction</td></tr>
</table>

- Each of these types of hand eczema is covered separately elsewhere in this book.
- Irritant hand eczema is most common, followed by atopic hand eczema.
- Allergic contact hand eczema accounts for perhaps 10% to 25% of cases.

HISTORY

- The epidemiology is as follows: female patients are affected more often than male patients.
- Occupational risks include irritant chemical exposure, frequent wet work, chronic friction, and work with sensitizing chemicals.

Exogenous Factors

- Irritants include chemical irritants (such as solvents), friction, cold air, and low humidity.
- Allergens include occupational and other types. Immediate type I allergy can involve reactions to latex and food proteins, and delayed type IV allergy can involve reactions to rubber additives, preservatives, fragrance, and nickel. Ingested allergens (i.e., nickel) may play a role.
- Infection can involve id reactions, including hand eczema as a reaction to a distant focus of fungal ("dermatophytid") or bacterial ("bacterid") infection.

Endogenous Factor

- Atopic diathesis (hay fever, asthma, atopic eczema) may be seen.

SKIN FINDINGS

- The entire skin should be examined for clues and contributing factors and for exclusion of other dermatoses (i.e., psoriasis).
- This condition is variable; acute, subacute, and chronic eczematous changes may be seen. Al-though there is no reliable association between clinical pattern and etiology, the following findings may prove useful:
  - Xerosis, erythema, burning more than itching on dorsal or volar hands: irritant factors should be suspected.
  - Nummular eczema, dorsal hands and fingers: allergy, irritation, or atopy can play a role; occasionally, contact urticaria (type I allergy) is the culprit.
  - Recurrent crops of intensely pruritic vesicles on lateral fingers and palms: pompholyx, otherwise called *dyshidrotic eczema*, should be suspected.
  - Fingertip eczema (dryness, splitting, tenderness, no itch): an irritant, an endogenous factor (atopy during the winter), or frictional eczema should be suspected.
  - In fingertip eczema, the skin is hyperkeratotic with minute vesicles, if there is itching, atopy or contact allergic factors should be suspected.
  - Erythema, scaling, itching, in "apron" (base of the fingers) area of palm: atopy should be suspected.

NONSKIN FINDINGS

- Atopic patients may have a personal or family history of atopy, including eczema in childhood, hay fever, or asthma.

COURSE AND PROGNOSIS

- If exposures to irritants and allergens can be avoided early in the course, the prognosis is often good for complete recovery.
- Continued or long-standing exposure to irritants and allergens can result in chronic dermatitis.
- Avoidance and appropriate care often improve the condition, but in many patients, they do not resolve it entirely.

TREATMENT

- Treatment involves the identification and avoidance of irritants (i.e., frequent hand-washing and water exposure, soaps, detergents, solvents).
- Protective measures (i.e., vinyl gloves for wet work) can be taken.
- Topical medium- to high-potency corticosteroids twice daily are administered. Ointments are preferred over creams. Occlusion with plastic to increase penetration should be considered.

- For severe dermatitis, a superpotent topical corticosteroid is applied after wet compresses containing Burow's solution, twice a day for the initial 3 to 5 days of treatment, followed by the application of a medium-potency topical corticosteroid twice a day for several weeks.
- The following should be considered: topical tar hand soaks with Balnetar oil, two or three capfuls diluted in a basin of water for 15 to 30 minutes twice a day, followed by the application of topical corticosteroid.
- Systemic steroids may occasionally be required to bring a severe acute inflammation under control.
- Most patients' conditions improve with avoidance of irritants, treatment with topical corticosteroids, and frequent lubrication.

- If allergy is suspected (hand edema, vesiculation, itching, and particularly dorsal hand or fingertip eczema), patch testing should be done to evaluate for contributing or causal allergens.
- The patient should be referred to a dermatologist in chronic unresponsive cases.

DISCUSSION

- Chronic, endogenous vesicular hand dermatitis (pompholyx) represents a most difficult management problem.
- Patch testing to occupational and environmental allergens should be considered if hand eczema does not improve or resolve with simple measures.

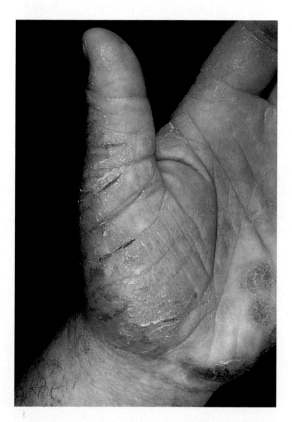

The skin is very dry, cracked, and painful. Long-standing hand eczema may be a continuous cycle of acute (vesicle), subacute (redness and scaling), and chronic (very dry, cracked) inflammation.

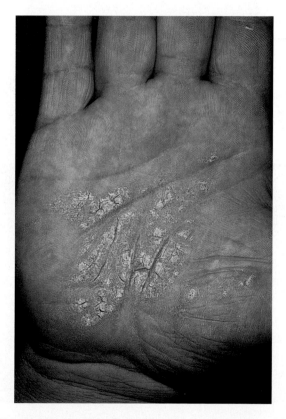

Dry, thick, fissured hyperkeratotic eczematous plaques are difficult to treat. They last for months and years and may be impossible to distinguish from psoriasis.

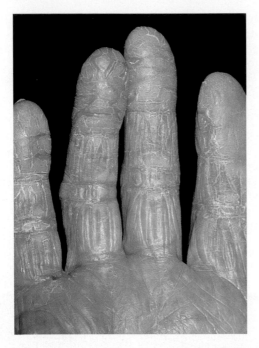

Long-standing severe subacute and chronic eczema may be atopic dermatitis, irritant dermatitis, or a contact allergy.

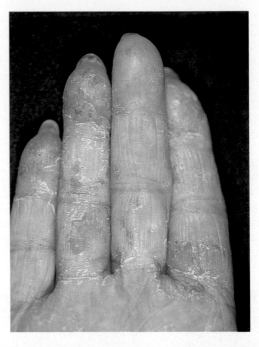

This dry, cracked, and chronic inflammation had been present for months. Inflammation of the fingertips is a poor prognostic sign indicating a difficult-to-manage form of eczema that may be long lasting.

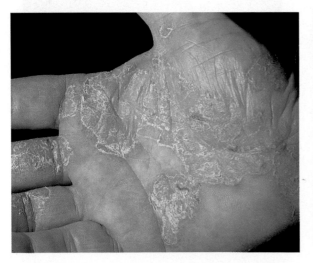

Psoriasis must always be in the differential diagnosis for chronic hand eczema. The differential diagnosis of hand eczema and psoriasis of the palms may not be possible even with a biopsy.

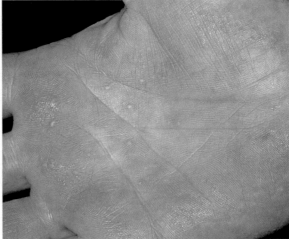

Isolated vesicles with erythema and minimal scale are the classic presentation for dyshidrotic eczema.

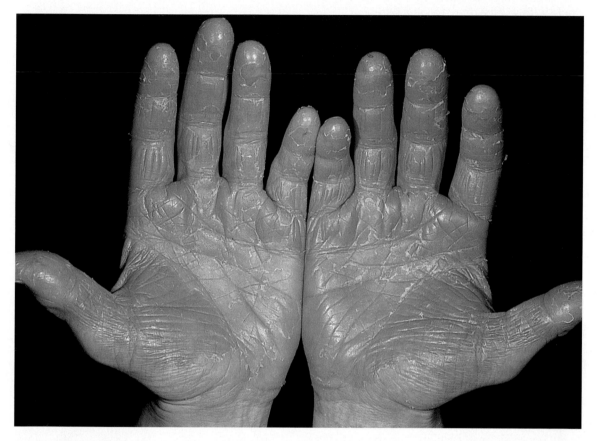

Severe subacute inflammation. The differential diagnosis includes irritant contact dermatitis, allergic contact dermatitis, atopic dermatitis, and psoriasis.

■ ASTEATOTIC ECZEMA

DESCRIPTION

- A distinctive clinical pattern of eczematous dermatitis is caused by excessive dryness and chapping of the skin.

HISTORY

- Asteatotic eczema is a form of subacute eczematous dermatitis that tends to be chronic and low grade with winter-time seasonal flares.
- Men and women are equally affected.
- It is more common in patients with the atopic diathesis (see section on atopic dermatitis), especially in later life.
- Most patients have a history of previous similar flares.
- The prevalence peaks in late winter and improves in summer, especially in colder, drier climates.
- The condition becomes symptomatic sometime after the early autumn and tends to improve late the following spring.
- Any cutaneous site may be affected, although the lower legs are most commonly involved.
- Early on, affected individuals often note that their skin looks and feels dry.
- With progression, itch, with increasing inflammation, becomes the most prominent symptom.
- Burning and stinging occur in advanced cases with fissures and crusting.

SKIN FINDINGS

- The clinical picture is that of subacute eczematous dermatitis.
- Xerosis with accentuated skin markings are constant features from the onset.
- Inflammation is at first subtle but becomes more pronounced over time.
- Faint, poorly defined erythema progresses to fiery red, acute eczematous papules that coalesce into broad plaques.
- Vesicles are not typically seen, although excoriations are nearly universal.
- Dry, thin desquamation progresses toward a pattern termed eczema craquele, with thin superficial fissures reminiscent of the cracked finish on porcelain or of a dried river bed.
- With progression, the eczema develops acute features with weeping, crusting, and intense erythema.

NONSKIN FINDINGS

- Fever is unusual and suggests cellulitis.

LABORATORY

- The clinical picture is distinctive enough that skin biopsy is rarely needed to establish the diagnosis.
- Skin biopsy confirms epidermal spongiosis with dermal inflammation and often secondary impetiginization.

COURSE AND PROGNOSIS

- Seasonal recurrence should be expected.
- Mild seasonal flares with itching and xerosis tend to improve with the changing seasons and lubrication.
- Active subacute inflammation generally responds with topical medium-potency corticosteroid ointments and also improves with the season.
- A severe localized flare with acute features such as weeping and crusting also responds to individualized topical therapy as outlined later.
- Severe flares should be treated aggressively because they may become generalized.

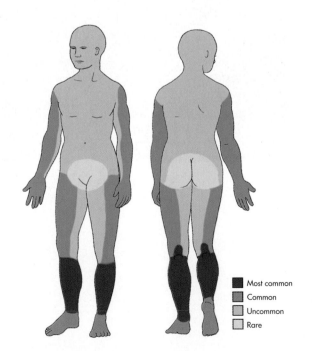

Most common
Common
Uncommon
Rare

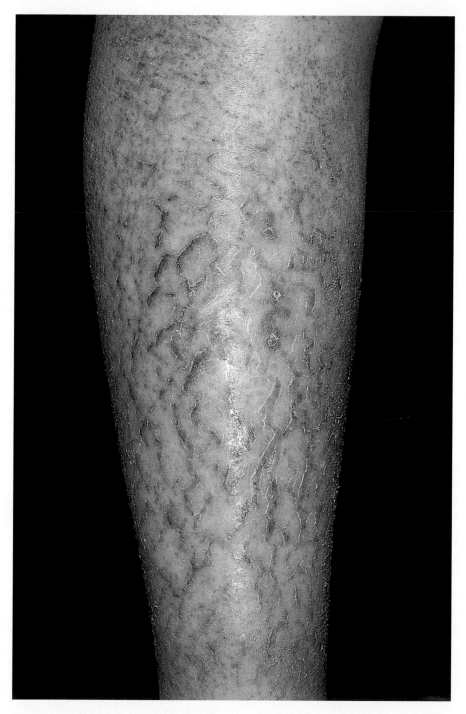

The skin is very dry, cracked, and fissured. This pattern evolved in an atopic patient who continued to wash excessively dry skin. The skin may be painful.

DISCUSSION

- The differential diagnosis includes other subacute eczematous dermatoses such as stasis dermatitis, irritant contact dermatitis, atopic dermatitis, allergic contact dermatitis, and cellulitis.
- More than one dermatosis may be present. The second dermatosis may mask or exacerbate the primary eczematous process.
- Irritant and allergic contact dermatitis may develop as a result the patient's own efforts at self-treatment.
- The patient should be asked about what he or she has been applying to the involved areas.
- Stasis dermatitis occurs, commonly on the lower legs, in older patients. There is usually a history of vascular insufficiency and leg edema and the presence of hemosiderin staining of the skin.

MANAGEMENT

- Therapy is determined by the stage of the asteatotic eczema and the degree of inflammation.
- For xerosis, therapy consists of sensitive skin measures, namely the limited use of mild superfatted soaps and the liberal use of emollients.
- Petrolatum offers a preservative-free choice as a lubricant, although patient compliance may be difficult.
- Moisturizers containing lactic acid, urea, or glycolic acid may also be useful.
- Early inflammation is best treated topically with a medium-potency corticosteroid, preferably in an ointment base.
- Therapy should be continued until the erythema and scaling resolve.
- The liberal use of emollients should then be continued as a prophylaxis against recurrence.
- Localized flares with acute eczematous features of weeping and crusting should be treated first as acute eczema.

- Patients require close follow-up during this stage because localized flares may become generalized (autoeczematization).
- Referral to a dermatologist should be considered for the management of acute flares and an evaluation for possible allergic contact dermatitis.
- Wet dressings with Burow's solution along with a medium-potency topical corticosteroids in a cream base are helpful for débridement and reducing inflammation.
- Oral antibiotics may be indicated for secondary impetiginization and the possibility of cellulitis.
- Once the weeping, induration, and crusting improve, the wet compresses should be stopped to avoid excessive drying of the involved areas.
- A medium-potency topical corticosteroid ointment should be continued until the redness and scaling resolve.
- Thereafter, sensitive skin care, including emollients, are helpful in limiting recurrence.
- Systemic steroid therapy is rarely indicated for asteatotic eczema and then only for generalized (autoeczematization) flares.

CAVEAT

- The patient should be asked what he or she is doing to treat the dermatitis.
- Home remedies might include household bleach, astringents, hot water, shake lotions, and other potential irritants that may be exacerbating the condition.
- Neomycin, corticosteroids, and preservatives in various medicaments are potential sources of allergens.
- Referral to a dermatologist should be considered for patients with refractory dermatitis.

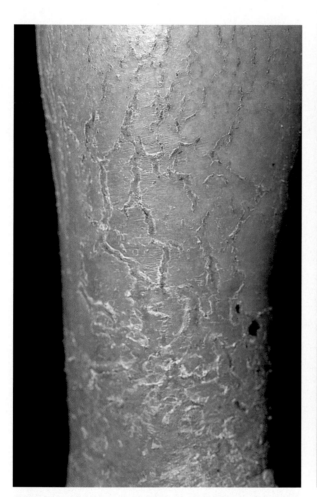

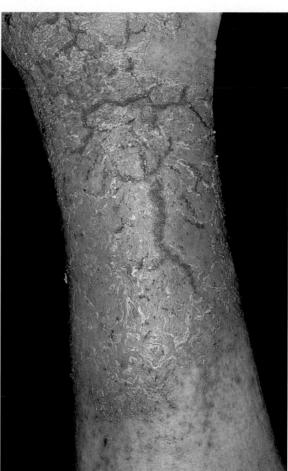

The skin has split into a cracked porcelain pattern that is the hallmark of asteatotic eczema.

Asteatotic eczema. Severe long-standing inflammation. There are large deep fissures and secondary infection.

■ CHAPPED, FISSURED FEET

DESCRIPTION

- Findings include scaling, erythema, and tender fissuring of the plantar feet.
- The tendency for severe chapping is age related; it is most common in prepubertal children.

HISTORY

- Chapped, fissured feet are most common in early autumn, when the weather becomes cold and heavy socks and impermeable shoes or boots are worn.
- Symptoms include soreness and pain.
- The mean age of onset is 7.3 years; the mean age of remission is 14.3 years.

SKIN FINDINGS

- The skin on the plantar feet, especially the weight-bearing skin of the toes and metatarsal regions, is dry, erythematous, scaly, and fissured. Fissuring may be deep and very tender.

- Chapping may extend to the sides of the toes.
- Eventually, the entire sole may be involved.

DISCUSSION

- The role of atopy is suspected but not yet well defined.

DIFFERENTIAL DIAGNOSIS

- Tinea pedis
- Allergic contact dermatitis
- Psoriasis

TREATMENT

- The feet should be kept dry; prolonged time in moist, occlusive shoes should be avoided.
- A thick emollient ointment should be applied several times each day.
- If the condition is pruritic, topical steroids provide some relief. Group II or III topical steroid ointments are applied twice a day, preferably with plastic-wrap occlusion at bedtime, for 2 to 3 weeks.

Dryness and scaling first appear about the toes and may spread to involve the entire surface of the soles.

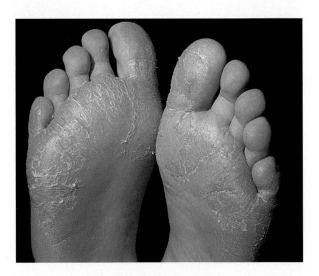

Symmetric involvement of the soles. Inflammation may be confined to just part of the soles. Tinea and contact dermatitis are in the differential diagnosis.

- A 15-minute tar-oil (Balnetar) soak is followed by the application of a lubricating ointment or topical corticosteroid.
- Preventative measures include changing into light leather shoes after the removal of wet boots, alternating footwear to allow complete drying, changing cotton socks frequently if moist.

CAVEAT

- Atopic dermatitis in children occurs mainly on the dorsal toes. Children with chapped, fissured feet complain of soreness and pain.

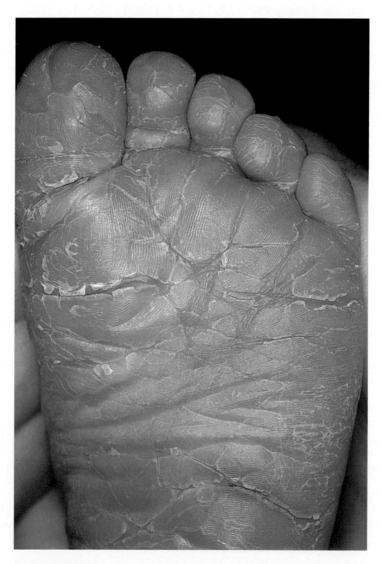

Cracks and fissures appear in cases of long duration. Pain becomes more intense than itching.

■ ALLERGIC CONTACT DERMATITIS

DESCRIPTION

- Allergic contact dermatitis is a delayed-type hypersensitivity reaction resulting in eczematous dermatitis.
- Poison ivy–induced dermatitis is a prototype of allergic contact dermatitis.
- Common causes of this type of allergy are nickel; rubber additives in items such as gloves and shoes (i.e., carbamates, thiurams, mercaptobenzathiazole); preservatives in water-based products such as toiletries, cosmetics, and cooling fluids (i.e., quaternium-15, imidazolidinyl urea, diazolidinyl urea, methylchloroisothiazolinone); fragrances and fragrance additives; dyes; formaldehyde and related chemicals; and topical medicaments (e.g., bacitracin, neomycin, hydrocortisone).

HISTORY

- Initial exposure and primary sensitization result in clinical inflammation generally 14 to 21 days after exposure.
- The time required for a previously sensitized person to develop clinically apparent inflammation is about 12 to 48 hours but may vary from 8 to 120 hours.
- Allergy to products (e.g., cosmetics, topicals) or other exposures can occur even when there is a history of prolonged use without difficulty.
- Multiple contact allergens are common.
- Points of interest for the history include the date of dermatitis onset, relationship to work (i.e., whether the condition improves during the weekend or vacations), work exposures, hobby and home exposures, and types of skin care products used.
- Individuals sensitized to topical medications or other allergens may develop generalized eczematous inflammation if those medications or chemically related substances are ingested. For example, raw cashew nut shell oil and poison ivy are chemically related.
- Some allergy-causing substances are photoallergins; sunlight and a chemical are required for the allergic reaction to occur.

SKIN FINDINGS

- The intensity of the inflammation depends on the degree of sensitivity, concentration, and quantity of antigen exposure.
- Allergic contact dermatitis is characterized by vesicles, edema, redness, and often, extreme pruritus. Strong allergens such as poison ivy result in bullae.
- Dermatitis distribution is usually first confined to the area of direct exposure.
- Dermatitis caused by plants is often distributed in linear streaks.
- Allergy to a topical product used on the face may be patchy and asymmetrically distributed.
- If exposure becomes chronic, allergic dermatitis may spread beyond the areas of direct contact.
- Strong sensitizers such as poison ivy may produce intense inflammation despite low concentration or exposure; weak sensitizers may cause only erythema.
- The hands, forearms, and face are common sites of allergic contact dermatitis. Allergic contact dermatitis may affect very limited skin sites such as the eyelids, dorsal hands, lips, and tops of the feet.
- Airborne particulate matter (i.e., burning poison ivy) can lead to dermatitis of the face (including the eyelids and postauricular skin), the neck, and other exposed skin surfaces.
- Photoallergic contact dermatitis typically affects the exposed skin of the face, neck, forearms, and dorsal hands; there is usually submental, upper eyelid, and postauricular sparing.
- Most occupational allergic contact dermatitis affects the hands; the face and eyelids may be affected if there is an airborne allergen.

LABORATORY

- Patch testing is performed by physicians trained in the technique and is indicated for cases of persistent or recurrent dermatitis despite appropriate topical therapy.
- Patch testing should be performed to screen for allergens, items of occupational or avocational relevance, and personal care products.
- Photopatch testing should also be performed in patients with photodistributed dermatitis.

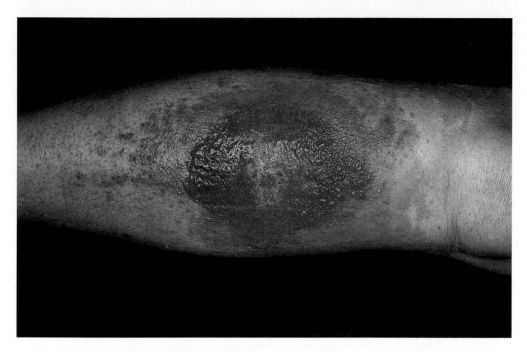

Poison ivy–induced dermatitis. Severe acute inflammation with confluent vesicles.

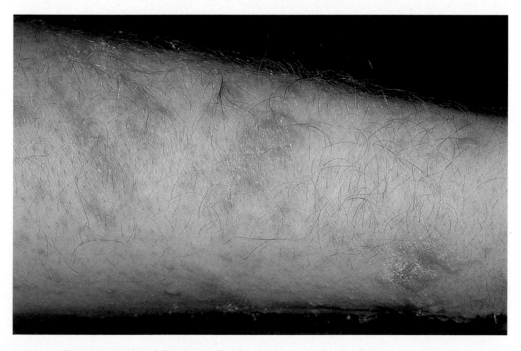

Poison ivy–induced dermatitis. The distribution is confined to the area of exposure.

DIFFERENTIAL DIAGNOSIS

- Irritant contact dermatitis (Patch testing is not performed for irritant type dermatitis.)
- Atopic dermatitis

TREATMENT

- Avoidance of the allergenic substance is essential to recovery.
- Identification of the cause is essential. If the cause is not obvious, treatment should be begun, and further evaluation and patch testing should be planned.
- Topical treatment involves a corticosteroid twice a day for 2 weeks.
- Corticosteroid potency is based on the body site affected: low potency for the face; medium potency for the arms, legs, and trunk; and high potency for the hands and feet.
- When possible, corticosteroid ointment rather than cream should be prescribed because additives in creams may be allergenic.
- The patient's skin regimen should be simplified to avoid further possible allergen exposure. No other topical products (except plain petrolatum or the prescribed corticosteroid) should be used during treatment.
- For severe or generalized allergic contact dermatitis, a 3-week tapering course of oral corticosteroids is appropriate. This should not be relied on repeatedly.
- Some allergens (such as hair-dye chemicals and glues) can penetrate rubber gloves, so protection may not be adequate.
- Some allergens, such as nickel and chromate, are associated with chronic dermatitis, despite avoidance.
- Time should be spent on patient education, detailing potential sources of exposure.
- Once an allergen is determined, reviewing allergen exposure lists in depth and providing suitable alternatives is recommended.

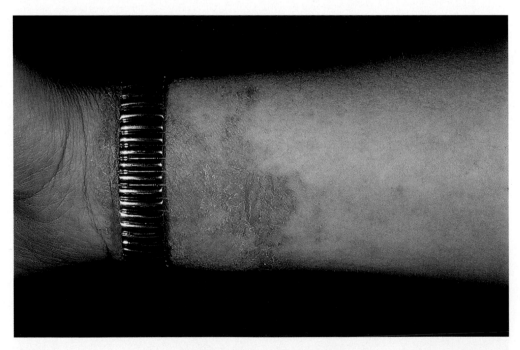

Allergic contact dermatitis to nickel.

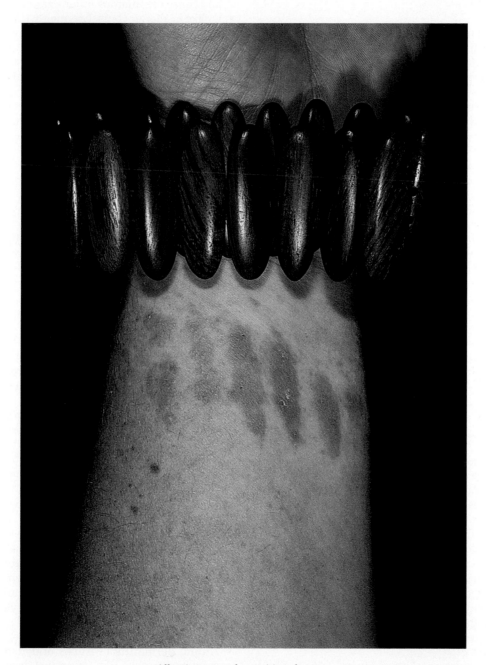

Allergic contact dermatitis to lacquer.

■ IRRITANT CONTACT DERMATITIS

DESCRIPTION

- Some 80% of cases of contact dermatitis involve irritant contact dermatitis.
- Irritant contact dermatitis is an eczematous dermatitis often caused by repeated exposure to mild irritants such as water, soaps, heat, and friction.
- The intensity of the inflammation is usually related to the concentration of irritant and the exposure time. Mild irritants cause dryness, fissuring, and erythema; strong irritant chemicals may produce an immediate reaction characterized by burning, erythema, edema, and possibly, ulceration of the skin.

HISTORY

- A background of atopy (hay fever, asthma, or eczema) predisposes to an increased susceptibility to skin irritation.
- Irritant contact dermatitis is the most common type of occupational skin disease.
- Employment duties and household duties, including child care and hobbies, are critical parts of the history. Jobs characterized by repeated wet work such as food service, health care, child care, and hairstyling predispose the patient to irritant contact dermatitis.
- Common irritants include detergents, acids, alkaline chemicals, oils, organic solvents, oxidants, reducing agents, and water.
- Coarse fibers, such as particulate fiberglass, or wood dust can cause irritant contact dermatitis.
- Exposure may occur from direct contact or the airborne route.
- Examples of irritants that can cause an airborne irritant contact dermatitis include fiberglass, formaldehyde, epoxy resins, industrial solvents, glutaraldehyde, and sawdust.
- Repeated friction and mechanical irritation can result in irritant contact dermatitis.
- Irritant eczematous dermatitis may occur with continuous exposure to mild irritants. Once the irritation threshold is reached, persistent dermatitis may result from less exposure to mild irritants (even water).
- Low environmental humidity reduces the threshold for irritation.
- Continuous exposure to moisture and wet-and-dry cycles in areas such as the hands, the diaper area, or the skin around a colostomy may eventually cause eczematous inflammation.
- Unlike in allergic contact dermatitis, in irritant contact dermatitis, prior sensitization is not required.
- An irritant dermatitis may become complicated by allergy as the number of applied topical remedies increases and damaged skin allows better penetration of allergens.
- Atopic individuals are predisposed to irritant contact dermatitis and often have prolonged dermatitis that is more difficult to manage.

SKIN FINDINGS

- The hands are most often affected. Both dorsal and palmar surfaces can be affected.
- Erythema, dryness, painful cracking or fissuring, and scaling are typical. Vesicles may be present.
- Symptoms of tenderness and burning are common. Often, burning predominates over itch.
- Acute irritant dermatitis may show juicy papules and/or vesicles on an erythematous patchy background, weeping, and edema.
- Persistent, chronic irritant dermatitis is characterized by lichenification, patches of erythema, fissures, excoriations, and scaling.
- A hyperkeratotic form characterized by repeated scaling, cracking, and low-grade erythema may result from repeated mechanical trauma, such as paper handling.
- Open skin may burn on contact with topical products that are otherwise usually tolerated.

LABORATORY

- A potassium hydroxide examination may be performed to exclude tinea.
- Patch testing should be performed to evaluate the role of contributing allergic contact dermatitis if the history suggests it (i.e., exposure to allergens) or if the condition is refractory or persistent despite treatment and preventive measures.
- Skin biopsy, which is rarely performed, shows spongiosis, dermal edema, and an inflammatory infiltrate of predominantly lymphocytes.

DIFFERENTIAL DIAGNOSIS

- Atopic dermatitis (Vesicles and itch are often more common in allergic contact dermatitis than in irritant contact dermatitis.)
- Allergic contact dermatitis
- Tinea

TREATMENT

- Early diagnosis, treatment, and preventive measures can prevent the development of a chronic irritant dermatitis.
- The avoidance of or a decreased exposure to cutaneous irritants is critical for recovery of an effective skin barrier.
- The number of wet-and-dry cycles resulting from activities such as repeated hand-washing should be decreased.
- Cotton gloves under vinyl gloves may allow for a decreased frequency of hand-washing for wet work.

- The mildest soap possible should be used, and when appropriate, no soap should be used.
- Appropriate protective gloves should be worn for specific solvent or chemical exposure. (When the patient's occupation is deemed relevant, Material Safety Data Sheets are consulted for exposure and protection information.)
- Frequent application of a bland emollient such as Vaseline or Aquaphor to affected skin is essential.
- For irritant hand dermatitis, a medium- to high-potency topical steroid ointment applied twice a day for several weeks can be helpful in reducing erythema, itching, swelling, and tenderness.

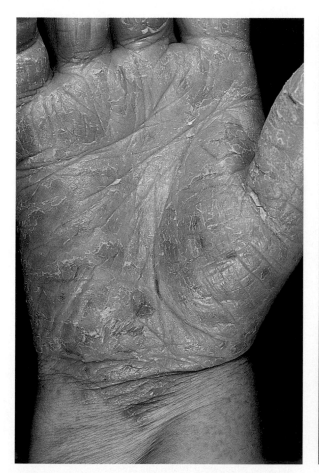

Erythema, dryness, painful cracking, or fissuring and scaling are typical. Psoriasis would be in the differential diagnosis.

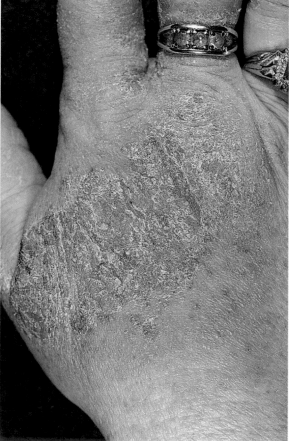

Erythema, dryness, and scaling are the characteristics findings in subacute irritant eczema.

■ FINGERTIP ECZEMA

DESCRIPTION

- This common form of eczema is limited to the fingertips.
- One finger or several can be affected.
- Itch is limited or is absent; often, tender or burning discomfort occurs.

HISTORY

- Usually, fingertip eczema is a winter problem, but it may occur year round.
- It is uncommon in children and occurs most frequently in adults.

ETIOLOGY

- Atopy may be a predisposing factor.
- Irritant chemicals or frictional contact may play a role.
- A less frequent etiology is allergic contact dermatitis to plants, resins, and glues.
- Occupational and hobby-related allergens, heat, repeated water exposure, repeated wet-and-dry cycles, and friction should be considered.

SKIN FINDINGS

- Dry, scaling, pink, and fissured fingertips are found.
- Peeling reveals red, tender skin.
- Vesiculation is not typically seen.
- The process stops before the distal interphalangeal joint is reached.

COURSE AND PROGNOSIS

- The condition may last for months or years and is often very resistant to treatment.
- Precipitating factors are often not easily and consistently avoided.

DISCUSSION AND DIFFERENTIAL DIAGNOSIS

- Allergy and psoriasis should be ruled out.
- An uncommon presentation of contact allergy should be considered in handlers of tulip bulbs, florists, and dentists or others who work with acrylate-type adhesives. An allergy to artificial nails must also be considered.
- If the nail is separated from the nailbed, candidal infection should be considered.

MANAGEMENT

- Management involves the avoidance of repeated wet-and-dry cycles, irritating detergents or solvents, heat, and friction.
- This condition should be managed as a subacute or chronic eczema; irritants should be avoided, and affected areas must be lubricated frequently.
- A bland emollient such as Vaseline should be applied frequently.
- Tar creams such as Fototar or MG217 should be applied twice each day.
- A lactic acid cream (Lac-Hydrin 12% cream) may be of some help.
- Medium-potency topical steroids with or without occlusion give temporary relief.

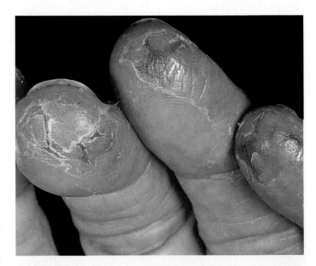

The tips are very dry, smooth, red, and fragile. The inflammation tends to be chronic. Spontaneous improvement occurs, but it is often of short duration. Patients manipulate and pick at the scale, which perpetuates this process.

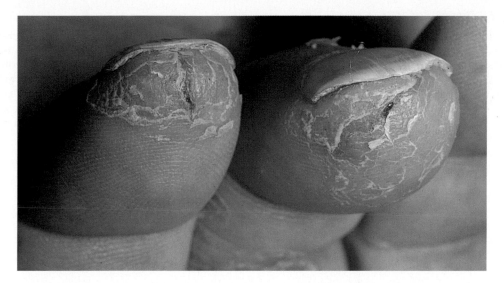

Patients protect these deep, painful cracks with bandage strips. They wear cotton gloves and heavy moisturizers to bed in an attempt to control this highly resistant form of eczema.

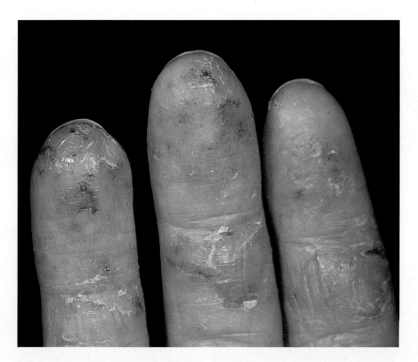

Inflammation may start on the fingertips but eventually may slowly spread to involve the fingers and palms.

■ KERATOLYSIS EXFOLIATIVA

DESCRIPTION

- Keratolysis exfoliativa is a common, chronic, asymptomatic, noninflammatory, bilateral peeling of the palms of the hands and soles of the feet; its cause is unknown.

HISTORY

- Keratolysis exfoliativa occurs most commonly during the summer.
- It is often associated with sweaty palms and soles.
- Some people have repeated episodes, and others experience this phenomenon only once.

SKIN FINDINGS

- Scaling starts simultaneously from several points on the palms or soles with 2 or 3 mm of round scale that appears to have originated from a ruptured vesicle; however, vesicles are never seen.
- The scales continue to peel and extend peripherally, forming larger, roughly circular areas resembling ringworm, and the central area becomes slightly red and in a few cases, tender.
- Scaling borders may coalesce.

COURSE

- This condition resolves in 1 to 3 weeks but may recur.

TREATMENT

- No therapy other than lubrication is required.

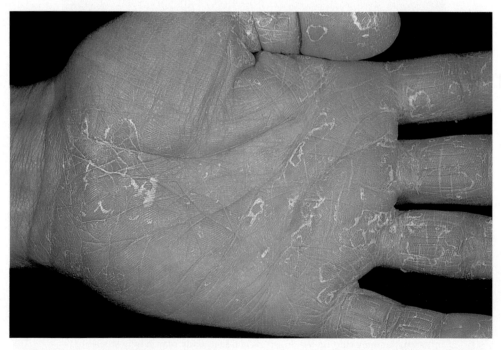

Spontaneous peeling of the palms is common and unexplained. It may be seasonal and asymptomatic. Moisturizers are usually sufficient, and the process resolves with age.

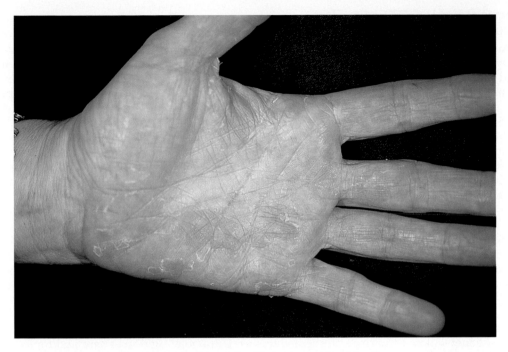

Some cases persist and the skin becomes red and fragile.

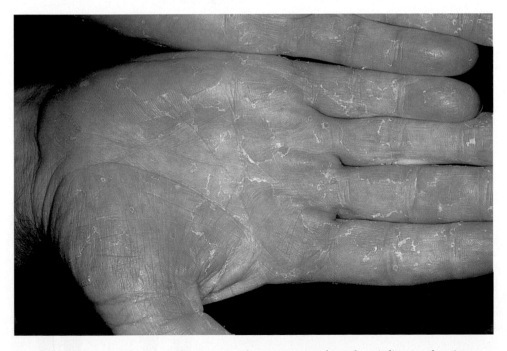

Extensive long-standing cases do not respond to treatment and may be misdiagnosed as tinea.

■ NUMMULAR ECZEMA

DESCRIPTION

- Nummular eczema is a form of eczema characterized by often generalized, exceedingly pruritic, round (coin-shaped) lesions of eczematous inflammation.

HISTORY

- Adults are most often affected.
- The onset is usually gradual, with no clear precipitant.
- Nummular eczema often begins with a few isolated lesions on the legs; with time, multiple lesions occur, seemingly without any particular distribution.
- Lesions often resolve or improve after the administration of topical corticosteroids, only to recur in the same area after corticosteroid withdrawal.

SKIN FINDINGS

- Sharply demarcated, scaling, round plaques appear on the trunk and extremities.
- A yellow honey–colored crust indicates secondary impetiginization.
- Weeping of lesions and vesiculation can characterize flares.
- Secondary infection may result in disease flares.

LABORATORY

- Patch testing reveals a relevant positive result in a fourth to a third of cases.
- A culture of the lesion may reveal *Staphylococcus aureus.*

DIFFERENTIAL DIAGNOSIS

- Psoriasis (often more obviously symmetric with silvery scales)
- Tinea (possible central healing and peripheral scaling)

COURSE AND PROGNOSIS

- The course is variable and unpredictable; this condition may be chronic, relapsing for years.
- Once lesions are established, they tend to remain the same size and reoccur on previously affected skin.
- This is one of the most difficult forms of eczema to treat.

TREATMENT

- See the section on the treatment of subacute or chronic eczema.

- Active tinea pedis should be sought; tinea is treated with antifungal agents if it is present, since occasionally, generalized nummular eczema may be an id reaction to a distant site of tinea infection.
- The use of a medium- to high-potency topical steroids and bland emollients (Aquaphor, Eucerin, Vaseline) should be aggressive. A topical steroid is applied to affected skin twice a day for 2 to 3 weeks.
- The efficacy of topical steroid is increased by using occlusion with plastic wrap or a sauna suit, by hydrating the skin with a bath before medication application, or by using both techniques.
- A secondary infection is treated with systemic antistaphylococcal antibiotics (e.g., dicloxacillin, 250 mg four times a day; cephalexin, 250 mg four times a day).
- Antihistamines are prescribed for itching.
- Systemic corticosteroids should be avoided for long-term management.
- Refractory cases should be referred to a dermatologist.
- Ultraviolet light treatment and topical tar emollients can be helpful.

DISCUSSION

- The cause is unknown. Environmental changes (such as soap and detergent) usually make no difference.

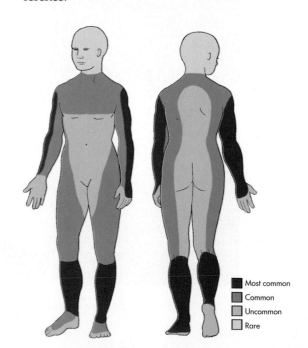

■	Most common
■	Common
■	Uncommon
☐	Rare

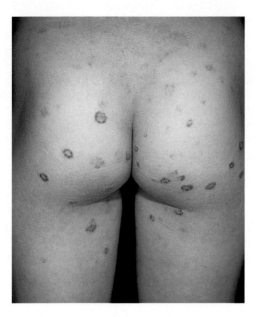

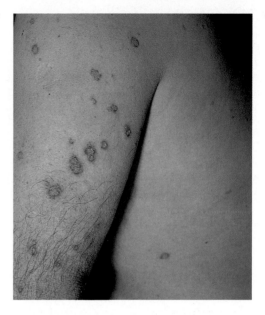

Lesions last for months and years and unlike other forms of eczema are treatment resistant. The cause is unknown.

The most common areas are the dorsum of the hands, the lower legs, the upper extremities, and the trunk. Men are most commonly affected.

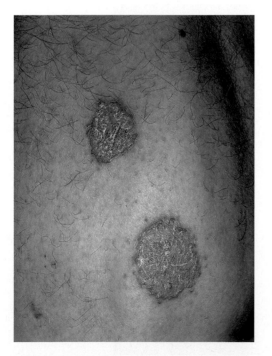

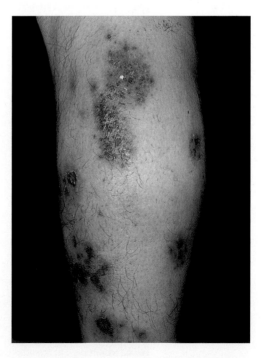

Coin-shaped lesions appear as vesicles and papules that enlarge and become confluent. They are 1 to 5 cm in diameter and are often confused with fungal infections.

Lesions may be acute with exudate and crusts or chronic with erythema and scale. Itching is of variable intensity.

■ POMPHOLYX

DESCRIPTION

- Pompholyx is also referred to as *dyshidrosis* or *dyshidrotic eczema*.
- A distinctive, typically recurrent eczematous dermatitis of unknown etiology, pompholyx is characterized by sudden eruptions of usually highly pruritic, symmetric vesicles on the palms, lateral fingers, or soles.

HISTORY

- Affected patients frequently have an atopic background (personal or family history of asthma, hay fever, or atopic eczema).
- Moderate to severe itching precedes a flare.

SKIN FINDINGS

- Vesicles are 1 to 5 mm in diameter, are monomorphic, are deep seated, are filled with clear fluid, and resemble tapioca. Vesicles erupt suddenly and symmetrically on the palms or lateral fingers or on the plantar feet.
- Rings of scale and peeling follow the eruption as itch diminishes.

COURSE AND PROGNOSIS

- Vesicles resolve slowly over 1 to 3 weeks.
- Chronic eczematous changes with erythema, scaling, and lichenification may follow.
- Waves of vesiculation can recur indefinitely.
- For unknown reasons, the chronic, recurring eruption variably ceases with time.

DIFFERENTIAL DIAGNOSIS

- Pustular psoriasis of the palms and soles (Vesicles of psoriasis rapidly become cloudy with purulent fluid; pain more than itch is often the chief complaint.)
- Id reaction resulting from a distant focus of tinea infection
- Inflammatory tinea
- Acute allergic contact dermatitis

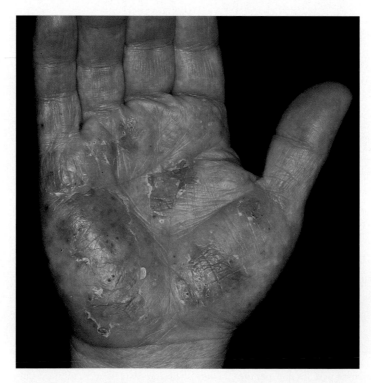

The acute process ends as the skin peels, revealing a red, cracked base with brown spots. The brown spots are sites of previous vesiculation.

MANAGEMENT

- The initial treatment consists of cold, wet compresses twice a day with either tap water or Burow's solution, followed by the application of a medium- to high-potency steroid cream.
- For severe flares, short courses of oral corticosteroids (e.g., methylprednisolone [Medrol Dosepak] or prednisone, 0.5 to 1 mg/kg/day tapered over 1 to 2 weeks) are prescribed.
- Corticosteroids should not be relied on for repeated or chronic treatment.
- Oral antihistamines can alleviate pruritus.
- Topical psoralen plus ultraviolet A (PUVA) is a treatment option for frequent, refractory eruptions.
- In individuals allergic to nickel, attempts to control pompholyx with elimination diets (such as a nickel-reduced diet) may be worth a trial in difficult cases. The administration of disulfiram (Antabuse, 200 mg/day for 8 weeks) may be helpful in patients with nickel sensitivity and pompholyx hand dermatitis.
- Moderating or eliminating stress can be helpful and is anecdotally curative in some.

DISCUSSION

- The causes of this recurrent, sometimes disabling dermatitis is unknown; provoking factors seem heterogenous.
- Systemic contact allergens may play a role, since some individuals with positive patch tests show vesicular reactions on the hands when challenged orally with nickel, cobalt, or chromium.
- A relationship to stress is postulated but poorly studied.
- *Dyshidrosis* is a misnomer; the sweat glands are uninvolved and are not dysfunctional.

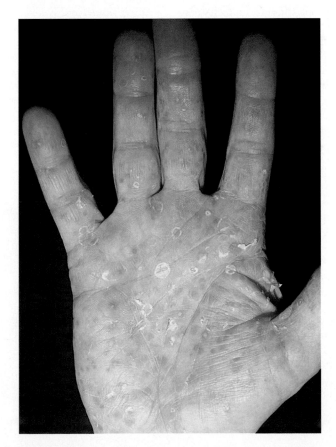

Pustular psoriasis. Differentiation from dyshidrotic eczema is sometimes impossible.

■ PRURIGO NODULARIS

DESCRIPTION

- In prurigo nodularis, there are very pruritic papules and nodules on easily accessed skin; it may be considered an idiopathic, nodular form of lichen simplex chronicus.
- Lesions are secondary to repeated, localized scratching and picking.

HISTORY

- The onset is usually gradual and in the setting of pruritus.
- Prurigo nodularis occurs primarily in adults.
- Stress is often anecdotally implicated.
- Individuals with atopy and diabetes may be predisposed.
- Affected patients may be compulsive "pickers."

SKIN FINDINGS

- Few to numerous dull, erythematous to hyperpigmented nodules distribute randomly. Extensor arms and legs are typically affected; the lumbosacral area, nape of the neck, and dorsal hands are other reachable areas typically involved.
- Lesions are created by repeated rubbing and scratching.
- The 1- to 2-cm nodules are red or brown, hard, and often dome shaped with a smooth, crusted, or warty surface.

LABORATORY

- Skin biopsy is rarely necessary.
- In generalized prurigo of recent onset (<1 year), systemic causes of pruritus should be evaluated and excluded.

DIFFERENTIAL DIAGNOSIS

- Causes of generalized pruritus should be excluded in recent and generalized cases; these include drug reactions, hypothyroidism, occult liver disease (including hepatitis C), infection with the human immunodeficiency virus, occult malignancy (including solid organ metastatic disease and leukemia or lymphoma [i.e., Hodgkin's disease]).

COURSE AND PROGNOSIS

- Prurigo nodularis is often resistant to treatment and lasts for years.
- Cessation of itching, digging, and scratching is critical to lesion resolution and successful treatment.

TREATMENT

- Medium- to high-potency topical corticosteroids (e.g., triamcinolone acetonide, fluocinonide, desoximetasone) can be used with plastic-wrap occlusion to enhance penetration and provide a barrier to scratching.
- Treatment options include corticosteroid-impregnated tape (Cordran), applied to lesions every day.
- Topical superpotent steroids (e.g., betamethasone [Diprolene], halobetasol [Ultravate], clobetasol [Cormax]) can be applied twice a day to individual lesions for 2 weeks.
- Intralesional steroid injections (Kenalog, 5 to 10 mg/ml) can be given and repeated every 4 to 6 weeks if needed. Caution should be used when there is hypopigmentation in dark skin.
- Pramoxine with hydrocortisone (Pramasone ointment) or Sarna lotion may help relieve intense pruritus.

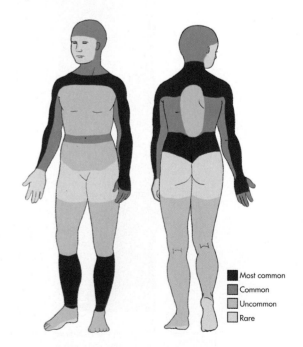

■ Most common
■ Common
□ Uncommon
□ Rare

- Light therapy (ultraviolet B, narrow-band ultraviolet B, psoralen plus ultraviolet A [PUVA]) can be considered for severe, generalized cases.
- Cryotherapy is sometimes successful.
- Excision of individual nodules is rarely performed but sometimes helpful.

DISCUSSION

- Complaints of pruritus vary. Few patients claim there is no itching. Scratching is habitual; for most, pruritus is intense.

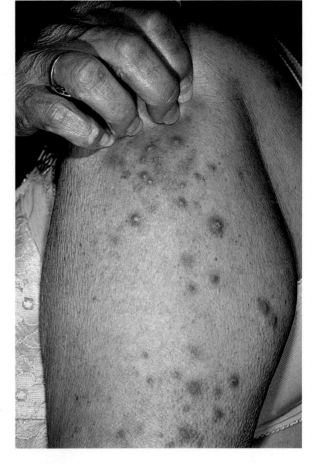

Thick, hard nodules are typically found on the extensor surfaces of the forearms and legs. Chronic picking causes them.

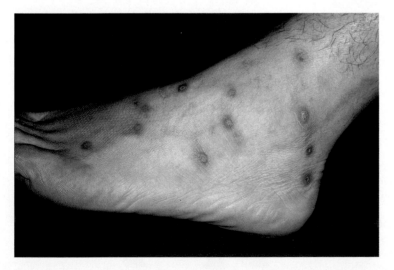

Lesions measure 0.5 to 1 cm and are red to dark brown. They persist, are difficult to treat, and recur if habitual picking is not controlled.

■ STASIS DERMATITIS

DESCRIPTION

- Stasis dermatitis is an eczematous dermatitis of the legs; it is associated with varicose and dilated veins, edema, hyperpigmentation, and thickening of the skin (lipodermatosclerosis).

HISTORY

- There is often a prior history of deep venous thrombosis or a history of surgery or trauma to the leg or of ulceration.
- There is often a family or personal history of varicose veins.
- The patient complains of heaviness or aching in the leg that is aggravated by prolonged standing or walking.
- The legs are swollen at the end of the day.
- Dermatitis and itching often occur for weeks.
- Stasis dermatitis is a chronic problem with common relapses.

SKIN FINDINGS

- Subacute and chronic eczematous dermatitis appears on lower legs or surrounding a venous ulcer.
- The dermatitis (often dramatic) is associated with dry, fissured skin.
- The dermatitis can be generalized (id reaction).
- Edema, brown discoloration (hemosiderosis), ulceration, or erosion occurs.
- Excoriation occurs from the incessant scratching.
- White scars on the medial calf indicate previous ulceration.
- Dilated and tortuous veins appear.
- Stasis papillomatosis (elephantiasis nostra) is found in chronically congested limbs; it occurs with local lymphatic disturbances (e.g., chronic venous insufficiency, primary lymphedema, trauma, recurrent erysipelas).
- Secondary infection (impetiginized) with staphylococci is common.

LABORATORY

- If indicated, the veins are studied.
- A Doppler ultrasound is performed.
- An ankle brachial index is obtained to check for arterial disease; results of less than 0.8 indicate significant arterial disease.
- In patients with a strong family or personal history of multiple deep vein thrombosis, the clotting cascade (protein S, protein C, activated protein C resistance) should be checked.

TREATMENT

- Cool water compresses are applied for 10 to 20 minutes twice a day for acute exudative inflammation
- Group II to V topical steroids are applied twice a day (cream if acute, ointment if chronic).
- Domeboro compresses and an oral antibiotic (e.g., dicloxacillin) are administered if infected
- For generalized dermatitis (id reaction), an oral steroid is administered with a 2-week taper.
- Oral antihistamines (e.g., hydroxyzine), 10 to 25 mg every 4 fours as needed, may help control itching.
- Lubrication (creams better than lotions) can help dryness.
- Compression (20 to 30 mm Hg) is accomplished with stockings (Venosan [support socks], Sigvaris [Sampson and Delilah], or Jobst [lightweight support hose]) or Ace wraps.
- More aggressive compression (30 to 40 mm Hg at the ankle) may be more beneficial.
- Superficial venous incompetence may benefit from vein stripping or sclerotherapy.

DIFFERENTIAL DIAGNOSIS

- Contact dermatitis (especially neomycin)
- Cellulitis

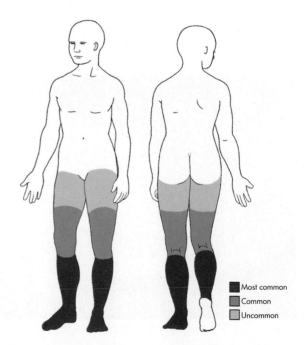

■ Most common
■ Common
□ Uncommon

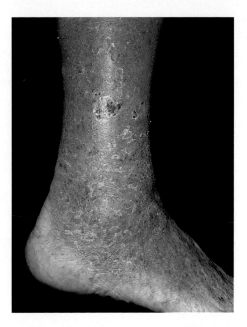

Ulcers heal with ivory white sclerotic scars.

Recurrent ulceration and fat necrosis are associated with loss of subcutaneous tissue and a decrease in leg circumference. Chronically inflamed skin of the lower legs becomes diffusely red, thickened and bound down by fibrosis. Ulceration occurs with the slightest trauma and takes months to heal.

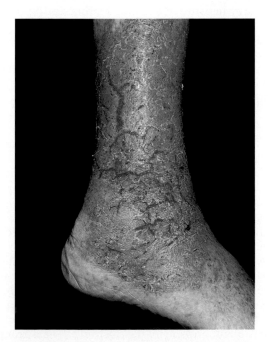

Infection or irritation from washing can precipitate severe acute exacerbations of stasis dermatitis.

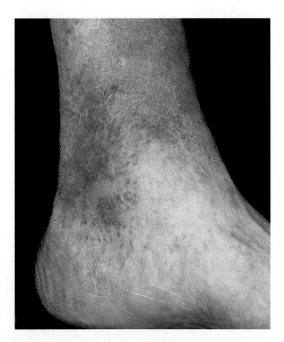

The skin is further compromised each time ulceration and inflammation recur and the cycle continues.

■ VENOUS LEG ULCERS

DESCRIPTION

- A venous leg ulcer is a chronic nonhealing lesion located on the medial aspect of the leg.
- It is associated with chronic venous insufficiency.

HISTORY

- Venous leg ulcers often occur in middle-aged to elderly patients.
- They are more common in women than in men.
- Ulcer formation often occurs suddenly after slight trauma.
- Patients complain of aching and swelling legs; the pain is worse with standing and better in the morning.
- Ulcers may be asymptomatic or may ache slightly.
- Severe pain may indicate other pathologic conditions (e.g., infection, arterial disease).
- Healing is slow, taking weeks or months.
- Venous leg ulcers are a chronic, recurring problem.

SKIN FINDINGS

- Edema, usually pitting, is common; it disappears at night with elevation of the legs.
- Chronic edema, trauma, infection, and inflammation lead to subcutaneous tissue fibrosis where the skin has a firm, nonpitting, "woody" quality.
- Ultimately, a loss of subcutaneous tissue and a decrease in the lower leg circumference (lipodermatosclerosis) occur.
- Advanced disease is represented by an "inverted bottle leg"; when the proximal leg swells, the lower leg shrinks.
- Vein varicosities are often prominent.
- The patient may have secondary eczematous dermatitis (stasis dermatitis).
- The ulcer remains small or enlarges rapidly without any further trauma.
- Ulcers have sharp or sloping border and are deep or superficial.
- Removing crust and debris reveals a moist base with granulation tissue.
- Ulcers are replaced with ivory-white sclerotic scars.

LABORATORY

- Ultrasound identifies the presence and source of significant venous reflux.
- Chronic lesions are biopsied to rule out cancer (basal cell or squamous cell).

- Cultures are not usually helpful; ulcers are often contaminated, not infected.
- If infection is a concern, a biopsy should be done and the tissue submitted for bacterial identification and quantification. (More than 10^6 organisms per square centimeter indicates infection.)

DIFFERENTIAL DIAGNOSIS

- Arterial ulcers
- Neuropathic ulcers
- Infectious ulcers
- Neoplastic ulcers
- Metabolic causes
- Pyoderma gangrenosum
- Antiphospholipid syndrome

TREATMENT

Control of Chronic Venous Insufficiency

- Compression is achieved with Ace wraps, graded compression stockings, or external pneumatic compression devices.
- Unna's boots are also helpful.
- The routine use of systemic antibiotics does not increase healing rates.
- Group III to V topical steroids are used (7 to 14 days) for stasis dermatitis.
- Heavy moisturizers (e.g., Eucerin cream) protect the skin.
- Neomycin-containing antibiotics, which may sensitize the skin, should be avoided.
- Pentoxifylline (Trental), 400 mg three times a day, increases fibrinolytic activity and may reduce lipodermatosclerosis.

Ulcer Therapy

- The crust and exudate are surgically or mechanically débrided.
- Proteolytic enzymes have little benefit in débriding.
- The application of occlusive film promotes rapid healing by suppressing crust formation and enhancing epidermal migration.
- Metronidazole gel (MetroGel) applied before dressing helps decrease odor.
- A variety of synthetic dressings are now available.
- Hydrocolloid dressings (e.g., DuoDerm CGF) are effective and easy to use as the initial treatment.
- The dressing type is changed if healing is slow.
- Exudative and draining ulcers are treated with absorbent dressing of the calcium alginate group.

- Continuous wet saline compresses the macerate crust in deep ulcers and promotes granulation tissue.
- Signs of malnutrition (e.g., low serum albumin level) should be noted.
- Vitamin and mineral supplementation should be considered. This includes ascorbic acid (1 to 2 gm/day), zinc sulfate (220 mg three times a day), and vitamin E (200 mg twice a day).
- Skin grafting should be considered for difficult cases; it is most successful when applied to granulation tissue free of exudate and when edema has been controlled.
- "Artificial" skin (e.g., Apligraft , Dermagraft, Integra Artificial Skin) is now available.

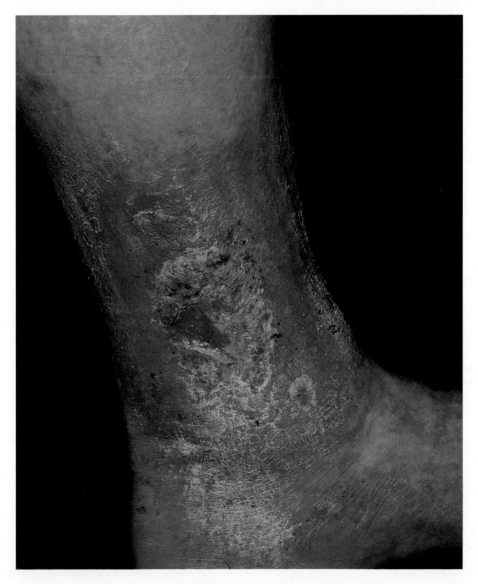

The skin is diffusely red, thickened, and bound down by fibrosis. Ulceration occurs with the slightest trauma.

■ ATOPIC DERMATITIS

DESCRIPTION

- Atopic dermatitis is an eczematous eruption that is distressingly itchy, recurrent, often flexural, and symmetric.
- It generally begins early in life and is characterized by periods of remission and exacerbation. The distribution of affected skin varies with age.
- Major and minor diagnostic criteria have been proposed.

Major Criteria (Four Required for Diagnosis)

- Pruritus
- Young age at onset
- Typical morphology and distribution
- Flexural lichenification and linearity in adults, facial and extensor involvement in infants
- Chronic or chronic and relapsing course
- Personal or family history or atopy (asthma, allergic rhinoconjunctivitis, atopic dermatitis)

Minor or Less-Specific Features

- Xerosis
- Ichthyosis
- Palmar hyperlinearity
- Keratosis pilaris
- Immediate type I skin test responses
- Dermatitis of the hands and feet
- Cheilitis
- Nipple eczema
- Increased susceptibility to cutaneous infections
- Perifollicular accentuation

HISTORY

- The incidence is 7 to 24 per 1000.
- The highest incidence is in children.
- Some 70% of patients have a family history of one or more of the following: asthma, hay fever, or eczematous dermatitis.
- Atopic dermatitis is autosomal dominant, with variable penetrance suggested.
- Aggravating factors include contact irritants and allergens; perspiration; excessive heat; rough fibers (such as wool); tight clothing; cool, dry air with no humidity; and emotional stress.
- The role of dust mite and food allergies in cases of severe infantile atopic eczema and aeroallergens is controversial.
- The dermatitis becomes less severe in most children by the teen years. Most children outgrow atopic dermatitis, but some develop chronic relapsing disease, especially eyelid, hand, and retroauricular dermatitis.
- Most cases of atopic dermatitis are precipitated by environmental stress on genetically compromised skin, not by interaction with allergens.
- Atopic dermatitis seems to result from a vicious circle of dermatitis associated with elevated T-cell activation, hyperstimulatory Langerhans' cells, defective cell-mediated immunity, and B-cell overproduction of immunoglobulin B.

SKIN FINDINGS

- Atopic inflammation begins abruptly with erythema and severe pruritus.
- Typical lesions are papular, eczematous dermatitis with redness and scaling.
- Acute lesions may be oozing and vesicular, subacute lesions are scaly and crusted, and chronic lesions are often dull red and lichenified.
- Dermatitis distribution:
  - *Infantile phase (2 months to 2 years):*
    - In this phase, atopic dermatitis appears on the cheeks, perioral area, and scalp; around the ears; and on the body, sparing the diaper area.
    - The extensor tops of the feet and the elbows are often involved.
    - The lesions are often exudative.
  - *Childhood phase (2 to 12 years):*
    - There is flexural involvement (antecubital and popliteal fossae, neck, wrists, and ankles).
    - Scratching and chronicity lead to lichenification.
  - *Adult phase (12 years to adult):*
    - Flexural involvement is common.
    - Hand dermatitis may be the only manifestation.
    - Upper eyelid dermatitis is another frequent finding.
    - The dermatitis can be diffuse and patchy on the body.
    - Associated findings are dry skin, ichthyosis vulgaris, and keratosis pilaris.
- Complications:
  - Lesions are frequently colonized with *Staphylococcus aureus*; secondary infection resulting in another flare of dermatitis or persistence is common.

- Increased susceptibility to viral infections (i.e., herpes simplex, molluscum contagiosum, cutaneous fungal infections) occurs.
- Hypopigmentation and hyperpigmentation may result from previous inflammation.
- Emotional and behavior problems may be frequent in children affected by moderate to severe disease.

NONSKIN FINDINGS

- Often, there is a personal or family history of asthma, hay fever, or seasonal rhinitis.

LABORATORY

- Laboratory studies are not routinely indicated or performed.
- Culture and sensitivity testing of crusted or oozing lesions is performed if bacterial superinfection is suspected.
- Elevated immunoglobulin E levels (>200 IU/ml) occur in approximately 80% to 90% of patients.
- The incidence of eosinophilia correlates roughly with disease activity.
- Routine allergy testing, dietary testing, and environmental or dietary manipulation are often not productive.

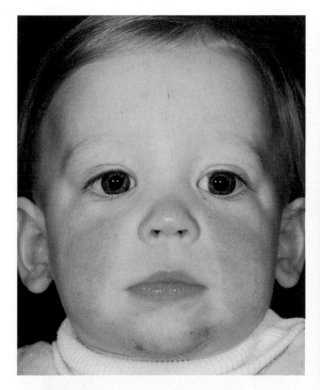

A common appearance in children with erythema and scaling confined to the cheeks and sparing the perioral and paranasal area.

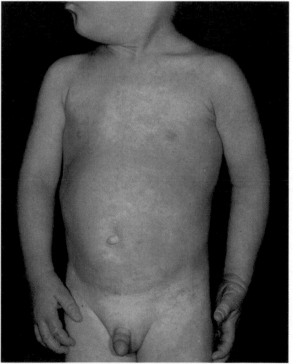

Generalized infantile atopic dermatitis sparing the diaper area, which keeps the skin hydrated and protected from scratching.

DIFFERENTIAL DIAGNOSIS

- Contact dermatitis, irritant or allergic type
- Nummular eczema and seborrheic dermatitis
- Scabies (considered in new-onset disease)
- Cutaneous T-cell lymphoma
- Tinea infections
- Uncommon: congenital disorders, metabolic disorders (i.e., zinc deficiency) immune deficiency disorders (e.g., Wiskott-Aldrich syndrome, hyperimmunoglobulinemia E syndrome, severe combined immunodeficiency)

TREATMENT

Inflammation and infection should be controlled or eliminated.

- Topical corticosteroids of appropriate strength for the patient's age and the affected area are applied twice daily to inflamed skin for 10 to 21 days.
- Oral antibiotics (e.g., dicloxacillin, cephalexin [Keflex]) are administered for secondary infection.
- For acute lesions and severe flares, a compress with Burow's solution is applied for 20 minutes three times a day, followed by the application of a topical steroid.

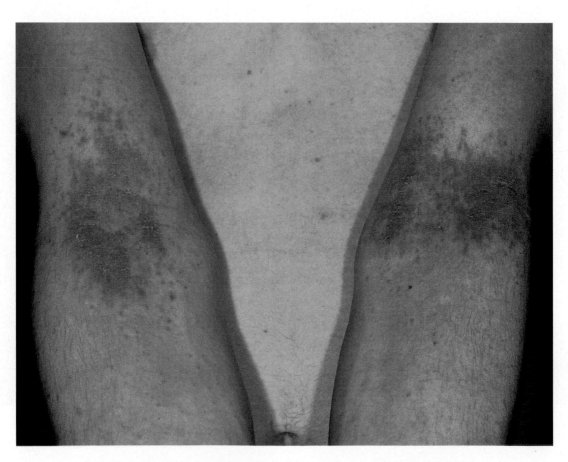

Classsic appearance of confluent papules forming plaques in the antecubital fossa.

The skin barrier should be restored and preserved.

- Bland emollients such as Vaseline petroleum, Aquaphor, or Unibase are used at least once a day after a hydrating bath.
- A plain, thick, greasy moisturizer works much better than a lotion or a cream.

Aggravating factors must be eliminated or controlled.

- Activity that results in sweating, which is irritating to the skin should be avoided.
- Soft, light, cotton clothing is best. Wool or other coarse fibers are to be avoided.
- The environment should be cool and well ventilated.
- Stress-reduction techniques may be helpful.

Pruritus must be controlled. Oral antihistamines with sedative effect (e.g., diphenhydramine [Benadryl], hydroxyzine [Atarax], and doxepin) are helpful, especially at night to allow more restful sleep.

- A dermatologist is consulted for the management of severe, refractory disease.

The options for treating severe atopic dermatitis follow:

- A *short* course of oral corticosteroids can break the cycle of inflammation.
- Tacrolimus ointment 0.1 is a new agent. It is very effective when applied twice a day.
- Hospitalization can be considered for rest, environmental control, and wet compresses three times a day, followed by the application of a medium-potency topical steroid.
- A medium-potency topical steroid with vinyl-suit occlusion can be applied 2 hours twice a day for 1 to 2 weeks.
- Ultraviolet light therapy includes ultraviolet A, ultraviolet B, and psoralen plus ultraviolet A (PUVA).
- Other immunomodulating therapy includes an oral cyclosporin, azathioprine, and interferon gamma.

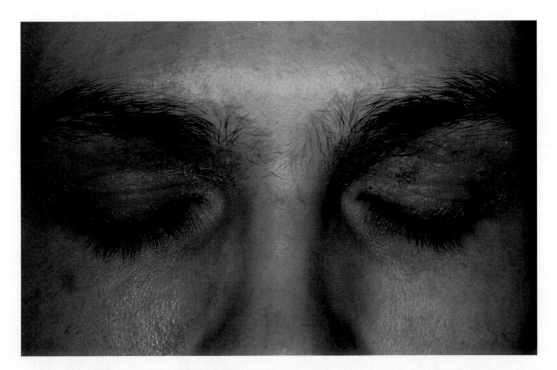

Atopic dermatitis of the upper eyelids, an area that is often rubbed with the back of the hand.

◼ DOMINANT ICHTHYOSIS VULGARIS

DESCRIPTION

- Dominant ichthyosis vulgaris is a is a disorder of keratinization characterized by dry, rectangular scales resembling cracked pavement; these scales appear most prominently on the extensor extremities.
- It is associated with the atopic diathesis in 50% of cases.

HISTORY

- The onset is in early to middle childhood.
- The condition may improve with age or may persist throughout life.
- The scales are more noticeable and often pruritic in the winter, when the humidity is low.
- Ichthyosis vulgaris is autosomal dominant: 1 in 300 have the disorder.

SKIN FINDINGS

- Findings are often mild.
- Dry, small, rectangular scales appear on the extensor extremities.
- The lower extremities, particularly the anterior shins, are often more noticeably affected.
- Affected skin has the appearance of cracked pavement or fish scales.
- This condition characteristically spares the flexor surfaces.
- It is usually asymptomatic but may become pruritic or chapped in the winter.
- Palmar creases may be accentuated.
- Keratosis pilaris may also be present.
- Scaling rarely involves the entire cutaneous surface.
- Scaling of the skin results from the retention of scale rather than increased proliferation.
- The condition may result from a defect in the skin protein, filaggrin.

LABORATORY

- No tests are indicated.
- Skin biopsy is rarely performed; when performed, it shows a decreased or an absent granular layer.

DIFFERENTIAL DIAGNOSIS

- Dry skin
- Acquired ichthyosis (more sudden and later onset, generalized, as a manifestation of systemic disease [i.e., infection with the immunodeficiency virus, malignancy, drugs, autoimmune disease])
- Sex-linked ichthyosis vulgaris

TREATMENT

- Ichthyosis vulgaris often improves with age; infrequently, it resolves completely.
- Increased environmental humidity and warmth often result in resolution or improvement.
- Regular application of moisturizing cream or lotion decreases pruritus and improves skin appearance.
- The optimal time for applying moisturizer is immediately after bathing and hydrating the skin.
- Emollients containing lactic acid, urea, or alpha hydroxy acids are helpful for treating severe dryness and scaling. Ammonium lactate 12% (LacHydrin) lotion or cream is very effective. They should be applied daily.

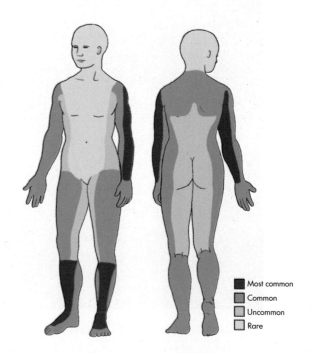

Most common
Common
Uncommon
Rare

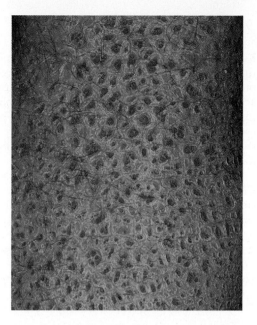

Dominant ichthyosis vulgaris. White, translucent quadrangular squares on the extensor aspects of the arms and legs. This form is significantly associated with atophy.

Sex-linked ichthyosis vulgaris. Patients have dry skin in the summer months that evolves into large, brown, quadrangular scales during the dry winter months.

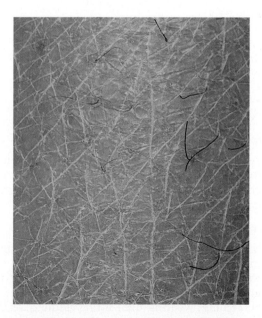

Ichthyosis is a disorder of keratinization characterized by the development of dry, rectangular scales. The skin on this patients lower leg show features of ichthyosis and asteatotic eczema (eczema craquele).

This patient has severe dry skin that has cracked and resembles ichthyosis.

■ KERATOSIS PILARIS

DESCRIPTION

- Keratosis pilaris consists of rough, monomorphic, tiny, follicle-based scaling papules most commonly on the posterolateral aspects of the upper arms but occasionally more widespread, including the anterior and lateral thighs and the buttocks.
- It results from mild follicular plugging and perifollicular inflammation.

HISTORY

- Keratosis pilaris is very common in young children, peaking in adolescence.
- It is probably more common in atopic individuals.
- It is usually asymptomatic but may be somewhat pruritic.
- Treatment is often sought for a troubling cosmetic appearance.
- The unusual adult diffuse pattern persists indefinitely.

SKIN FINDINGS

- Small, pinpoint follicular papules and occasionally pustules remain in the same areas for years.
- A red halo appears at the periphery of the keratotic papule.
- The skin feels rough, like sandpaper.
- Lesions most commonly appear on the posterolateral upper arms and anterior thighs. Occasionally, the condition is generalized.

LABORATORY

- No laboratory tests are performed.

DIFFERENTIAL DIAGNOSIS

- Acne (Facial lesions may be confused with it; uniform small size and association with dry skin and chapping differentiate keratosis pilaris from pustular acne.)

TREATMENT

- Many patients seek treatment for cosmesis, since most often, the lesions are asymptomatic.
- Keratosis pilaris often improves or resolves with age and by the adult years.
- Scratching, wearing tight-fitting clothing, or undergoing treatment with abrasive washes or gritty scrubs may aggravate the condition.
- Tretinoin (Retin-A) may induce temporary improvement, but irritation is usually unacceptable.
- Lac-Hydrin 12% cream or lotion twice a day can reduce roughness.
- Low-potency topical steroids may be used in limited courses to temporarily reduce the redness but should not be used on a long-term basis.
- The recognition of keratosis pilaris helps avoid inappropriate treatment.

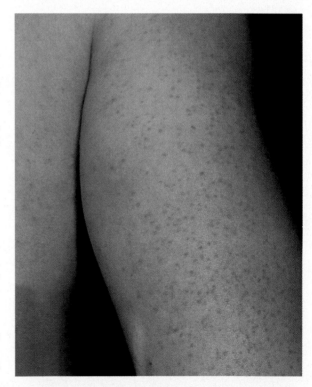

Small, follicular papules are most commonly found on the posterolateral aspects of the upper arms. Most lesions are not this red.

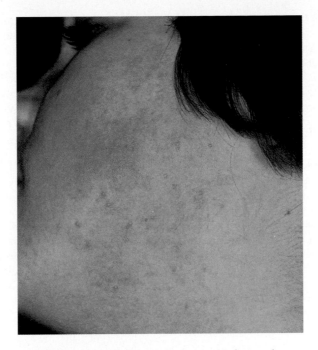

This is common on the face of children and is frequently confused with acne.

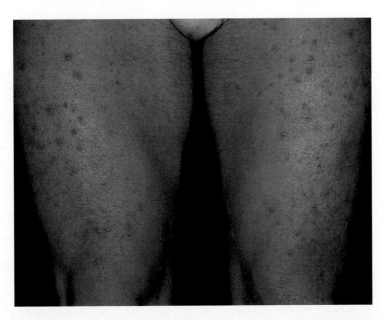

Infected lesions in a uniform distribution. Typical bacterial folliculitis has a
haphazard distribution.

■ PITYRIASIS ALBA

DESCRIPTION

- There are common, asymptomatic, hypopigmented, slightly elevated, fine, scaling patches with indistinct borders.
- Pityriasis alba affects the lateral cheeks, lateral upper arms, and thighs; it occurs more often in young children and usually resolves by early adulthood.

HISTORY

- Pityriasis alba is asymptomatic.
- Children and young adults are affected.
- There is no history of prior rash, trauma, or inflammation.
- Affected individuals are often atopic.
- Loss of pigment is often more noticeable and distressing in darkly pigmented individuals.

SKIN FINDINGS

- White, round-to-oval macules vary in size; they are generally 2 to 4 cm in diameter.
- A fine surface scale may be seen with close inspection.
- Lesions are most common on the lateral cheeks, lateral upper arms, and thighs.
- The condition is more obvious in the summer, when affected skin does not tan.

LABORATORY

- A potassium hydroxide examination of the fine scale is negative.

DIFFERENTIAL DIAGNOSIS

- Tinea versicolor (very rare on the face)
- Vitiligo (more sharply demarcated, often over joints, symmetric, and more widespread)
- Chemical leukoderma

TREATMENT

- No treatment is usually recommended.
- The patient should be reassured that the loss of pigment is not permanent.
- Hypopigmentation usually fades with time.
- Hydrocortisone cream 1% applied for a limited time (a few weeks) on affected skin may help the patients most distressed by the pigment irregularity.

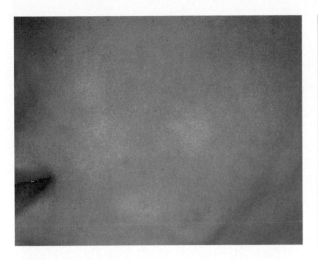

Hypopigmented round spots are a common occurrence on the faces of atopic children.

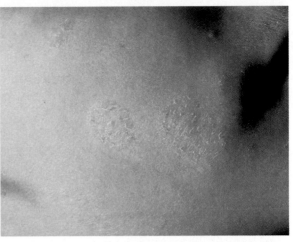

The superficial hypopigmented plaques become scaly and inflamed as the dry winter months progress.

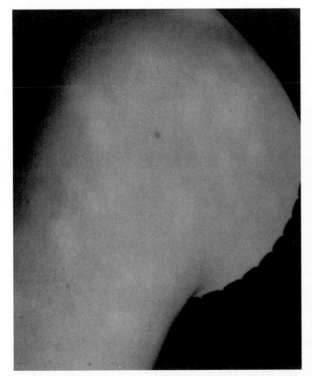

Irregular hypopigmented areas are frequently seen in atopic patients and are not to be confused with tinea versicolor or vitiligo.

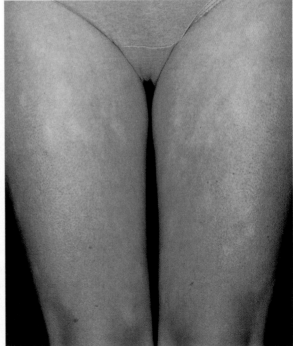

Lesions present here are more numerous than are typically seen.

3

Urticaria

■ ACUTE URTICARIA (HIVES)

DESCRIPTION

- Acute urticaria is a variably pruritic, common, distinctive reaction pattern. Transient, edematous, red plaques vary in size and shape. Individual lesions last less than 24 hours. Urticaria is classified as acute (<6 weeks' duration) or chronic (>6 weeks' duration).

HISTORY

- Acute urticaria may occur at any age.
- It is more common in atopic individuals.
- The etiology is determined in many cases.
- Histamine release by allergens (e.g., drugs, foods, pollens) is mediated by immunoglobulin E.
- Hives itch, but the intensity varies.
- The pruritus is milder in deep hives (angioedema).

SKIN FINDINGS

- Erythematous or white, nonpitting, edematous plaques occur.
- The plaques change size and shape by peripheral extension and regression.
- This is a dynamic process; new lesions evolve as old ones resolve.
- The lesions vary in size and are round or oval; when confluent, they become polycyclic.
- The lesions may be uniformly red or white, Thicker plaques have a more uniform color.
- The lesions may be surrounded by a clear or red halo.
- Bullae or purpuric lesions appear with intense swelling.
- The distribution is usually haphazard.
- Linear lesions suggest dermagraphism (physical urticaria).

LABORATORY

- There are no routine studies.

DIFFERENTIAL DIAGNOSIS

- Urticaria vasculitis in lesions lasting more than 24 hours
- Drug eruption
- Viral exanthem
- Bites (papular urticaria)
- Bullous pemphigoid in an elderly patient
- Hereditary angioedema

TREATMENT

- All suspected triggers (e.g., drugs, aspirin, food, drink) should be stopped.
- Antihistamines are administered; this includes H_1 blockers (e.g., hydroxyzine, 10 to 25 mg every 4 to 6 hours [sedation may be a problem]). Nonsedating H_1 blockers do not work as well, but they are useful for the daytime hours to prevent somnolence; these include loratadine (Claritin, 10 mg), cetirizine (Zyrtec, 5 mg, 10 mg), and fexofenadine (Allegra, 60 mg, 180 mg).
- Prednisone (e.g., 60 mg for 2 days, 40 mg for 5 days, and then 20 mg for 7 days) can work in patients whose condition is difficult to control with antihistamines.
- Epinephrine is administered for extensive cases.
- Generally, keeping the patient cool physically and emotionally is advisable.
- Cool, soothing baths (e.g., with Aveeno) can be suggested.
- Hot showers should be avoided because they only worsen the pruritus.
- Topical steroids are not effective.

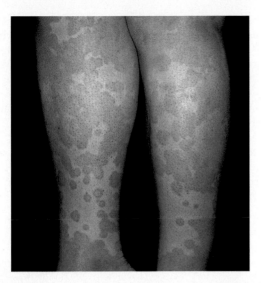

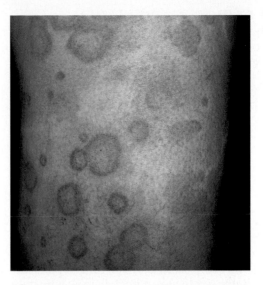

Circumscribed, raised, edematous, red plaques involve the superficial portion of the dermis. The itch varies in intensity. Lesions vary from a few to numerous and vary in configuration

Urticaria resolves spontaneously in less than 14 days in most patients. It persists for months and sometimes years in about 5% of patients. These lesions have a clear center, and the surrounding skin is diffusely red and less swollen.

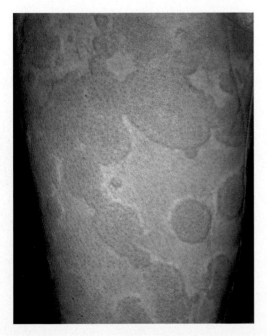

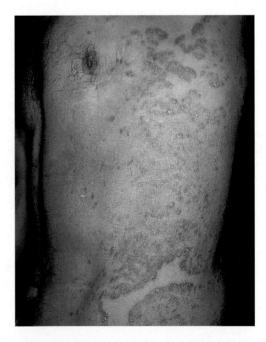

Lesions occur on any skin surface, including the palms and soles. They appear in many forms and last 24 to 48 hours. The most characteristic presentation is a red, raised plaque surrounded by a faint white halo. When confluent, they become polycyclic.

Plaques have become confluent on the trunk.

■ CHRONIC URTICARIA

DESCRIPTION

- Chronic urticaria is a case of the hives lasting more than 6 weeks.

HISTORY

- The cause is determined in only 5% to 20% of cases.
- Chronic urticaria presents a major problem in diagnosis and management.
- The course of the disease is unpredictable; the condition can last months or years.
- The five *I*s should be sought:
  - Inhalants (uncommon): dust, molds, feather, pollen
  - Ingestants (common): foods, additives, dyes, drugs
  - Injectants: drug or bug
  - Infection: bacterial, viral, fungal, parasitic
  - Internal disease: thyroid disease, lupus, another autoimmune disease

SKIN FINDINGS

- Red or white, nonpitting edematous plaques are formed.
- Changes in size and shape occur over time.
- As old lesions disappear, new ones appear.
- Each lesion lasts less than 24 hours.

LABORATORY

- If the etiology remains undetermined during the history and physical examination, there is little chance of it being determined by laboratory testing.
- Tests to consider include sinus films to rule out sinusitis, dental x-ray films to rule out dental abscess, and a thyroid microsomal antibody test to rule out autoimmune thyroid disease.

DIFFERENTIAL DIAGNOSIS

- Physical urticaria, which is ruled out by the history, physical examination, and testing
- Urticarial vasculitis if individual lesions last more than 24 hours (A skin biopsy confirms the diagnosis.)
- Bullous pemphigoid in elderly patients

TREATMENT

- An antihistamine is the drug of first choice. Hydroxyzine, 10 to 25 mg, is administered every 4 hours, working up to 100 mg every 4 hours as needed.
- Nonsedating antihistamines should be considered for daytime use; these include loratadine (Claritin, 10 mg), cetirizine (Zyrtec, 5 mg, 10 mg), and fexofenadine (Allegra, 60 mg, 180 mg). These drugs may be less effective than hydroxyzine.
- Oral steroids are of questionable benefit.
- Environmental changes should be made to reduce the number aeroallergens.
- A salicylate-free diet may be tried.
- A highly restricted diet (lamb, rice, sugar, salt, water) may be tried for 5 days.
- Empiric antibiotic therapy seldom tried for occult infection.

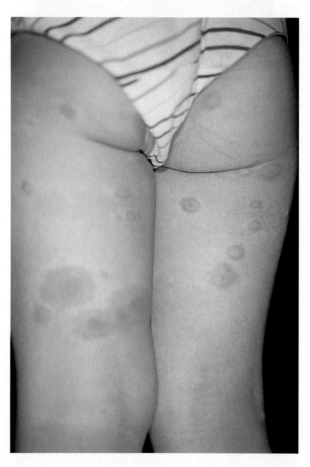

Urticaria is common, occurring in up to 25% to 50% of the population. People of all ages are affected, but the highest incidence is in young adults.

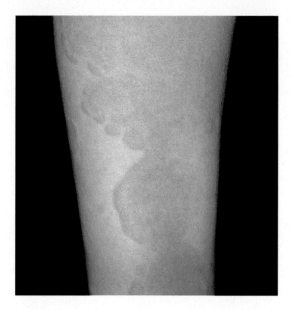

Lesions may become confluent and sometimes cover an entire extremity.

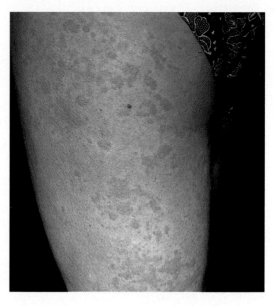

A portion of the border may be reabsorbed, giving the appearance of incomplete rings. A variation in color is usually present in superficial hives. Thicker plaques have a uniform color.

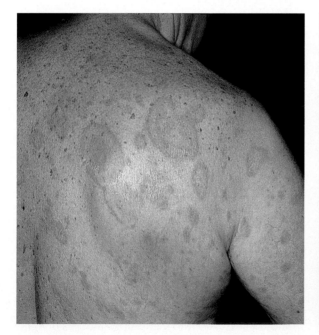

The presentation is highly variable. Here, the lesions resemble the targets of erythema multiforme.

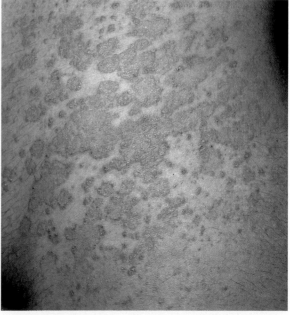

Some patients with extensive involvement have systemic symptoms such as shortness of breath, wheezing, nausea, abdominal pain, diarrhea, and headache.

■ PHYSICAL URTICARIAS

DESCRIPTION

- Physical urticarias are brief attacks of hives induced by physical stimuli (e.g., scratching, pressure, heat, cold, sunshine).

HISTORY

- The major distinguishing feature is that the attacks are brief.
- The attacks last 30 to 60 minutes; however, in pressure urticaria, they last several hours.
- Dermographism is the most common physical urticaria; hives are produced by rubbing and stroking the skin. The onset is sudden and is preceded by viral infection, antibiotic therapy (penicillin), or emotional upset; most often, the cause is unknown. Attacks last weeks to years.
- Pressure urticaria occurs 4 to 6 hours after a pressure stimulus and lasts 8 to 72 hours. Deep, itchy, burning, or painful swelling occurs. The hands, feet, trunk, buttocks, lips, and face are commonly affected. Lesions are induced by standing, walking, wearing tight garments, or sitting on a hard surface for long time. This condition is disabling for those performing manual labor. The mean duration is 9 years.
- In cholinergic urticaria, hives begin within 2 to 20 minutes after overheating from exercise, exposure to heat, or emotional stress. They last for minutes to hours (median, 30 minutes). This condition presents between 10 and 30 years of age. It is chronic.
- Cold urticaria occurs with a sudden drop in air temperature or exposure to cold water. This condition often begins after infection, drug therapy, or emotional stress. The age of onset is 18 to 25 years. There are severe reactions with generalized urticaria; angioedema can occur.
- In solar urticaria, hives occur minutes after exposure to the sun and disappear in 1 hour. Several different wavelengths cause solar urticaria. This condition is persistent.

SKIN FINDINGS

- Itchy wheals from scratching and friction define dermagraphism.
- Repeated deep swelling is a clue to the diagnosis of pressure urticaria.
- Round, papular wheals, 2 to 4 mm in diameter and surrounded by slight to extensive red flare, are diagnostic of cholinergic urticaria.
- Classic hives are seen after exposure to cold; they are typically noted on the hands.
- Typical hives develop after exposure to ultraviolet light in solar urticaria.

LABORATORY

- The diagnosis is confirmed by the patient's history. Laboratory evaluation is unnecessary.
- In dermagraphism, a tongue blade drawn firmly across the arm or back produces whealing within 1 to 3 minutes.
- In pressure urticaria, testing with localized pressure points confirms the diagnosis.
- In cholinergic urticaria, the patient runs in place or uses an exercise bicycle for 10 to 15 minutes; then he or she is observed up to 1 hour to detect typical micropapular hives.
- In cold urticaria, hives are induced with an ice cube held against the skin for 1 to 5 minutes.
- In solar urticaria, phototesting identifies the wavelength involved.

DIFFERENTIAL DIAGNOSIS

- For solar urticaria: polymorphous light eruption, connective tissue disease, porphyria

TREATMENT

- In dermographism, treatment is often unnecessary. Symptomatic dermographism is treated with antihistamines (e.g., hydroxyzine); low dosages (10 to 25 mg every 4 hours) provide adequate relief. The conditions of many patients are controlled for long periods with very low doses of hydroxyzine.
- In cholinergic urticaria, strenuous exercise is limited. Hydroxyzine (10 to 50 mg) can be taken 1 hour before exercise.
- In cold urticaria, the patient should be protected from sudden decreases in temperature. Cyproheptadine (Periactin) is effective but sedating. The dosage is adjusted to control symptoms. Doxepin and ketotifen are also effective.
- In solar urticaria, antihistamines are administered, sunscreens should be used, and the patient should be exposed to increasing amounts of light.

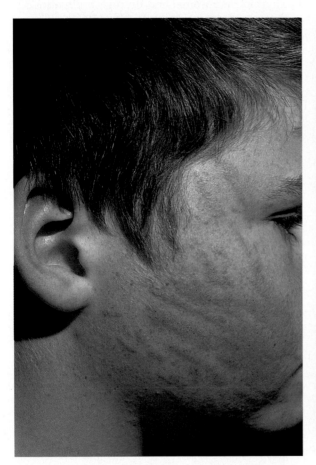

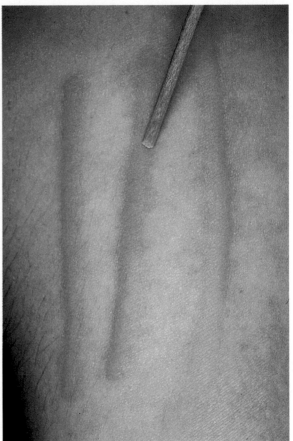

Dermographism. The onset is usually sudden; young patients are affected most commonly. The degree of response varies. Young patients may be highly reactive for months and then appear to be in remission, only to have symptoms recur.

Dermographism is the most common form of physical urticaria. Scratching produces a linear wheal that fades in 15 to 60 minutes. Itching is mild to intense. The skin should be stroked in any patient who complains that scratching creates itching and swelling.

■ ACQUIRED ANGIOEDEMA

DESCRIPTION

- Angioedema is an acute or chronic hivelike swelling in the subcutaneous tissue of the skin and mucosa.

HISTORY

- Hives and angioedema commonly occur simultaneously.
- The deeper reaction (angioedema) produces a more diffuse swelling.
- Itching is usually absent. Symptoms consist of burning and painful swelling.
- The lips, palms, soles, limbs, trunk, and genitalia are most commonly affected.
- Involvement of the gastrointestinal and respiratory tracts produces dysphagia, dyspnea, colicky abdominal pain, and attacks of vomiting and diarrhea.
- There are two forms of this disease: acute and chronic.
- In acute angioedema, there is a severe allergic type 1 immediate hypersensitivity immunoglobulin E-mediated reaction. The disease is usually self-limited. Identification and removal of the offending agent (e.g., drugs, contrast dyes) resolves the problem. Most attacks resolve within 24 to 48 hours.
- Most cases of chronic angioedema are idiopathic. This condition is most common in the 40- to 50-year-old age group. Women are most frequently affected. The pattern of recurrence is unpredictable, and episodes can occur for 5 or more years.
- Late-onset, recurrent angioedema may indicate an acquired deficiency of C1q esterase inhibitor. Two types of acquired angioedema are described. One form is associated with malignancy (B-cell lineage); the other is defined by the presence of an autoantibody directed against the C1-inhibitor molecule. Both are very rare.

SKIN SYMPTOMS

- The reaction is similar to that of hives, but there also is deeper edema (swelling) of the subcutaneous tissues of the skin and mucosa.

LABORATORY

- Thyroid microsomal and thyroglobulin antibodies are present in some patients with chronic angioedema.
- Patients with acquired C1-inhibitor deficiency have low levels or the absence of functional C1-inhibitor activity and low levels of CH_{50}, C1q, C1, C4, and C2.

TREATMENT

- Acute severe attacks are treated with epinephrine and high dosages of antihistamines.
- EpiPen or EpiPen Jr. is prescribed for patients who experience severe reactions. Affected patients should wear a bracelet that identifies the diagnosis.
- For chronic disease, antihistamines such as hydroxyzine are administered.
- Corticosteroids may be required for suppression.
- The use of levothyroxine should be considered if patients are hypothyroid or euthyroid.

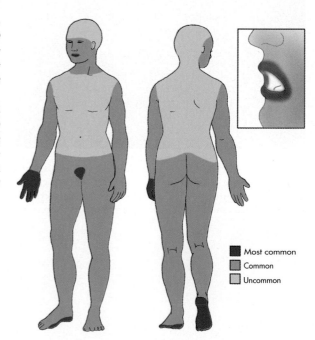

Most common
Common
Uncommon

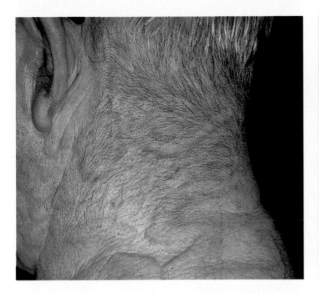

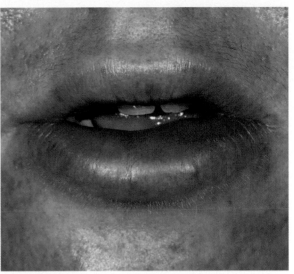

Angioedema affects the face, lips, palms, soles, or a portion of an extremity. It may become confluent and cover wide areas. The color is uniform. Hives vary in color.

Angioedema is a hivelike swelling cause by increased vascular permeability in the subcutaneous tissue of the skin and mucosa. Hives and angioedema may occur simultaneously. Itching is usually absent. Symptoms consist of burning and painful swelling.

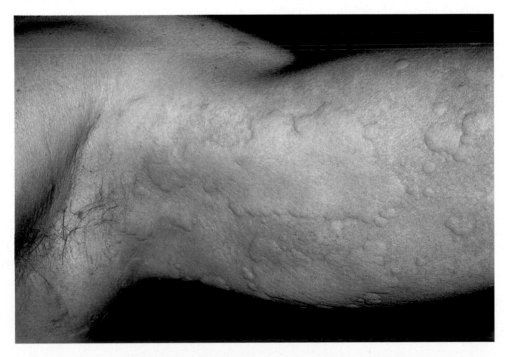

Angioedema. Urticarial plaques are confluent and cover wide areas.

■ MASTOCYTOSIS

DESCRIPTION

- Mastocytosis is a rare disease in which the skin is excessively infiltrated by mast cells.
- There are several clinical presentations; the pediatric cutaneous form is the most common.

HISTORY

- The incidence is 1 in 1000 to 1 in 8000 live births.
- Mastocytosis is usually confined to the skin in young children.
- Adults are more likely to develop systemic forms.
- The cause is unknown; familial occurrence is rare.
- The onset occurs between birth and 2 years in 55% of cases; an additional 10% of cases occur before age 15.
- The condition gradually improves and usually clears spontaneously by puberty.
- Disease that begins after age 10 usually persists for the patient's life.
- When this disease is systemic, the gastrointestinal tract and the skeletal system are most commonly involved. There can be an associated mast cell leukemia.
- Itching, minimal with localized disease, is troublesome when large numbers of lesions are present.

SKIN FINDINGS

- There are two main types: localized and generalized. The generalized forms are rare.
- The typical presentation is pediatric-onset localized cutaneous disease.
- Findings consist of red-brown, slightly elevated plaques averaging 0.5 to 1.5 cm in diameter.
- Plaques typically form in small groups on the trunk.
- The plaques are often dismissed as variations of pigmentation.
- A larger, solitary collection is called a *mastocytoma*.
- Large numbers can occur on any body surface.
- Erythema and blisters (often after scratching) are common in the first 2 years of life.

- Stroking any lesion induces intense erythema and a wheal (Darier's sign); such a reaction is highly characteristic of the disease and is as reliable as a biopsy.

LABORATORY

- A skin biopsy is obtained; special metachromatic stains (i.e., Giemsa, toluidine blue) stain cytoplasmic mast cell granules deep blue.
- Overproduction of mast cell mediators (e.g., histamine) occurs with systemic disease.
- Quantitation of urinary *N*-methylimidazoleacetic acid (a major metabolite of histamine) and other metabolites is used as a measure of systemic disease.

DIFFERENTIAL DIAGNOSIS

- Urticaria
- Dermagraphism
- Bites
- Café-au-lait spots

TREATMENT

- Topical steroids, often under occlusion, or injectable corticosteroids are useful for limited areas.
- Recognition helps parents limit unintentional scratching and trauma of the lesions.
- In children, more generalized disease is treated with antihistamines and cromolyn.
- Systemic disease is managed in a stepwise manner:
  - An H_1 antihistamine for flushing and pruritus
  - An H_2 blocker or proton-pump inhibitor for gastric and duodenal manifestations
  - Oral cromolyn sodium for diarrhea and abdominal pain
  - Nonsteroidal antiinflammatory agents or aspirin (to block mast cell biosynthesis of prostaglandin D2) for severe flushing
  - Photochemotherapy (psoralen plus ultraviolet A [PUVA]), which can be useful in extensive cases
  - Avoidance of mast cell stimulators (e.g., morphine, codeine, cough remedies containing dextromethorphan)

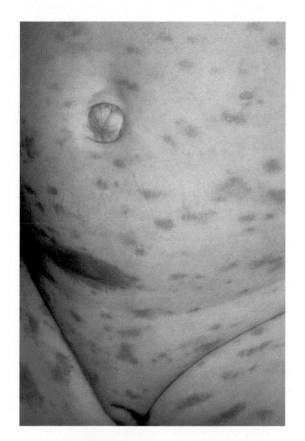

A few to many red-brown , slightly elevated plaques typically occur between birth and 2 years of age. The trunk is the most common site.

Stroking a lesion produces a wheal surrounded by intense erythema (Darier's sign). The reaction occurs within minutes.

■ PRURITIC URTICARIAL PAPULES AND PLAQUES OF PREGNANCY (PUPPP)

DESCRIPTION

- PUPPP is the most common gestational dermatosis.
- It is characterized by itching and papules that start on the abdomen late in the third trimester.

HISTORY

- The average age of onset is 25 (range, 16 to 40 years).
- The incidence is 1 in 160 pregnancies.
- Some 42% of cases involve primigravidas, 28% involve women who are pregnant for the second time, and 16% involve women who are pregnant for the third time.
- Most problems begin late in the third trimester but may occur in the first or second trimester. A postpartum onset (3 to 5 days) is rare.
- The mean duration is 6 weeks, but the rash is usually not severe for more than 1 week.
- Recurrence with future pregnancies is unusual.

SKIN FINDINGS

- The problem begins on the abdomen in 90% of patients.
- In those with striae, the problem most often presents in or around the striae.
- The rash spreads in a few days in a symmetric fashion to involve the buttocks, upper and lower extremities, chest, and back. The hands, feet, palms, soles, and face may be involved.
- Itching is moderate to intense; excoriations are rarely seen.
- Lesions begin as red papules that are often surrounded by a narrow, pale halo. They increase in number and may become confluent, forming edematous urticarial plaques.
- In other patients, erythematous patches that are discrete or confluent are surmounted by tiny papules or vesicles.

LABORATORY

- Biopsy reveals a slight to moderate perivascular infiltrate of mononuclear cells, some eosinophils, and variable epidermal spongiosis.
- There are no laboratory abnormalities; the results of direct immunofluorescence of lesional and perilesional skin are negative.

COURSE AND PROGNOSIS

- There are no associated complications during pregnancy and delivery.
- Recurrences in subsequent pregnancies are unusual.
- Infants do not develop the eruption.

DISCUSSION

- Congenital abnormalities are absent or unrelated to PUPPP.
- Unlike urticaria, the eruption remains fixed and increases in intensity, clearing in most cases before or within 1 week after delivery.

TREATMENT

- Treatment is supportive. The expectant mother can be assured that the pruritus will quickly terminate before or after delivery.
- Itching can be relieved with group V topical steroids; cool, wet compresses; oatmeal baths; antipruritic lotions (Sarna lotion); and antihistamines. Prednisone (30 to 40 mg/day) may be required if the pruritus becomes intolerable.

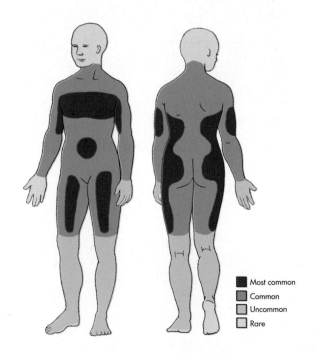

Most common
Common
Uncommon
Rare

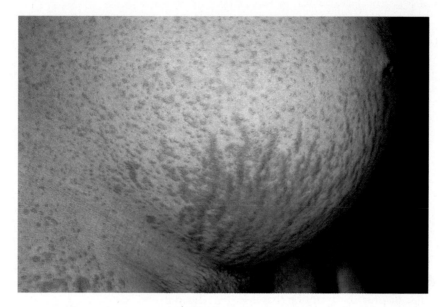

Lesions begin as red papules surrounded by a narrow, pale halo. They increase in number and become more confluent. Unlike urticaria, these lesions remain fixed and may not disappear until after delivery.

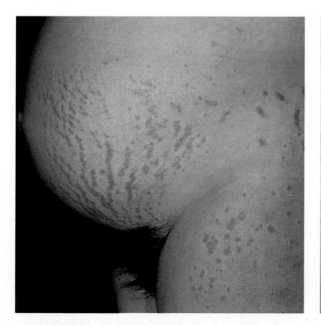

The abdomen is often the initial site of involvement. Initial lesions may be confined to striae.

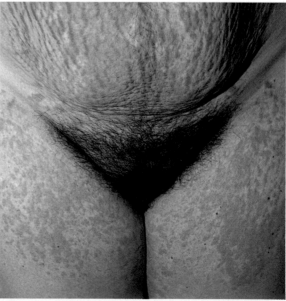

Lesions spread in a symmetric fashion to involve the buttock, legs, arms, and back of the hands. The face is not involved.

4

Acne, Rosacea, and Related Disorders

■ ACNE

DESCRIPTION

- Acne is a papular or pustular eruption that is located on the face, chest, and back.
- Acne occurs with variable severity. Sometimes, just comedones appear; at other times, it is cysts.

HISTORY

- Acne is common in the teenage years but may persist well into adulthood.
- Male patients have more severe disease than female patients.
- Women typically complain of premenstrual flares.
- Areas where the skin is rubbed, such as under the hat or the chin strap, may have accentuated acne.
- There are several variants of acne, including acne fulminans (severe cystic acne with arthralgias, fever, weight loss), steroid acne (comedonal and pustular acne on the chest 2 to 5 weeks after a steroid has been taken), neonatal acne (acne at birth), acne necrotica (itchy acne of the scalp,) and acne excoriée (acne that has been manipulated, leaving erosions and scars).
- Greasy foods cause obesity, not acne.
- The propensity to form scars varies from patient to patient.
- The redness and pigmentation after acne lesion resolution may take months to fade.

SKIN FINDINGS

- Acne lesions are divided into inflammatory and noninflammatory lesions.

- Noninflammatory lesions consist of open comedones (whitehead) and closed comedones (blackheads).
- Inflammatory acne lesions are characterized by the presence of papules, pustules, and nodules (cysts).
- Papules are smaller than 5 mm in diameter.

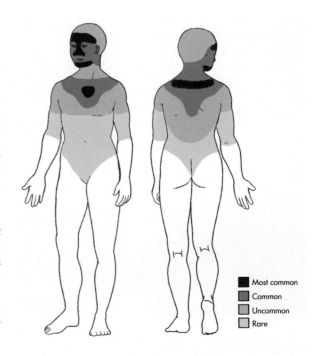

Most common
Common
Uncommon
Rare

- Pustules have a visible central core of purulent material.
- Nodules are larger than 5 mm in diameter. They may become suppurative (cysts) or hemorrhagic.
- Recurring rupture and reepithelialization of cysts lead to epithelial-lined sinus tracks, often accompanied by disfiguring scars.

DIFFERENTIAL DIAGNOSIS
- Rosacea (which has flushing and blushing but no comedones)

TREATMENT
- A program can be established in three visits for most patients.
- Most treatment is continual and prolonged, since it is control, not cure, that is most often achieved.
- Excessive washing interferes with most treatment programs.
- A framework that helps in acne therapy is thinking about the disease as oily skin, blocked pores, and infected pores.

Approach to Therapy
- It takes a least 2 months for most topical programs to show their full effect, so patience must be exercised.
- The patient's propensity to scar should be determined. Patients who show evidence of scarring may be given a 2-month trial of topical therapy and oral antibiotics. Isotretinoin (Accutane) can be considered if there is no substantial improvement after this time. Patients with nodulocystic acne may be started on isotretinoin as initial therapy. Treatment should be aggressive; scarring should not be allowed.

Oily Skin
- Washing (not scrubbing) is useful.
- In female patients, oral contraceptives (e.g., Ortho Tri-Cyclen) can be of benefit. Spironolactone should be considered for women in their twenties and thirties.
- Low-dose isotretinoin is useful for patients with very oily skin. Dermatologists have various treatment schedules for this use.

Blocked Pores (Comedones [Blackheads, and Whiteheads])
- Agents that induce a continuous mild drying and peeling are used. These agents are used alone or combined with tretinoin and related drugs.
- Prescription and over-the-counter products used for this purpose contain sulfur, salicylic acid, resorcinol, and benzoyl peroxide.
- Some examples of benzoyl peroxide preparations are water-based gel (Benzac AC 2.5%, 5%, and 10%), alcohol-based gel (Benzagel 5% and 10%), and acetone-based gel (Persa-Gel 5% and 10%). A new formulation is Triaz 6% or 10%, which adds a hydroxy acid and zinc.
- Azelaic acid (Azelex cream) is comedolytic and antibacterial.
- Tretinoin and related drugs are comedolytic. Tretinoin (Retin-A) is available in several preparations. Retin-A solution (0.05%) is the strongest and most irritating. Retin-A gel (0.025% and 0.01%) is drying and is for oily skin. Retin-A cream (0.1%, 0.05%, and 0.025%) is lubricating and is for dry skin. A new formulation (Retin-A micro) is less irritating. Avita cream (0.025%) and gel are new formulations of tretinoin. Adapalene (Differin) 0.1% gel, pads, or solution may be less irritating.

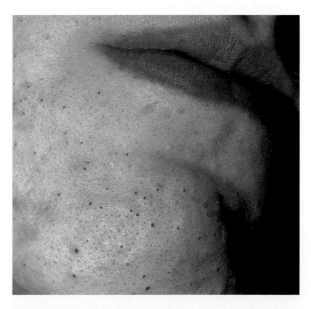

Open comedones (blackheads). Impacted sebum and cellular debris distend the follicular orifice.

Infected Pores (Papules, Pustules)

- Many patients have a combination of comedones, papules, and pustules.
- Tretinoin plus benzoyl peroxide is administered for comedones, papules, and pustules. Tretinoin is applied at bedtime and benzoyl peroxide in the morning.
- Topical antibiotics or benzoyl peroxide plus sulfacetamide or sulfur is administered for papules and pustules. One preparation is applied in the morning and the other in the evening.
- Antibiotics
  - Topical antibiotics can be prescribed initially or as adjunctive therapy after the patient's condition has adapted to tretinoin, benzoyl peroxide, or both agents.
  - Topical antibiotics include clindamycin (Cleocin T pads, solution, gel, and lotion), erythromycin (A/T/S, EryDerm, Erygel, Erycette pads, Staticin, T-Stat pads), and 3% erythromycin with 5% benzoyl peroxide (Benzamycin).
  - Sulfacetamide- and sulfur-containing products (Sulfacet-R, Novacet) can be administered; Klaron contains sulfacetamide.
  - With oral antibiotics, better clinical results and a lower rate of relapse are achieved by starting at higher dosages and tapering only after control is achieved.
  - Typical starting dosages are tetracycline, 500 mg twice a day; erythromycin, 1 gm/day in divided doses; doxycycline, 100 mg twice a day; and minocycline, 100 mg twice a day.
  - Antibiotics must be taken for weeks to be effective and are used for months to achieve maximal benefit.

Nodulocystic Acne

- Isotretinoin (Accutane) is very effective.
- A steroid (triamcinolone, 3 to 10 mg/ml) can be injected into individual cysts.
- Oral prednisone is sometimes used as initial therapy for very severe acne.
- For scarring, referral to a dermatologic surgeon for plastic surgery is advisable only after the acne is quiescent for at least a year. This allows for maximal normal healing before any invasive procedure.

Women Over the Age of 25

- Women over the age of 25 are a special problem in the treatment of acne. They tend to have long-term, low-grade acne.
- Conventional topical therapy, oral antibiotics, oral contraceptives, spironolactone, and isotretinoin (Accutane) are treatment options.

LABORATORY

- Laboratory workup is indicated for female patients with persistent acne and evidence of a hyperandrogenic state.
- Tests include measurements for testosterone, follicle-stimulating hormone, luteinizing hormone, and dehydroepiandrosterone sulfate (DHEA-S).

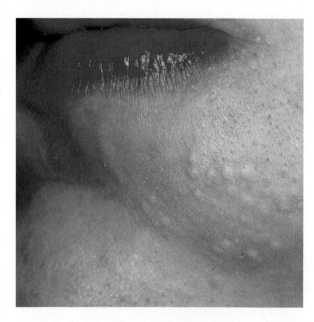

Closed comedones (whiteheads). Tiny white, dome-shaped papules have a very small follicular orifice.

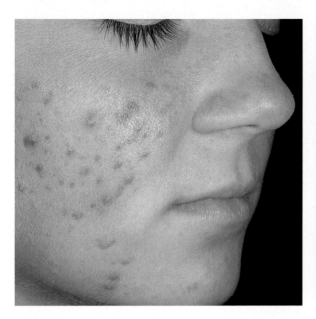

Papular acne. Red papules may be the only type of lesion. Topical medications and oral antibiotics are usually effective for control.

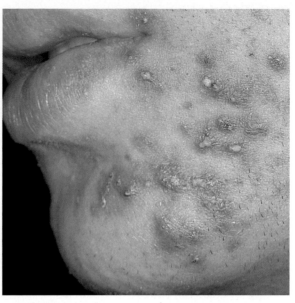

Pustular acne. The classic inflamed acne lesion. Scarring is possible. Topical medications and oral antibiotics are the treatments of first choice. Patients who have the potential to scar and in whom conventional treatment fails are candidates for isotretinoin.

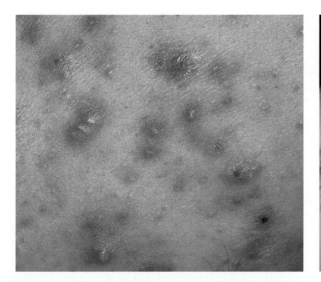

Cystic acne. Cysts are deeper in the skin than papules and pustules. They have the potential for extending and destroying surrounding follicular structures that result in scarring.

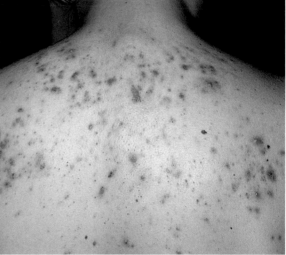

Cystic acne. The face, chest, and back are frequently involved. Some patients heal with extensive keloidal or atrophic scars. Cystic acne resists conventional topical medications and oral antibiotics. Isotretinoin is often required for control.

■ PERIORAL DERMATITIS

DESCRIPTION

- Perioral dermatitis is a distinctive eruption around the mouth, nose, and eyes.
- Perioral dermatitis typically occurs in young women.
- It resembles acne.
- Isolation of a fusobacterium suggests a bacterial etiology.
- The routine use of moisturizers may be a cause.

HISTORY

- A persistent eruption continues for months.
- The eruption may start around the mouth but may also involve the perinasal and periocular regions.
- This condition is asymptomatic.
- Patients may have tried topical steroids, which causes temporary improvement.
- This condition is reported in children, but typically, it occurs in young female patients.
- Untreated, the disease persist for months.
- With oral treatment, most problems clear in 2 weeks.
- Relapse is uncommon.

SKIN FINDINGS

- Pinpoint papules and pustules on a red and scaling base are confined to the chin and nasolabial folds.
- There is a clear zone around the vermilion border.
- There are varying degrees of involvement.
- Pustules on the cheeks adjacent to the nostrils are common.
- Sometimes, perioral dermatitis remains confined perinasally. Sometimes, it occurs lateral to the eyes.
- Children often have periocular and perinasal lesions.

DIFFERENTIAL DIAGNOSIS

- Acne
- Seborrheic dermatitis
- Atopic (eczematous) dermatitis

TREATMENT

- Tetracycline (500 mg twice a day), erythromycin (500 mg twice a day), doxycycline (100 mg twice a day), or minocycline (100 mg twice a day) is given for a 2- to 4-week course. The condition of many patients responds to lower doses.
- Treatment is predictably effective.

- Once the condition is resolved, the antibiotic is stopped or tapered over 4 to 5 weeks.
- Patients are retreated with renewed activity.
- Long-term maintenance is sometimes required.
- Topical treatment involves twice-a-day use of 1% metronidazole cream (MetroGel), sodium sulfacetamide 10% plus sulfur 5% (Sulfacet-R), clindamycin (Cleocin T pads, solution, and lotion) or erythromycin 2% solution (A/T/S) or gel (Emgel). Topical antibiotics are not predictably effective. Oral antibiotics are used if a 4- to 6-week course of topical treatment fails.
- Short courses of hydrocortisone (0.5% or 1%) along with cool compresses help suppress erythema and scaling.
- Stronger steroids should be avoided.
- The patient should not routinely use moisturizers.
- Warn patients that prolonged use of topical steroids on the face creates this disease.

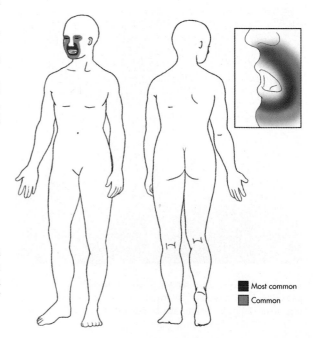

Most common
Common

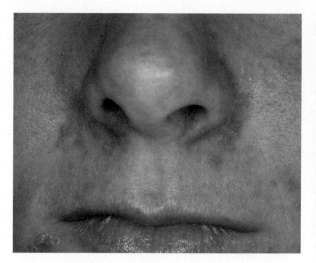

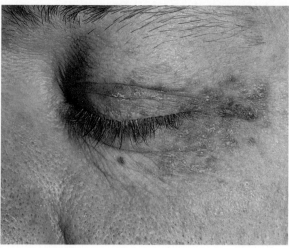

Pinpoint pustules next to the nostrils may be the first sign or only manifestation of the disease.

Pinpoint papules and pustules similar to those seen next to the nostrils are sometimes seen lateral to the eyes.

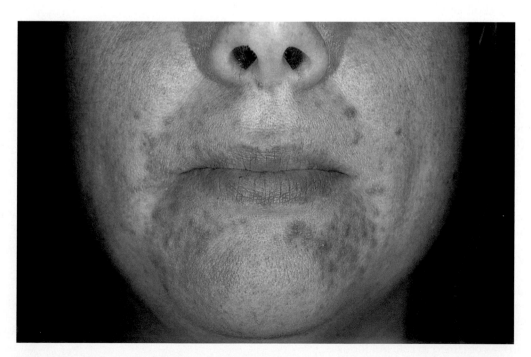

Long-term treatment with topical steroids should be suspected in a patient with perioral dermatitis of this intensity.

■ ROSACEA (ACNE ROSACEA)

DESCRIPTION

- Rosacea is a common facial eruption.
- Patients are usually over age 30 and of most often of Celtic origin.
- It has dual components: one vascular (redness, telangiectasia, flushing, blushing) and one eruptive (papules, pustules).

HISTORY

- The typical patient is 30 to 50 years old.
- The patient complains of redness and pimples.
- There is flushing or facial redness.
- Rosacea is exacerbated by the ingestion of hot foods and drinks, the ingestion of alcohol (red wines), or exposure to the sun and other heat sources.
- Ocular symptoms include mild conjunctivitis with soreness, grittiness, and lacrimation.
- The condition is chronic (years), with episodes of activity followed by quiescence.

SKIN FINDINGS

- Eruptions appear on the forehead, cheeks, and nose and about the eyes.
- Erythema, telangiectasias, or both conditions are present.
- Usually, there are fewer than 10 papules and pustules at any one time.
- Severe cases have numerous pustules, telangiectasia, diffuse erythema, oily skin, and edema (cheeks and nose).
- Chronic, deep inflammation of the nose leads to an irreversible hypertrophy called *rhinophyma.* This is more common in men.
- Ocular signs include conjunctival hyperemia, telangiectasia of the lid, blepharitis, superficial punctate keratopathy, chalazion, corneal vascularization and infiltrate, and corneal vascularization and thinning.

LABORATORY

- The diagnosis is usually made clinically; tests are usually unnecessary.
- Bacterial culture is obtained to rule out folliculitis.
- A potassium hydroxide test is performed to rule out tinea.
- A biopsy is obtained to rule out lupus.

DIFFERENTIAL DIAGNOSIS

- Acne (no comedones in rosacea)
- Pustular tinea
- Perioral dermatitis
- Folliculitis (staphylococcal, gram negative)
- Lupus erythematosus

TREATMENT

- The patient should avoid physically hot food and drinks, spicy foods, red wines, and sunlight.
- Green-based cosmetic foundations mask the redness.
- Sunscreens are recommended.
- The pustular component is treated topically or systemically.
- For topical treatment, metronidazole (MetroGel, MetroCream, Metrolotion, Noritate) and sulfacetamide plus sulfur lotion (Sulfacet-R, Novacet) are the most effective. Sulfacet-R is especially useful for oily skin; it is available tinted or tint free. Clindamycin (Cleocin T solution, pads, or lotion) and erythromycin (Erycette pads, Emgel, T-Stat lotion or pads) are less effective.

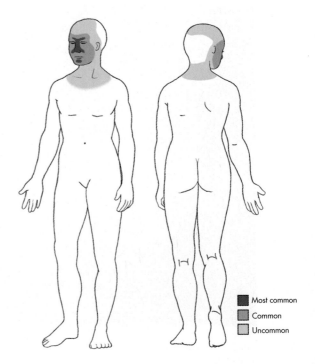

■ Most common
☐ Common
☐ Uncommon

- Systemic therapy is more effective. Tetracycline (500 mg twice a day), erythromycin (500 mg twice a day), doxycycline (100 mg twice a day), or minocycline (100 mg twice a day) in a 2- to 4-week course usually controls the pustules. In many patients, this condition then responds to lower doses.
- Bactrim DS, twice a day, or metronidazole, 250 mg/day, may be used for resistant cases.
- Ocular symptoms are treated with systemic antibiotics.

- Medication is stopped or tapered after the condition resolves.
- The response after therapy is unpredictable.
- Recurring disease is retreated; then medication is tapered to the minimum dosage that provides adequate control.
- For chronic relapsing cases or failure to respond, isotretinoin (Accutane), 0.5 mg/kg/day for 20 weeks, should be considered.
- Rhinophyma benefits from electrosurgery, carbon dioxide laser surgery, and plastic surgery.

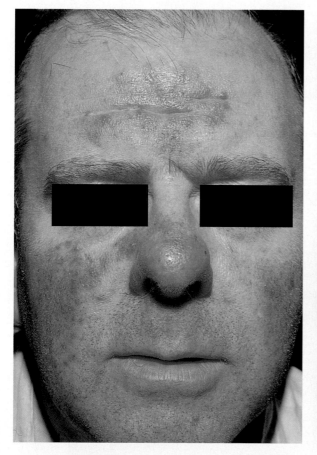

Erythema is intense on the nose and cheeks. Inflammation of the nose must be controlled to prevent permanent changes (rhinophyma) from occurring.

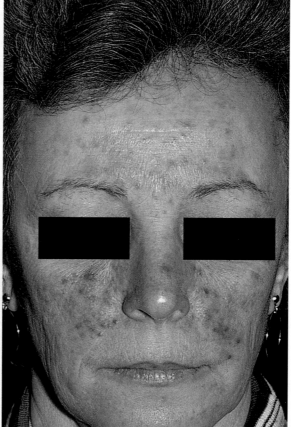

An extensive case with many papules and pustules. Rosacea may consist of three components (erythema, papules, and pustules). The diagnosis may be difficult to establish in patients without papules and pustules.

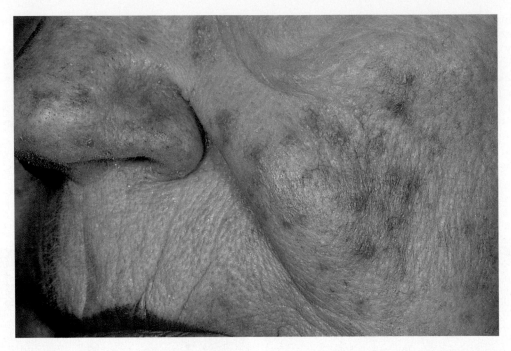

The classic presentation for rosacea is a patient with papules and pustules on the forehead, nose, and cheeks. Papules and pustules are not usually found on the nose in acne patients.

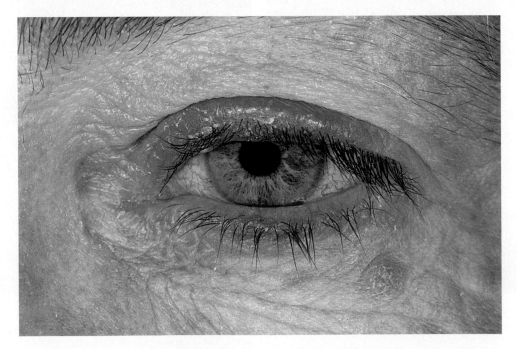

Ocular signs occurs in up to 50% of patients with rosacea. Mild conjunctivitis with soreness, grittiness, and lacrimation are the most common complaints.

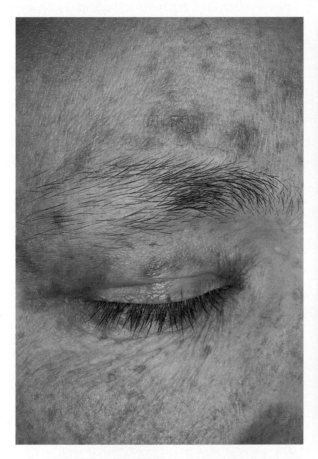

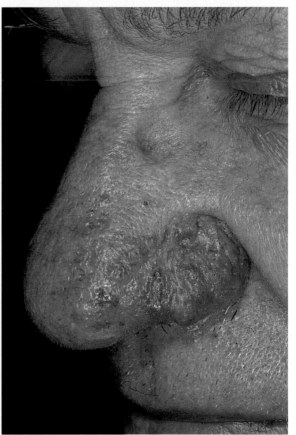

Rosacea can involve the entire face. Withdrawal from long-term topical steroid therapy can produce an identical picture.

Chronic inflammation of the nose results in irreversible hypertrophy (rhinophyma) in predisposed individuals.

■ HIDRADENITIS SUPPURATIVA

DESCRIPTION

- Hidradenitis suppurativa is a chronic suppurative and scarring disease occurring in the axillae, in the anogenital regions, and under the female breast.

HISTORY

- Hidradenitis suppurativa is more common in female patients.
- It presents with a painful "boil."
- Systemic symptoms are uncommon.
- It is worse in the obese.
- It does not appear until after puberty. Most cases appear in the second and third decades of life.
- There is clustering in families.
- The disease is progressive and self-perpetuating.
- There is great variation among patients in the clinical severity.

SKIN FINDINGS

- The hallmark is the double comedone (blackhead with two or more surface openings).
- Sinus tracts are common.
- Extensive, deep, dermal inflammation results in large, painful abscesses.
- Cordlike bands of scar tissue crisscross the site.
- Sebum excretion is not an important factor, and this may explain the unsatisfactory therapeutic effect of conventional acne treatment and retinoids.

LABORATORY

- Biopsy shows follicular occlusion by keratinous material, folliculitis, and secondary destruction of the skin adnexa (apocrine glands) and subcutis.

DIFFERENTIAL DIAGNOSIS

- Acne
- Furuncle or carbuncle

TREATMENT

- Large fluctuant cysts are incised and drained.
- Intralesional triamcinolone acetonide (Kenalog), 2.5 to 10 mg/ml, is administered for smaller cysts.
- Weight loss sometimes is helpful.
- Long-term oral antibiotics are the mainstay of treatment. Agents include tetracycline (500 mg twice a day), erythromycin (500 mg twice a day), doxycycline (100 mg twice a day), and minocycline (100 mg twice a day). Lower dosages are tried for maintenance.
- Second-line antibiotics include trimethoprim/sulfamethoxazole Bactrim DS (1 by mouth twice a day), metronidazole (375 mg twice a day), and clindamycin (150 mg twice a day).
- Oral contraceptives are sometimes helpful, especially with premenstrual flares.
- Isotretinoin (1 mg/kg/day for 20 weeks) is effective in selected cases (best in early nonscarred sinus tract lesions).
- Surgical excision is often the only solution.
- Local opening of the sinus tract can be helpful.

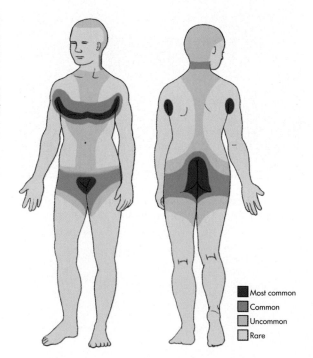

Most common
Common
Uncommon
Rare

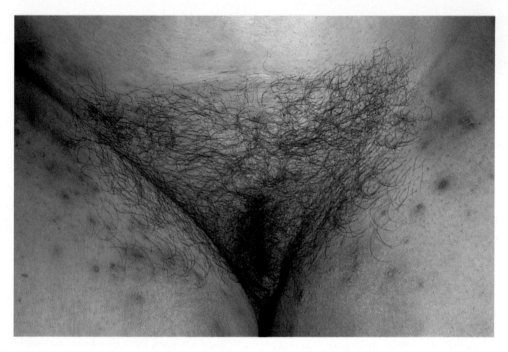

Hidradenitis should be suspected when a patient complains of boils in the groin. Comedones, which are markers for this disease, should be carefully sought.

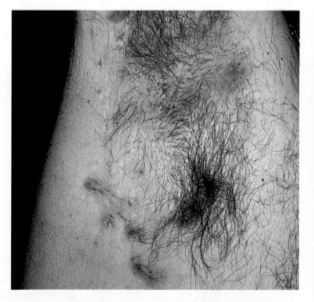

These large deep cystic lesions heal with scarring. Intralesional cortisone injections may help abort and contain an active lesion.

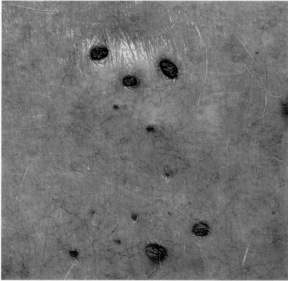

Double and triple comedones are blackheads with two or more surface openings that communicate under the skin. They are a hallmark of hidradenitis. The axillae, the area under the breast, the groin, and the buttock area should be examined for markers of the disease.

5

Psoriasis and Other Papulosquamous Diseases

■ PSORIASIS

DESCRIPTION

- Psoriasis is one of the papulosquamous diseases (scaly, papules, plaques).
- It affects the skin, the nails, and joints.
- There are many forms, but the common presentation is scaly plaques involving the elbows, knees, and scalp.

HISTORY

- Psoriasis affects 1% to 3% of the population worldwide.
- It is transmitted genetically; its etiology is unknown. Men and women are equally affected.
- This condition is lifelong and is characterized by chronic, recurrent exacerbations and remissions.
- Stress may precipitate an episode.
- Environmental influences modify the course, severity, and age of presentation.
- The extent and severity of the disease vary widely.
- This condition is most severe when associated with disease caused by the human immunodeficiency virus (HIV).
- It can develop at the site of physical trauma.
- In childhood, the first episode may be stimulated by streptococcal pharyngitis.
- In general, late-onset disease tends to be milder.
- This condition is worse in the dry winter weather.
- The amount of pruritus varies.
- Psoriatic arthritis (rheumatoid factor negative) occurs in 5% to 8% of the population with psoriasis.

The onset may precede, accompany, or follow skin manifestations.
- Drugs that precipitate or exacerbate psoriasis include lithium, beta blockers, antimalarials, and systemic steroids.

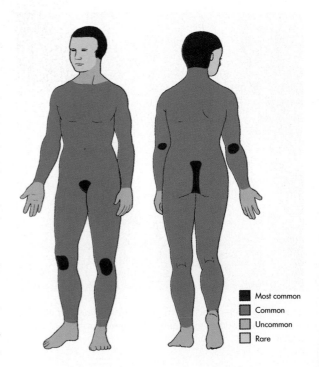

Most common
Common
Uncommon
Rare

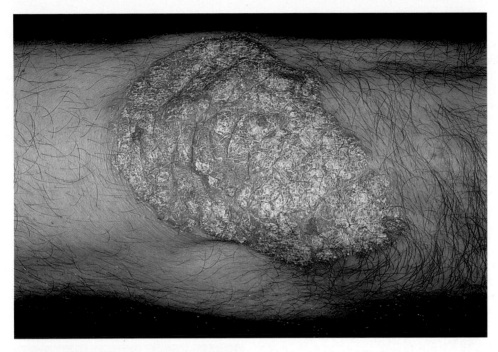

Plaque psoriasis. The classic presentation. Thick red plaques have a sharply defined border and an adherent silvery scale.

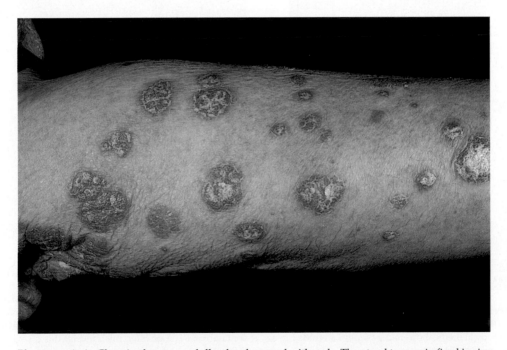

Plaque psoriasis. Chronic plaques are dull red and covered with scale. They tend to remain fixed in size and position for long periods.

Skin Findings

Plaque

- This form begins as red, scaling papules that coalesce to form round-to-oval plaques.
- It usually spares the palms, soles, and face.
- It affects the extensor more than the flexor surfaces.
- The deep, rich, red color is a characteristic feature that remains constant.
- The scale is adherent and silvery white and reveals bleeding points when removed (Auspitz's sign).
- The scale may become extremely dense, especially on the scalp.

Guttate (associated with group A streptococcus)

- This form is associated with a sudden appearance of scaly papules.

Localized pustular (palmoplantar pustulosis)

- Localized recurrent crops of small, sterile pustules evolve from the red base, commonly on the palms and soles. The pustules do not rupture but turn dark brown and scaly as they reach the surface.

Inverse (intertriginous)

- Psoriasis inversus occurs in flexural or intertriginous areas in the groin and under the breasts.
- Psoriatic plaques of skinfolds appear as smooth, red plaques with a macerated surface.

Generalized pustular

- Sterile pustules are localized or generalized. Generalized pustular psoriasis is a serious disease.

Erythrodermic

- Erythrodermic psoriasis presents as total body redness and is a serious disease.

Nail disease

- Pitting, onycholysis (separation of nail from nail bed), subungual debris, and nail-plate deformity occur in some cases.
- These changes offer supporting evidence of the diagnosis when skin changes are equivocal or absent.
- Also, total nail dystrophy or oil-drop sign occurs.

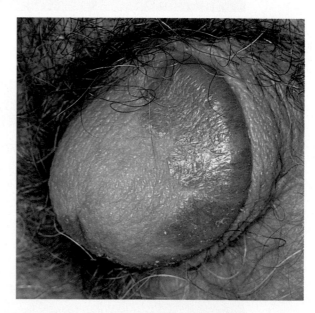

Plaque psoriasis. A fixed red plaque with a sharp border on the glans is a common presentation for psoriasis. It may be the only cutaneous lesion. The plaques often last for months and years. Topical steroids provide temporary relief but should not be used constantly. Most other topical medications are too irritating. Patients should be reassured that this disease is not contagious. Patients often misinterpret this disease as a yeast infection.

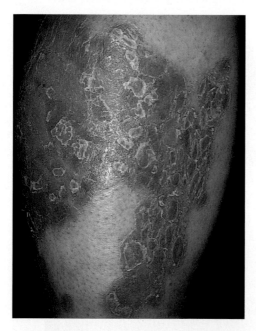

Plaque psoriasis. Plaques may become red and inflamed. Inflamed plaques need to be treated carefully with topical medication. All topical medications except topical steroids can aggravate these active lesions.

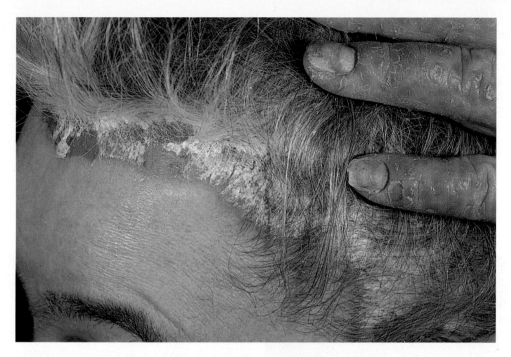

Scalp psoriasis. Dense scale covering a part or the entire scalp surface is highly characteristic of psoriasis. The scalps of all patients with psoriasis should be checked.

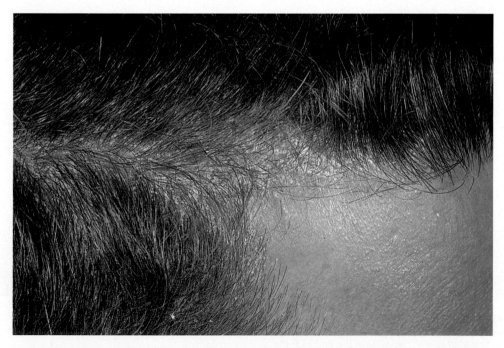

Scalp psoriasis. Sometimes, it is impossible to distinguish between scalp psoriasis and seborrheic dermatitis. The ears and faces of patients with seborrheic dermatitis are often involved.

LABORATORY

- In guttate psoriasis, the presence of streptococci is confirmed with an antistreptolysin-O titer or throat culture.
- In inverse disease, a potassium hydroxide test is performed to rule out candidal infection.
- In severe flares, HIV infection should be sought.
- When the diagnosis is uncertain, a biopsy should be performed.

DIFFERENTIAL DIAGNOSIS

- Seborrheic dermatitis
- Eczema (dyshidrotic hand and foot eczema)
- Tinea capitis, tinea manus, tinea pedis
- Lichen simplex chronicus
- Candidal infection
- Syphilis
- Pityriasis rosea
- Drug eruption
- Acute generalized exanthematous pustulosis

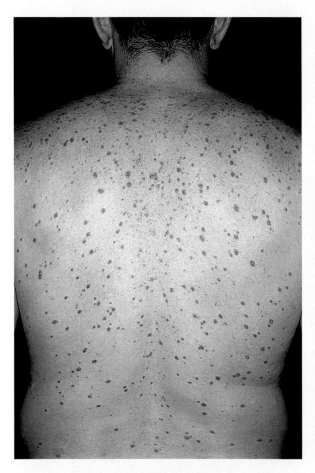

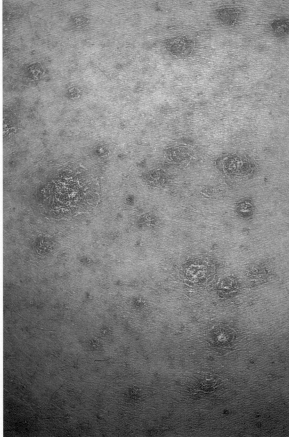

Guttate psoriasis. An acute or chronic streptococcal pharyngitis should be suspected in when there is a sudden onset of uniform, small, round plaques. This is often the first sign that a patient has the psoriatic diathesis.

Guttate psoriasis. Lesions become larger after the acute phase, and the acute disease may evolve into chronic plaque psoriasis.

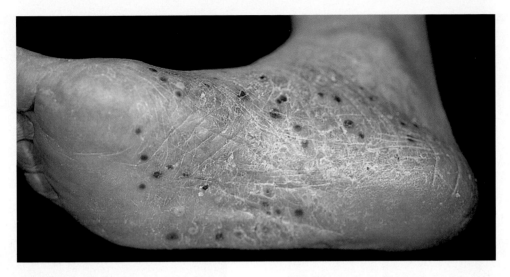

Pustular psoriasis of the soles. Extensive involvement is painful. Systemic medication is sometimes required for extensive cases.

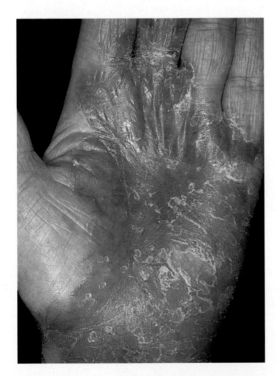

Psoriasis of the palms. This deep red, smooth plaque is painful.

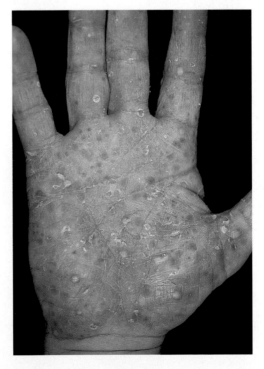

Pustular psoriasis of the palms. This unique form of psoriasis is long lasting and difficult to control. Differentiation from dyshidrotic eczema is sometimes difficult.

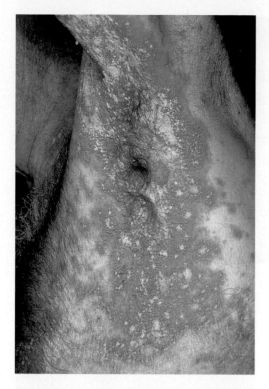

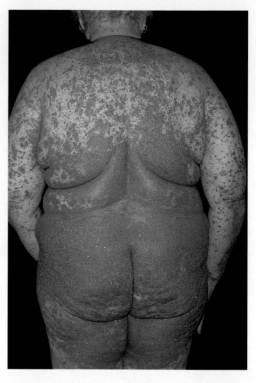

Pustular psoriasis. This rare form of psoriasis can be extensive and serious. It responds to cyclosporine, methotrexate, and acitretin.

Erythrodermic psoriasis. Generalized intense inflammation can occur and often requires systemic medications for control.

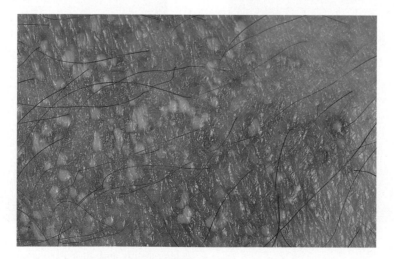

Pustular psoriasis.

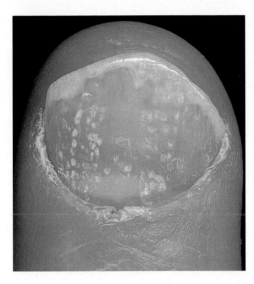

Psoriasis. Pitting. Foci of inflammation of the proximal nail matrix results in the accumulation of parakeratotic cells on the nail surface. These are shed as the nail grows out, leaving depressions or pits in the nail surface.

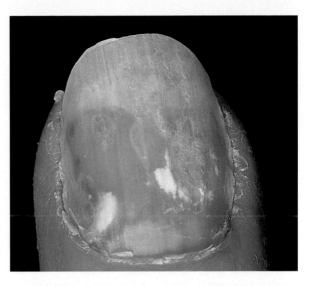

Psoriasis. Oil spot lesion. Accumulation of parakeratotic debris and serum under the nail produces the yellow nail spot lesion.

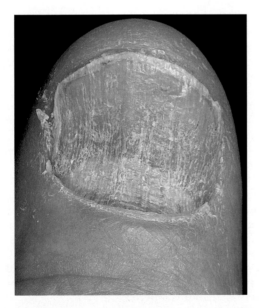

Psoriasis. Nail deformity. Inflammation of the proximal nail matrix causes nail-plate surface deformity

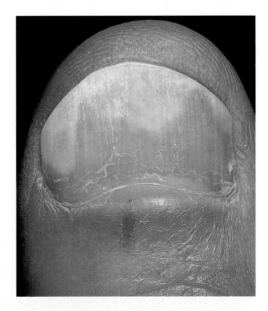

Psoriasis. Onycholysis and nail deformity. Inflammation of various parts on the nail matrix produces a bizarre pattern of nail deformity. Clinical differentiation from onychomycosis is sometimes difficult.

TREATMENT
Topical Therapy

Calcipotriol (Dovonex) is a vitamin D_3 analogue in a cream, ointment, and scalp solution.

- It is applied once or twice a day as tolerated in amounts up to 100 gm/wk.
- The medication should be confined to the plaque.
- Side effects include mild or transient local irritation and erythema.
- Group II to V topical steroids (applied at a different time of day) can be used to control irritation. They are used less frequently once irritation is controlled.

Topical steroids (group I to V) give fast but temporary relief.

- They are best for reducing inflammation and itching (e.g., intertriginous disease).
- A few, small, chronic plaques are treated with an intralesional steroid (triamcinolone [Kenalog], 10 mg/ml).
- Steroids becomes less effective with continued use.
- Side effects include atrophy and telangiectasia with long-term use.
- Steroids are best used in cycles (e.g., twice a day for 7 to 14 days followed by a "rest" for 7 to 14 days).

Anthralin (Drithocreme 0.1%, 0.25%, 0.5%, 0.1% HP; Micanol 1% cream) is useful for chronic extensor surface plaques and scalp problems.

- In the short-contact method the patient applies the medication and washes off in 20 minutes.
- The patient should leave the medication on for a longer duration if it is tolerated.
- The medication should be confined to the plaque.
- Side effects include irritation and staining.

Tazarotene (Tazorac) gel 0.05% and 0.1% is used topically once per night.

- The medication should be confined to the plaque.
- Group II to V topical steroids are applied once a day to control irritation; they are less frequently once irritation is controlled.
- Severe irritation is the only side effect.

There are several medications for the scalp.

- The scalp is difficult to treat; the goal is to provide symptomatic and cosmetic relief.

- Scales are removed first to facilitate penetration of medicine.
- Superficial scales are removed with salicylic acid (T/Sal) or tar (T/Gel, Reme-T, Pentrax) shampoos.
- Diffuse scalp scale is removed with fluocinolone (Derma-Smoothe/FS) lotion applied to the entire scalp at bedtime and washed out in the morning. This regimen should be repeated for 5 to 10 days. It removes the scales and controls inflammation.
- Phenol, sodium chloride, and liquid paraffin (Baker's P & S) is applied at bedtime and washed out in the morning.
- Hot olive-oil turbans help remove very thick scaling.
- Steroid solution or foam (e.g., clobetasol [Cormax scalp solution], betamethasone valerate [Luxiq]) penetrates through the hair.
- Steroid gels (e.g., fluocinonide [Lidex], clobetasol [Temovate], desoximetasone [Topicort]) penetrate through the hair and into the scales.
- Smaller plaques are treated with intralesional steroids.

Phototherapy

- Phototherapy is usually effective treatment; ultraviolet light may be used in combination with topical treatment. In some people, this condition does not respond to phototherapy; in others, it gets worse.
- Ultraviolet B (UVB) is typically given three to five times a week.
- Tanning booths (ultraviolet A [UVA]) sometimes help.
- Tar and lubricants enhance the effectiveness of UVB.
- Topical steroid use diminishes the length of remission.
- Side effects include sunburning, premature skin aging, and skin cancer.
- Narrow-band UVB is more effective but is not generally available.
- Psoralen plus ultraviolet A (PUVA) requires therapy three times a week until the condition resolves; then it is tapered.
  - Patients take photosensitizing psoralen $1\frac{1}{2}$ to 2 hours before exposure to UVA.
  - This is an effective method of controlling but not curing psoriasis.

- This treatment is used for symptomatic control of severe, recalcitrant, disabling, plaque psoriasis.
- Side effects include gastrointestinal intolerance of the drug, sunburning, photodamaged skin, cataracts, and skin cancer.

Systemic Therapy

- Patients who have psoriasis involving more than 20% of the body surface or who are very uncomfortable should consider systemic therapy. Such therapy is complicated and best managed by a dermatologist.
- A rotational approach to therapy minimizes the long-term toxic effects from any one therapy and allows effective long-term treatment.

Methotrexate (MTX) is the gold standard.
- It is most effective in erythrodermic and generalized pustular psoriasis.
- It is also useful for plaque disease and effective for arthritis.
- It is given orally, intramuscularly, or subcutaneously.
- The regimen should be "worked up" to a dose of 12.5 to 50 mg/wk.
- Folic acid, 1 mg/day, is administered but not on the day that MTX is administered.
- This medication requires close follow-up, including monitoring of the complete blood count and liver function and a periodic liver biopsy.
- Drug interactions can occur after the administration of salicylates, many nonsteroidal antiinflammatory agents, trimethoprim-sulfamethoxazole, penicillins, and other agents.
- Side effects include nausea, anorexia, fatigue, oral ulcerations, mild leukopenia, thrombocytopenia, and hepatic fibrosis or cirrhosis.

Cyclosporine (Neoral) is best administered for severe inflammatory psoriasis.
- The dosage is 2.5 to 5.0 mg/kg/day.
- The dosage is tapered after control is achieved.
- This medication requires close monitoring of blood pressure, the complete blood count, and creatinine, magnesium, cholesterol, and triglyceride levels.
- The dose is decreased if the creatinine level increases by 30% from the baseline.

- Drug interactions can occur.
- Side effects include hypertension and nephrotoxicity.

Acitretin (Soriatane) is highly effective for generalized pustular and erythrodermic psoriasis.
- It is useful in combination with PUVA and UVB.
- The regimen is begun at 10 to 25 mg/day as a single dose.
- Side effects (similar to those of isotretinoin [Accutane], which limits treatment for many patients) include teratogenicity, dry or sticky skin, myalgias, arthralgias, pseudotumor cerebri, depression, hair loss, hepatitis, pancreatitis, increased cholesterol and triglyceride levels, and bone marrow failure.

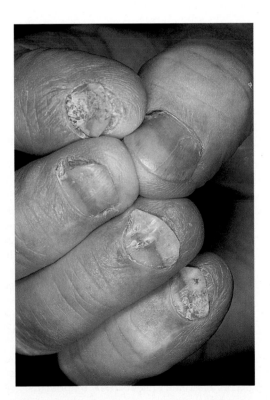

Psoriasis. Onycholysis and nail deformity. Inflammation of various parts on the nail matrix produces a bizzare pattern of nail deformity. Clinical differentation from onychomycosis is sometime difficult.

■ SEBORRHEIC DERMATITIS

DESCRIPTION

- Seborrheic dermatitis is a common, chronic, inflammatory dermatitis with a characteristic distribution in infants and adults.
- The extent of involvement among individuals varies widely, from mild dandruff to a more extensive inflammatory dermatitis.
- Pityrosporum ovale probably is a causative factor, but both genetic and environmental factors seem to influence the onset and course.

HISTORY

- Infants, teens, and adults can be affected.
- This condition is more severe and more difficult to control in patients with neurologic disease (e.g., head trauma, spinal cord injury, Parkinson's disease, stroke), or infection with the human immunodeficiency virus (HIV) or acquired immunodeficiency syndrome.

SKIN FINDINGS

Infants

- A yellow, greasy adherent scale commonly develops on the vertex of the scalp (cradle cap).
- The greasy scale may accumulate, thicken, and adhere over much of the scalp; it may be accompanied by redness.
- Dermatitis may affect the diaper area and axillary skin.
- Secondary infection can occur.

Adults

- Greasy scales and yellow-red coalescing macules, patches, and papules may be diffuse in characteristic locations, including the scalp and scalp margins, eyebrows, base of the eyelashes, nasolabial folds and paranasal skin, external ear canals, posterior auricular fold, presternal skin, and upper back.
- This condition may affect the flexural skin, including the inguinal folds, and submammary, anogenital, umbilical, and axillary skin.
- White scaling that adheres to the eyelashes and lid margins with variable amounts of erythema is characteristic of seborrheic blepharitis.

LABORATORY

- A skin biopsy is not usually necessary.
- Fungal culture and potassium hydroxide examination are indicated for atypical or resistant cases of scalp or facial scaling.

DIFFERENTIAL DIAGNOSIS

- Infants: atopic eczema, zinc deficiency, Langerhans' cell histiocytosis
- Adults: tinea faciei, lupus erythematosus, rosacea, psoriasis, pemphigus foliaceous

COURSE AND PROGNOSIS

- In infants, this self-limited condition requires little or no treatment.
- In adults, it tends to be a chronic condition with periods of remission and exacerbation.
- Flares are precipitated by stress, fatigue, or sunlight in some patients.
- Most cases are adequately controlled with treatment.

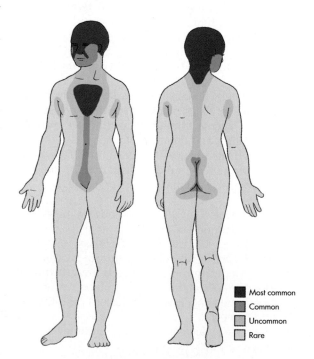

Most common
Common
Uncommon
Rare

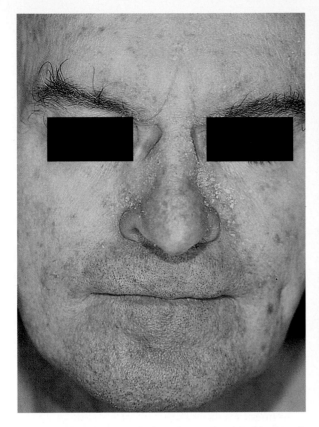

Older patients especially those with neurologic problems such as Parkinson's disease, are predisposed to extensive seborrheic dermatitis.

Erythema and scaling may be extensive and extend beyond the nasolabial folds.

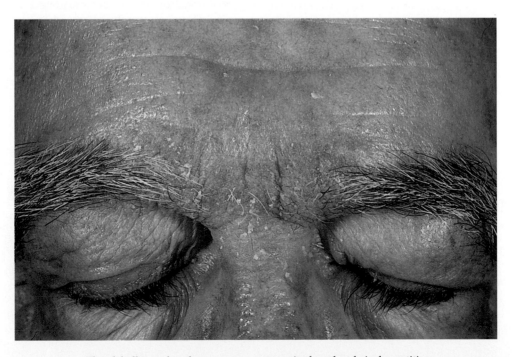

The glabellae and eyebrows are a common site for seborrheic dermatitis.

TREATMENT
General

- If there are heavy serum and a heavy crust, a course of oral antistaphylococcal antibiotics (dicloxacillin, cephalexin) may be considered.
- Ketoconazole (Nizoral cream) or ciclopirox applied once a day is effective in patients with widespread disease.
- Severe seborrhea is treated using the following:
  - A short course of oral ketoconazole (200 mg/day) or fluconazole [Diflucan] (150 mg/day) to eradicate *Pityrosporum ovale*
  - UVB phototherapy if there is no history of photoaggravation
  - A short course of oral corticosteroids

Facial and Intertriginous Involvement

- Mild facial seborrheic dermatitis may respond well to ketoconazole cream (Loprox Gel) applied daily to the affected skin or an antidandruff shampoo diluted with water and used as a daily facial wash. (The patient should avoid prolonged use of topical corticosteroids on facial skin.)
- A group VI or VII topical steroid cream or lotion (i.e., hydrocortisone, desonide) is applied twice a day initially and then two or three times a week as necessary. Long-term use must be avoided.

Scalp

- Mild scale is easily removed by frequent shampooing with products containing sulfur, salicylic acid, or both agents (e.g., Sebulex shampoo). Prolong remissions can be stimulated with the frequent use of salicylic acid, sulfur, zinc pyrithione (Head & Shoulders, ZNP Bar Soap), selenium (Selsun lotion, Selsun Blue), or tar shampoos (T/Gel, Reme-T, Pentrax).
- Dense, thick, adherent scaling is removed by applying warm mineral or olive oil to the scalp and washing several hours later.
- At bedtime, the patient applies liquor carbonis detergens 10% (coal-tar solution) in Nivea oil (compounded by a pharmacist) or Derma-Smoothe/FS lotion (peanut oil, mineral oil, fluocinolone acetonide 0.01%); it is washed out in the morning. Wetting the scalp before application and using a shower cap help penetration. This regimen should be repeated each night until the scalp no longer has scaling (1 to 3 weeks).

Blepharitis

- Scaling may be suppressed by lid massage and frequent washing with zinc- or tar-containing antidandruff shampoos.

DISCUSSION

- HIV infection should be considered in individuals with severe or widespread seborrheic dermatitis.

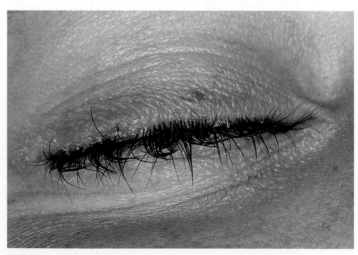

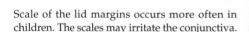

Scale of the lid margins occurs more often in children. The scales may irritate the conjunctiva.

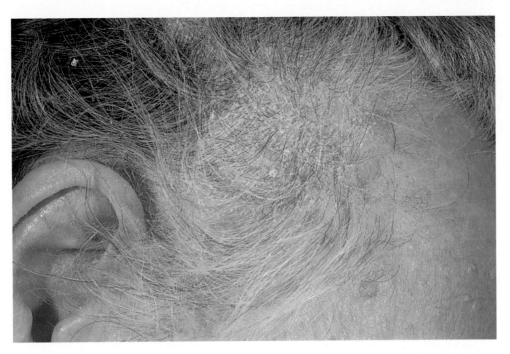

Fine to dense scale is the most common presentation for seborrheic dermatitis. Psoriatic scalp plaques are usually thicker and contain dense scale.

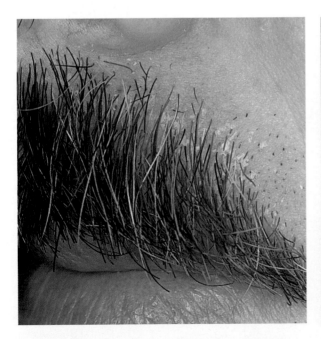

Scale forms in hair-bearing areas of the beard and scalp. Spontaneous clearing would be expected to follow shaving.

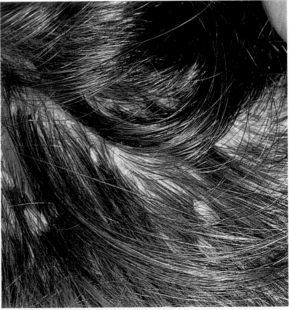

Dense patches of quadrangular scale occur in children. The scale adheres to the hair.

■ GROVER'S DISEASE (TRANSIENT ACANTHOLYTIC DERMATOSIS)

DESCRIPTION

- Grover's disease is an uncommon, acquired, persistent, papulovesicular eruption.
- Its cause is unknown. Often, it is a reaction to excessive heat or sweating.
- It may occur after a steam bath, hot tub use, or ionizing or ultraviolet radiation.

HISTORY

- Most cases involve white men older than 40.
- The male-to-female ratio is 3:1.
- Grover's disease has a self-limited course.
- There is mild to moderate itching. The itching may precede the onset of the eruption.
- This condition lasts for weeks, months, or years.

SKIN FINDINGS

- Findings include 1- to 3-mm, red-brown papulovesicles or keratotic papules.
- The lesions appear primarily on the chest, lower ribcage, upper back, and lumbar area. They may spread to the deltoids, lateral neck, and thighs.
- Lesions may heal with postinflammatory hyperpigmentation or hypopigmentation.

LABORATORY

- A biopsy is helpful. Microscopically, there are acantholysis (separation of cells in the epidermis) and dyskeratosis (changes in epidermal cells), like that seen in Darier's disease. Spongiotic changes (fluid in the epidermis), as occurs in eczema, is present when there is an associated eczematous component. Hyperkeratosis is common. The dermis may contain lymphocytes and eosinophils.
- Biopsy for immunofluorescence is usually negative.

COURSE AND PROGNOSIS

- Grover's disease is self-limited; its duration is correlated with age.
- Older patients are likely to have extensive eruptions of longer duration. Most cases last a few weeks or months. Some cases persist for years.
- The extent and severity fluctuate. Some cases are persistent or recurrent (sometimes seasonal).

DIFFERENTIAL DIAGNOSIS

- Acne
- Candidiasis
- Eczema
- Dermatitis herpetiformis
- Drug eruptions
- Viral exanthems
- Pityriasis rosea
- Miliaria (heat rash)
- Seborrheic dermatitis
- Seborrheic keratosis
- Impetigo
- Bites

TREATMENT

General Measures

- The patient should avoid strenuous exercise and exposure to sunlight. Colloidal oatmeal baths relieve itching. The use of soap should be minimized. Emollients are applied after washing to treat dry skin. Wet compresses with cool water or calamine lotion relieve itching. Mentholated lotions (Sarna) or pramoxine-containing preparations (Prax, Pramosone, Aveeno antipruritic cream) provide relief.

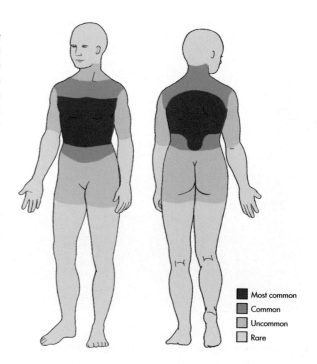

Most common
Common
Uncommon
Rare

- Antihistamines are of limited value in controlling itching.
- Antibiotics and dapsone are not effective.

Other Treatments

- A group I to V topical steroid may be used for initial control in most cases; then it is used as needed for recurrences.
- Oral vitamin A, 50,000 IU three times a day for 2 weeks then reduced to 50,000 IU a day for a maximum of 12 weeks, is effective for extensive and severely pruritic cases.

- Isotretinoin, 40 mg/day, is administered for 2 to 12 weeks. Once the patient's condition improves, the dosage is tapered to 10 mg/day, and the 12-week course is completed.
- Prednisone, 20 mg twice a day, controls extensive inflammation and itching. Then the dosage is tapered. The medication is discontinued once control is achieved.

CAVEAT

- Grover's disease mimics many other diseases. Biopsy establishes the diagnosis. Evaluating the effect of treatment is difficult because this disease often resolves spontaneously.

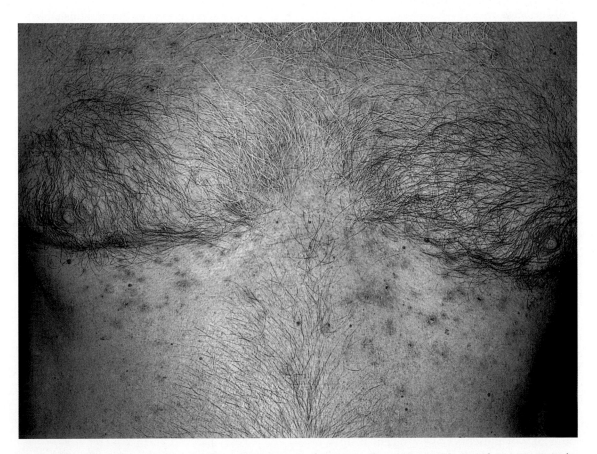

There are few too many papules or papulovesicles. Pruritus is often intense. Some cases are transient, but most persist for months.

■ PITYRIASIS ROSEA

DESCRIPTION

- Pityriasis rosea is a common, benign, usually asymptomatic, distinctive, skin eruption that may be viral in origin.
- It is typically confined to the trunk and begins with a single, red oval plaque, the herald patch, that is followed in about 1 week by a number of similar, smaller plaques.
- Pityriasis rosea clears spontaneously in 1 to 2 months.

HISTORY

- There is some evidence that pityriasis rosea is viral in origin.
- Small epidemics have occurred in fraternity houses and military bases.
- More than 75% of patients are between the ages of 10 and 35 years.
- Some 2% of patients have a recurrence.

SKIN FINDINGS

- A single, 2- to 10-cm oval lesion, the herald patch, is most frequently located on the trunk.
- Within 7 to 14 days, smaller lesions appear and reach their maximum number in 1 to 2 weeks.
- They are limited to the trunk and proximal extremities, but in extensive cases, they develop on the arms, legs, and face.
- Lesions are often concentrated in the lower abdominal area.
- The plaques are pink in Caucasians and dark brown in African-Americans.
- Early lesions are papular, and then oval plaques with a ring of scale located within the border (collarette scale) appear.
- Plaques oriented along skin lines on the back look like drooping pine tree branches.
- The number of lesions varies from a few to hundreds.
- Papular lesions are more common in young children, pregnant women, and African-Americans.
- Vesicular lesions are seen in infants and children. Most lesions are asymptomatic, but some patients complain of itching.

NONSKIN FINDINGS

- Some 20% of patients have a recent history of acute infection with fatique, headache, sore throat, lymphadentitis, and fever.

LABORATORY

- A serologic test for syphilis should be ordered if a clinical diagnosis cannot be made.
- A biopsy is useful in atypical cases.

COURSE AND PROGNOSIS

- The disease clears spontaneously in 1 to 2 months.

DISCUSSION

- The disease is benign and self-limited and does not appear to affect the fetus; therefore isolation is unnecessary.
- Variant patterns exist; these may create confusion between pityriasis rosea and secondary syphilis, guttate psoriasis, viral exanthems, tinea, nummular eczema, and drug eruptions.
- Tinea can be ruled out with a potassium hydroxide examination.
- Secondary syphilis may be indistinguishable from pityriasis rosea, especially if the herald patch is absent.

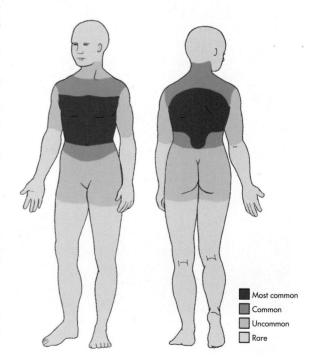

Most common
Common
Uncommon
Rare

TREATMENT

- Group V topical steroids and oral antihistamines may be used as needed for itching.
- Extensive cases with intense itching respond to a 1- to 2-week course of prednisone (20 mg twice a day).
- Direct sun exposure hastens the resolution.
- Ultraviolet light B, administered in five consecutive daily exposures, hastens the involution.

CAVEAT

- The herald patch is often misdiagnosed as ringworm.

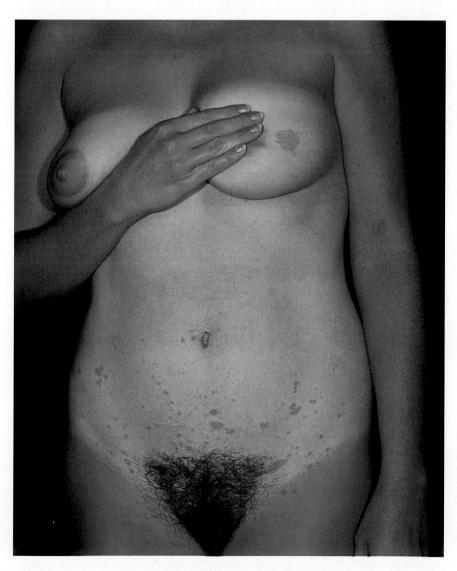

The herald patch is located on the left breast.

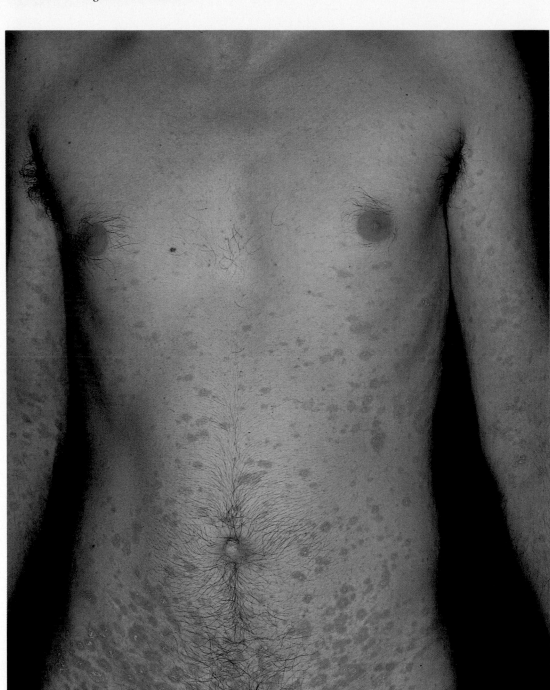

Fully evolved eruption of pityriasis rosea.

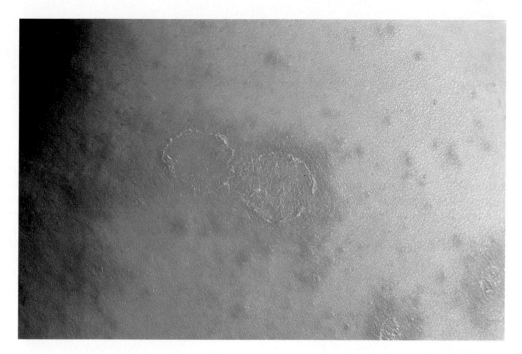

A ring of tissuelike scale (collarette scale) remains attached within the border of the oval plaque. This is almost pathognomonic of pityriasis rosea.

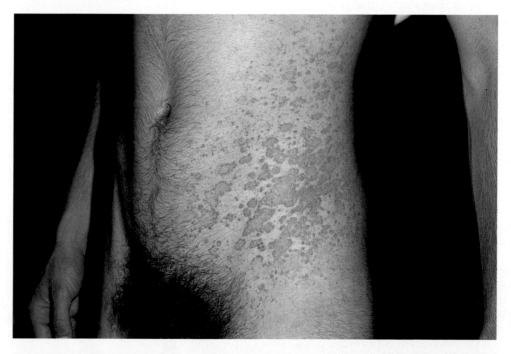

Lesions tend to be concentrated in the lower abdominal area and rarely extend lower than the upper thighs.

■ LICHEN PLANUS

DESCRIPTION

- Lichen planus is a distinctive inflammatory cutaneous and mucous membrane reaction pattern of unknown etiology.

HISTORY

- Lichen planus is rare in children under the age of 5 and is more common in women.
- Some 10% of patients have a positive family history.
- There are several clinical forms, including papular, hypertrophic, follicular, oral, and nail.
- Palmoplantar and vaginal lichen planus are rare conditions.
- The course is variable and unpredictable in all types.
- Itching is of variable intensity.
- This condition can occur abruptly as a generalized disease; it may be secondary to a drug.
- Severe oral lichen planus may degenerate to squamous cell carcinoma (3% of cases).

SKIN FINDINGS

- The primary lesion is a 2- to 10-mm, flat-topped papule with an irregular angulated border (polygonal papules). New lesions are pink-white but with time become purple.
- The surface has a lacy, reticular pattern of crisscrossed, whitish lines (Wickham's striae).
- The "five Ps" of lichen planus are pruritic, planar (flat-topped), polyangular, purple, and papules.
- This condition is most commonly located on the flexor surfaces of the wrists and forearms, the legs immediately above the ankles, and the lumbar region.
- Lesions that persist become thicker and dark red (hypertrophic lichen planus). They occur most often on the shins.
- Papules aggregate into different patterns (e.g., haphazard, annular, linear, guttate).
- Vesicles or bullae may appear.
- Persistent brown staining develops after the lesions resolve.
- On the scalp, hair loss is secondary to scarring in follicular lichen planus.
- Oral lichen planus can be seen on the tongue and lips but most commonly on the buccal mucosa. The most common form is nonerosive and has a white, lacy pattern. Oral erosive lichen planus is painful.

- Vaginal lichen planus has marked mucosal fragility and erythema.
- Nail changes often appear as an isolated finding. Proximal-to-distal linear depressions occur. Inflammation of the matrix results in adhesion of the proximal nailfold to the scarred matrix to form a pterygium.

LABORATORY

- Accumulation of mononuclear cells in the dermal-epidermal interface and a T cell–mediated cytotoxic reaction against basal keratinocytes are found when biopsy specimens are examined. Immunofluorescence done on a scalp biopsy helps rule out lupus.
- Anti–hepatitis C virus antibodies are detected in about 16% of patients with the cutaneous form and about 30% of patients with the oral form.

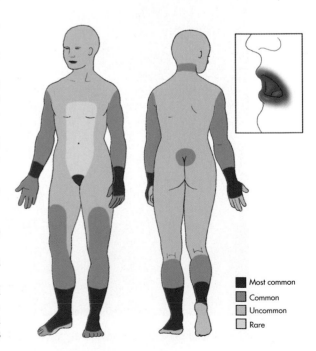

■ Most common
■ Common
□ Uncommon
□ Rare

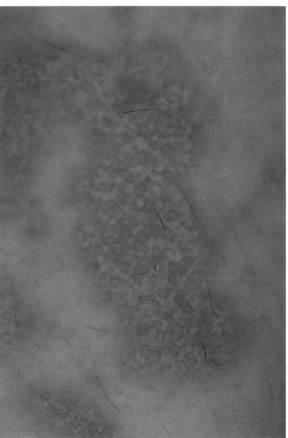

The primary lesion is a flat-topped papule with an irregular, angulated border (polygonal papules).

Close inspection of the surface show a lacy, reticular pattern of crisscrossed whitish lines (Wickham's striae), that can be accentuated with a drop of immersion oil.

DIFFERENTIAL DIAGNOSIS

- Papular lichen planus: chronic cutaneous (discoid) lupus, psoriasis, pityriasis rosea, papular eczema, superficial basal cell carcinoma, Bowen's disease
- Hypertrophic lichen planus: psoriasis, lichen simplex chronicus, prurigo nodularis, stasis dermatitis, Kaposi's sarcoma
- Oral lichen planus: leukoplakia, candidiasis (thrush), oral hairy leukoplakia, secondary syphilis, pemphigus, pemphigoid

TREATMENT

- Antihistamines (hydroxyzine, 10 to 25 mg every 4 hours) are administered for pruritus.
- Group I to III topical steroids are used as an initial treatment for localized disease.
- Intralesional triamcinolone acetonide (Kenalog, 5 to 10 mg/ml) is administered for hypertrophic lesions. This regimen may be repeated in 4 weeks.

- Prednisone is administered for generalized lichen planus. A 4-week course, starting at 1mg/kg/day, is used, and the dosage is gradually decreased.
- Corticosteroids (fluocinonide, fluocinolone acetonide, triamcinolone acetonide) in an adhesive base (benzocaine [Orabase]) is used as the initial treatment for oral lichen planus. The medication should be rubbed into the lesion.
- Inhaled corticosteroids (e.g., triamcinolone [Azmacort]) are an alternative to cream benzocaine (Orabase) preparations. They are simply sprayed onto lesions.
- Retinoids (acitretin), 1mg/kg/day, or cyclosporine, 5 or 6 mg/kg/day, may be considered for severe recalcitrant forms of lichen planus.
- Dapsone, azathioprine, and hydroxychloroquine have been used for severe recalcitrant oral lichen planus.

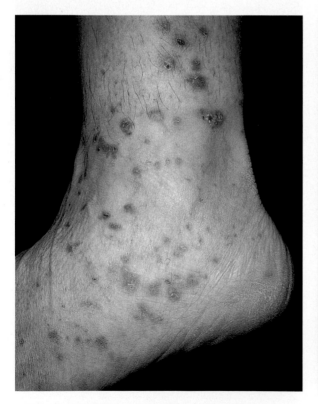

Lichen planus. Lesions are concentrated about the wrists and ankles. Itching varies in intensity and may not be present.

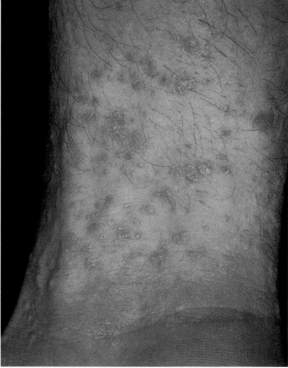

Localized lichen planus. Early lesions are present on the wrist, which is a common site for localized lichen planus.

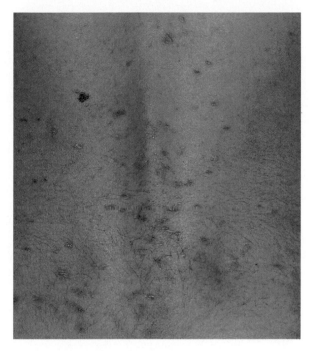

Generalized lichen planus. Papules are larger and are confluent in the lower back region.

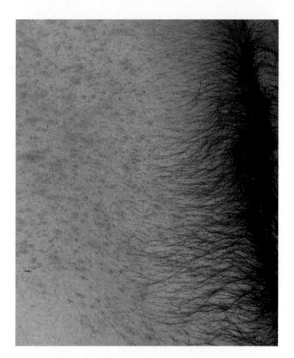

Generalized lichen planus.

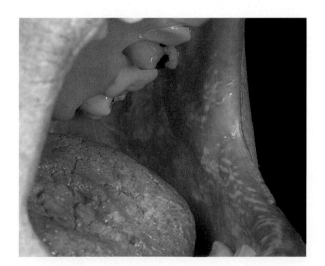

Mucous membrane lichen planus. A lacy, white pattern is present on the buccal mucosa.

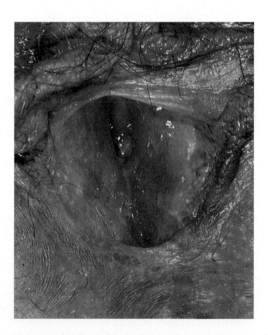

Erosive vaginal lichen planus. The entire vaginal tract is involved in this severe case.

◼ LICHEN SCLEROSUS ET ATROPHICUS

DESCRIPTION

- Lichen sclerosus et atrophicus is an uncommon chronic skin disease of unknown origin.
- It leaves the skin with a smooth, white, atrophic, and wrinkled surface.
- It most often occurs on the genitalia.

HISTORY

- The female-to-male ratio is 10:1.
- This disease has predilection for the vulva, perianal area, and groin.
- Female patients complain of pruritus, dysuria, or dyspareunia; this condition is chronic, is painful, and interferes with sexual activity.
- Male patients have recurrent balanitis leading to phimosis.
- Prepubertal lichen sclerosus et atrophicus occurs in infants and usually resolves without sequelae, other than hyperpigmentation.
- Skin lesions are often asymptomatic.
- Squamous cell carcinoma occurs in 3% of vaginal lesions.

SKIN FINDINGS

Vagina and Penis

- An ivory-white, atrophic plaque in the shape of an hourglass encircles the vagina and rectum.
- Delicate, thin, white, wrinkled, compromised mucosa may break down to become hemorrhagic and eroded.
- Atrophy can lead to shrunken and fused tissues.
- Purpura of the vulva is an occasional manifestation of pediatric lichen sclerosus et atrophicus (often misdiagnosed as child abuse).
- In the penile form the white atrophic plaques erode and heal with contraction, leading to severe phimosis.

Skin

- Early lesions are small, smooth, pink or ivory, flat-topped, slightly raised papules.
- White-brown, horny follicular plugs appear on the surface (delling).
- Papules coalesce, forming small, oval plaques with dull or glistening, smooth, white, atrophic, wrinkled surfaces.
- Skin may break down to become hemorrhagic and eroded.

LABORATORY

- Lesions are biopsied to make a diagnosis and to rule out squamous cell carcinoma of vulvar lesions that are white and raised (leukoplakia), fissured, ulcerated, and unresponsive to therapy.

TREATMENT

Topical Steroids

- Topical steroid creams (group V twice a day for 2 weeks) is the initial treatment for uncomplicated skin and mucosal lesions.
- Clobetasol propionate 0.05% (Cormax ointment) (short, intermittent courses) is effective for vaginal and penile disease. Dermatologists are experienced in the use of this superpotent steroid.
- Intralesional steroids (e.g., triamcinolone acetonide [Kenalog], 2.5 to 5.0 mg/ml) are useful for unresponsive areas.
- The liberal use of bland emollients (e.g., Vaseline creamy) soothes dry vaginal tissues and is used during and after treatment with topical steroids.

Other Treatments

- Acitretin (10 to 25 mg/day for 16 weeks) may be considered in severe disease.
- Selected refractory medical cases may benefit from surgery (e.g., circumcision, vulvectomy).

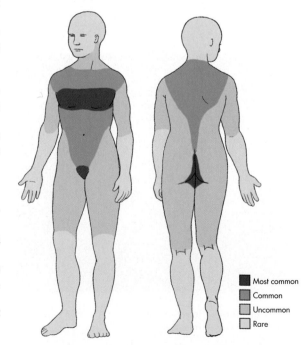

Most common
Common
Uncommon
Rare

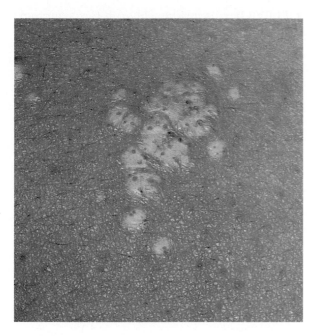

Early lesions are ivory-colored, flat-topped, slightly raised papules with follicular plugs.

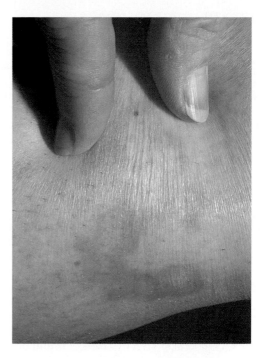

The epidermis is thin and atrophic and gives the appearance of wrinkled tissue paper when compressed.

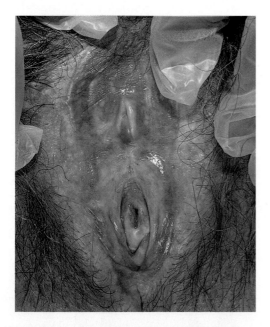

A white, atrophic plaque encircles the vagina and rectum. The skin is fragile and easily erodes.

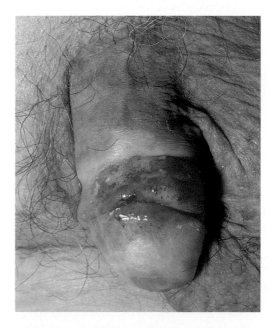

The glans is smooth, white, and atrophic. Erosions are present on the prepuce.

■ PITYRIASIS LICHENOIDES

DESCRIPTION

- Pityriasis lichenoides is a rare disease of unknown etiology with two variants: acute (pityriasis lichenoides et varioliformis acuta [PLEVA], or Mucha-Habermann disease), and chronic (pityriasis lichenoides chronica [PLC]).
- The terms *acute* and *chronic* refer to the characteristics of the individual lesions and not to the course of the disease.

HISTORY

- Pityriasis lichenoides can occur at any age; most cases occur in the second and third decades.
- PLEVA is usually a benign, self-limited papulosquamous disorder; its relationship to PLC is not clear.
- Some evidence suggests that PLEVA is a hypersensitivity reaction to an infectious agent.

SKIN FINDINGS
PLEVA

- PLEVA is characterized by crops of round or oval, red-brown papules, usually 2 to 10 mm singly or in clusters.
- Papules often have a violaceous center and a surrounding rim of erythema with or without psoriasis-like scaling.
- Lesions can become vesicular or pustular and undergo hemorrhagic necrosis, usually within 2 to 5 weeks, often leaving a postinflammatory hyperpigmentation.
- The distribution is on the trunk, thighs, and upper arms. The face, scalp, palms, and soles are involved in approximately 10% of cases.
- Although the lesions' onset, appearance, and evolution are acute, the disease tends to chronicity, with crops of lesions recurring over several months or years.

PLC

- PLC is characterized by an eruption consisting of brown-red papules with fine, micalike, adherent scaling; lesions occur primarily on the trunk and do not ulcerate or look necrotic.
- PCL may persist for years. Mild itching and irritation are common. Systemic symptoms are rare.

SYSTEMIC SYMPTOMS

- PLEVA begins insidiously, with few symptoms other than mild itching. Systemic symptoms are rare.

LABORATORY

- A biopsy is very helpful for confirming the diagnosis.
- Parakeratosis, regular acanthosis, and mild papillary dermal edema occur. A superficial and deep perivascular lymphocytic infiltrate, along with variable exocytosis of normal-appearing lymphocytes and erythrocytes, is seen.

DIFFERENTIAL DIAGNOSIS

- Pityriasis rosea
- Syphilis
- Lymphomatoid papulosis
- Pityriasis rosea
- Scabies
- Insect bite reaction
- Varicella

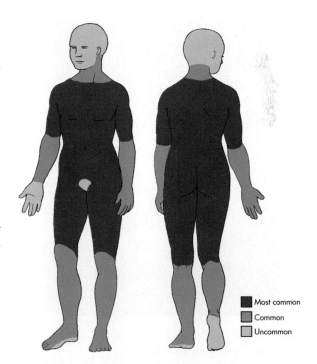

Most common
Common
Uncommon

TREATMENT

- No therapy is required, since the disease is self-limited.
- Erythromycin may produce remission in some cases. Clearing occurs with oral erythromycin, 30 to 50 mg/kg/day, in anecdotal reports; clearing may require 2 months. This medication is tapered over several months, since the disease may recur if the erythromycin is tapered too rapidly.
- Psoralen and ultraviolet light A (PUVA), ultraviolet light B (UVB) phototherapy, tetracycline, gold, methotrexate, oral corticosteroids, and dapsone have all been used with some success.

DISCUSSION

- The prognosis for both forms is good.
- Acute exacerbation is common, and disease may wax and wane for months or years. Individual lesions may resolve, although new lesions continue to erupt.
- High fever is a rare complication but may be associated with an ulceronecrotic type of lesion.
- Complications include a self-limited arthritis and superinfection of the skin lesions.

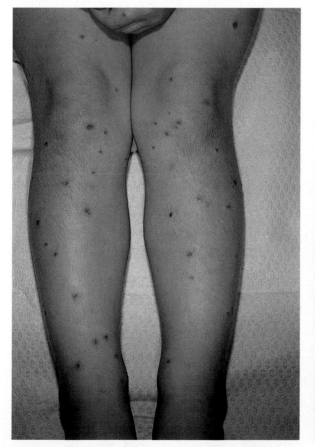

Crops of red-to-brown papules can become hemorrhagic, pustular, or necrotic. Acute exacerbations are common, and the disease may wax and wane for months or years.

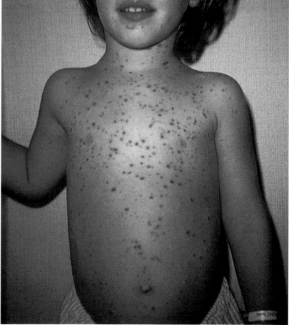

Lesions in children are vesicular or pustular and then undergo hemorrhagic necrosis. They appear on the trunk, thighs, and upper arms.

6

Bacterial Infections

■ IMPETIGO

DESCRIPTION

- Impetigo is a common, contagious, superficial skin infection produced by streptococci, staphylococci, or a combination of both bacteria. Bullous impetigo and nonbullous impetigo represent two clinical forms. Presently, *Staphylococcus aureus* is the primary pathogen.

HISTORY

- Impetigo may occur after a minor skin injury such as an insect bite or within lesions of atopic or another eczematous dermatitis; it often develops on normal skin.
- Children in close physical contact with one another have a higher rate of infection.
- Responsible staphylococci may colonize the nose and serve as reservoir for skin infection.
- Warm, moist climates and poor hygiene predispose people to this condition.

SKIN FINDINGS

- Lesions may be localized or widespread.
- Bullous impetigo
  - Thin-roofed bullae may turn from clear to cloudy. Bulla collapse, leading to an inner-tube shaped rim with a central thin, flat, honey-colored crust.
  - Lesions enlarge and often coalesce. There is minimal surrounding erythema. The thick crust accumulates in longer-lasting lesions.
- Nonbullous impetigo (crusted)
  - Vesicles or pustules rupture, exposing a red, moist base.

- The honey-yellow to white-brown, firmly adherent crust accumulates as the lesion extends radially; there is little surrounding erythema.
- Satellite lesions appear beyond the periphery.

NONSKIN FINDINGS

- Systemic symptoms are infrequent.
- Lesions are generally asymptomatic.

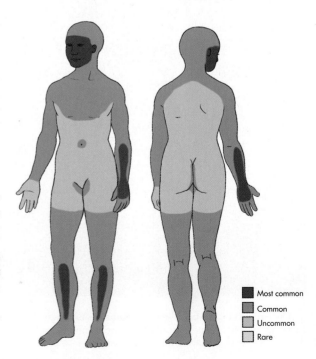

Most common
Common
Uncommon
Rare

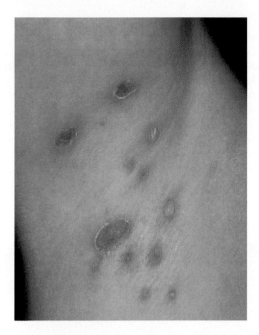

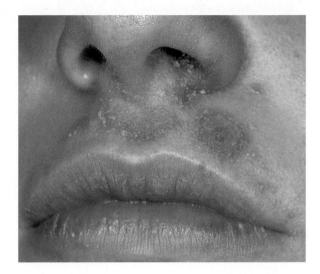

Bullous impetigo. Lesions are present in all stages of development. Bullae rupture, exposing a lesion with an eroded surface and a peripheral scale.

A tinea-like scaling border forms as the round lesions enlarge.

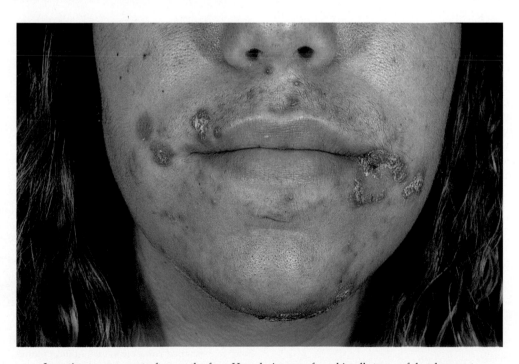

Impetigo occurs most often on the face. Here, lesions are found in all stages of development.

LABORATORY

- Cultures of lesions are not routinely indicated, since determining of the primary pathogen from culture may not be possible.

COURSE AND PROGNOSIS

- The disease is self-limiting, but untreated, it may last for weeks or months. Systemic complications are common.
- Poststreptococcal glomerulonephritis may follow impetigo, typically 1 and 5 weeks after infection and most commonly in children age 2 to 4.
- The incidence of acute nephritis is between 2% and 5%; in the presence of a nephritogenic strain of streptococci, the rate varies between 10% and 15%.
- Rheumatic fever has not been reported as a complication of impetigo.
- Serious secondary infections (e.g., osteomyelitis, septic arthritis, pneumonia) may follow seemingly trivial superficial infections in infants.

TREATMENT

- For limited, localized infections, mupirocin 2% ointment or cream (Bactroban) is used three times a day for 10 days.
- For widespread infections, oral antibiotics are administered. A penicillinase-resistant antibiotic such as dicloxacillin, 250 mg, or cephalexin (Keflex), 250 mg, is prescribed four times a day for 5 to 10 days. Antibiotic-resistant staphylococci are a concern with oral erythromycin.
- For recurrent impetigo, the presence of *S. aureus* is sought; the most common sites are the nares; less commonly, it can be found in the perineum, axillae, and toe webs.
- Recurrent disease may be stopped with mupirocin 2% ointment to nares twice a day for 5 days. This course is repeated monthly for several months to erradicate nasal carriers of *S. aureus.*

DISCUSSION

- Bullous impetigo is primarily a staphylococcal disease. Nonbullous impetigo was once thought to be primarily a streptococcal disease, but staphylococci are isolated from most bullous and nonbullous impetigo lesions. An epidermolytic toxin produced at the site of infection, most commonly by staphylococci of phage group II, causes intraepidermal cleavage below or within the stratum granulosum, resulting in bulla formation in bullous impetigo.

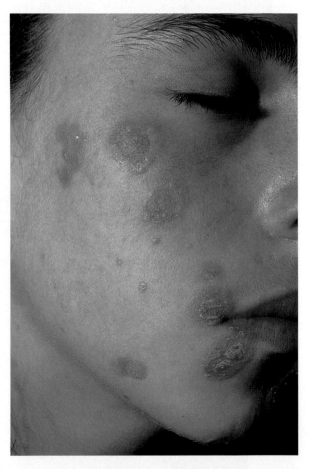

Vesicles enlarge rapidly to form bullae. The center collapses, but the peripheral area may retain fluid for many days in an inner tube–shaped rim. A thin, flat, honey-colored, "varnish-like" crust may appear in the center.

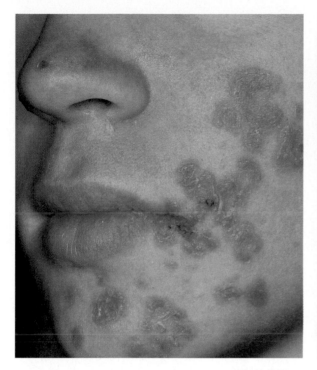

A thick, honey-yellow, adherent crust covers the entire eroded surface.

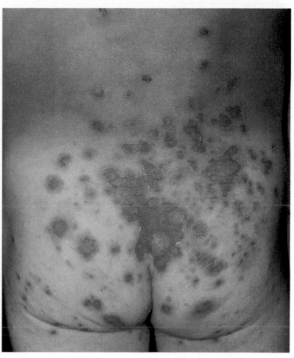

Widespread dissemination followed 3 weeks of treatment with a group IV topical steroid.

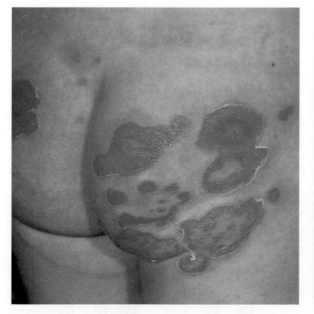

Bullous impetigo. Huge lesions with a glistening, eroded base and a collarette of moist scale.

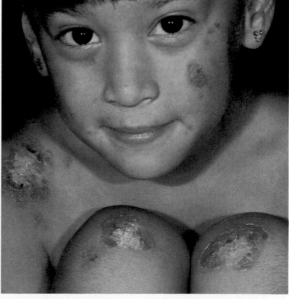

A bullous rim extended slowly for weeks. No topical or oral treatment had been attempted.

■ CELLULITIS

DESCRIPTION

- Cellulitis is an infection of the dermis and subcutaneous tissues characterized by erythema, edema, and pain.
- In adults, it is most common on the legs but can be seen on any body site.

HISTORY

- Localized pain and tenderness occur for a few days before presentation.
- The most susceptible populations are patients with diabetes, cirrhosis, renal failure, malnourishment, and human immunodeficiency virus. Patients who have cancer and are on chemotherapy and patients who abuse intravenous drugs and alcohol are also susceptible.
- Cellulitis typically occurs near surgical wounds and trauma sites (e.g., bites, burns, abrasions, lacerations, ulcers).
- It may develop in apparently normal skin or at sites of other dermatoses.
- Recurrent episodes occur with local anatomic abnormalities that compromise the venous or lymphatic circulation.
- The pinna and lower legs are particularly susceptible to this recurrent pattern.

SKIN FINDINGS

- A preexisting lesion such as an ulcer or erosion may act as a portal of entry for the infecting organism.
- Athlete's foot may be a common predisposing condition for cellulitis of the lower extremities.
- An expanding, red, swollen, tender-to-painful plaque with an indefinite border may cover a small or wide area.
- Palpation produces pain but rarely crepitus.
- Vesicles, blisters, hemorrhage, necrosis, or abscess may occur.
- Regional lymphadenopathy sometimes occurs.
- Repeated attacks on the legs can impair lymphatic drainage, leading to chronically swollen legs.
- The end stage of repeated infection of the leg includes dermal fibrosis, lymphedema, and epidermal thickening; it is called *elephantiasis nostras*.

LABORATORY

- Mild leukocytosis with a left shift and a mildly elevated erythrocyte sedimentation rate may be present.

- Cellulitis is most often caused by a group A streptococcus and *Staphylococcus aureus.* Many other bacteria can cause cellulitis.
- Culture of the lesion is a more predictable source of information than needle-aspirate cultures.

DIFFERENTIAL DIAGNOSIS

- Stasis dermatitis
- Thrombophlebitis
- Deep venous thrombosis
- Contact dermatitis
- Erythema nodosum

TREATMENT

- Pain can be relieved with cool Burow's compresses.
- Elevation of the leg hastens recovery.
- Empiric treatment with antibiotics aimed at staphylococcal and streptococcal organisms is appropriate.
- A penicillinase-resistant penicillin (e.g., dicloxacillin, 500 to 1000 mg orally every 6 hours), amoxicillin/clavulanate, a cephalosporin, or erythromycin (250 to 500 mg orally every 6 hours) is indicated.
- The mean time for healing after treatment is initiated is 12 days.

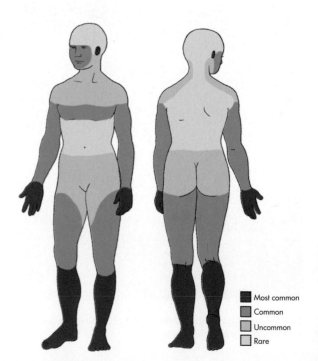

Most common
Common
Uncommon
Rare

- Most cases improve when the patient is on simple antibiotic therapy.
- Severe infections may require hospitalization and intravenous antibiotics.
- Prolonged antimicrobial prophylaxis may be effective in preventing recurrent episodes. This may be continued for months or years using erythromycin (250 mg twice a day) or phenoxymethyl penicillin (250 to 500 mg twice a day).

CAVEAT

- Interdigital athlete's foot may be a predisposing condition for cellulitis of the lower extremity. Cultures from the interdigital spaces may yield the pathogenic bacteria.

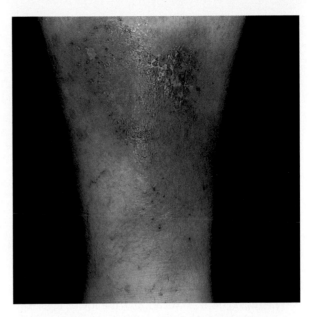

Cellulitis is characterized by erythema, edema, and pain. Patients with cellulitis of the leg often have a preexisting lesion, such as an ulcer or erosion, that acts as a portal of entry for the infecting organism.

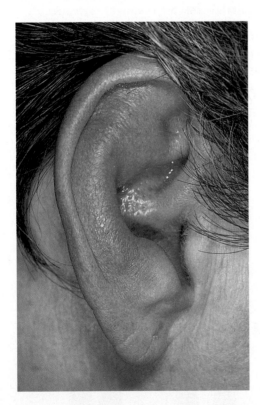

Cellulitis of the pinna may result from infection with *Pseudomonas* species or staphylococci and streptococci. The lymphatics may be permanently damaged during an attack, predisposing the patient to recurrent episodes of streptococcal erysipelas of the pinna. Recurrent attacks are brought on by manipulation or even the slightest trauma.

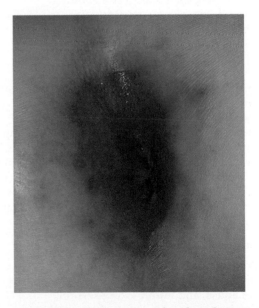

Perianal cellulitis. Cellulitis (group A beta-hemolytic streptococci) around the anal orifice is often misdiagnosed as candidiasis. It occurs more frequently in children. They are not systemically ill. Culture confirms the diagnosis. Systemic therapy is required.

■ ERYSIPELAS

DESCRIPTION

- Erysipelas is an acute, inflammatory form of cellulitis that differs from other types of cellulitis in that lymphatic involvement ("streaking") is prominent.
- It is more superficial and has margins that are more clearly demarcated from normal skin than does cellulitis.
- Infection may start at breaks in the skin, such as trauma, ulcers, bites, and superficial fungal infections. The site of entry is not always identified.

HISTORY

- Prodromal symptoms last from 4 to 48 hours and consist of malaise, chills, fever (101° to 104° F), and occasionally, anorexia and vomiting.

SKIN FINDINGS

- The most common location is the lower legs. The face, ears, and buttocks may also be involved.
- One or more red, tender, firm spots rapidly increase in size, forming a tense, red, hot, uniformly elevated, shining patch with an irregular outline and a sharply defined, raised border.
- The color becomes a dark and fiery red, and vesicles may appear at the advancing border and over the surface.
- Itching, burning, tenderness, and pain may be moderate to severe.
- Without treatment, the rash reaches its height in approximately 1 week and subsides slowly over the next 1 or 2 weeks.
- Red, sometimes painful streaks of lymphangitis may extend toward the regional lymph nodes.
- Repeated attacks can impair lymphatic drainage, which predisposes the patient to more infection and permanent swelling. This series of events takes place most commonly in the lower legs of patients with venous stasis and ulceration.

NONSKIN FINDINGS

- Predisposing diseases are lymphatic or venous circulatory problems, diabetes, renal failure, alcohol abuse, and immunosuppression.

LABORATORY

- Streptococci cause 80% of the cases; most often the culprits are group A streptococci, followed by group G and other non–group A streptococci. Group G streptococci may be a common pathogen, especially in patients older than 50 years.
- *S. aureus, Pneumococcus* organisms, *Klebsiella pneumoniae, Yersinia enterocolitica,* and *Haemophilus influenzae* are other causative agents.
- The diagnosis is based on the clinical findings; identification of the organism is difficult.
- Only a small percentage of cultures taken from the portal of entry and fluid from intact pustules or bullae are positive. The injection-aspiration method is unreliable.
- Blood cultures are sometimes positive if there is a high fever.
- The white blood cell count and erythrocyte sedimentation rate are frequently elevated.

COURSE AND PROGNOSIS

- Recurrences are common in patients suffering from local impairment of circulation.
- A relapse may occur in pharyngeal carriers of streptococci group A.

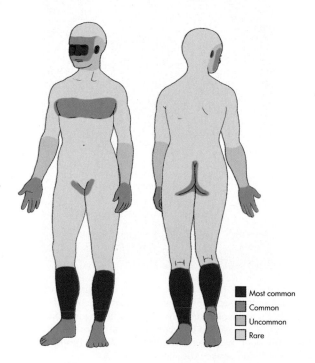

Most common
Common
Uncommon
Rare

DISCUSSION

- Erysipelas differs from cellulitis by exhibiting raised, clearly marginated borders and frequent lymphangitic streaking.

TREATMENT

- In acute episodes, penicillin V orally (250 to 500 mg four times a day) is the drug of choice. The diagnosis of the streptococcal origin should be reconsidered if the response to penicillin is not rapid. Azithromycin (Zithromax), 500 mg on day 1 and 250 mg on days 2 to 5, or clarithromycin (Biaxin), 250 to 500 mg every 12 hours for 7 to 14 days, are alternatives for patients who cannot take penicillin.
- Continuous antibiotic prophylaxis is indicated for patients with high recurrence rates. Daily administration of penicillin V orally (250 to 500 mg twice a day) or intramuscularly (i.e., benzathine penicillin, 2.4 mU every 3 weeks for 1 or 2 years) can help.

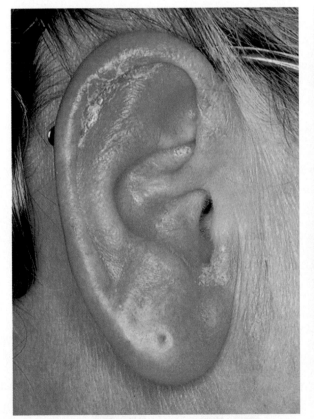

Recurrent episodes of infection have resulted in lymphatic obstruction and caused permanent thickening of the skin.

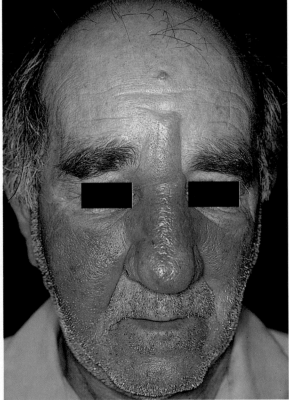

Erysipelas is an acute, inflammatory form of cellulitis in which lymphatic involvement ("streaking") is prominent. Erysipelas is more superficial than cellulitis and has margins that are more clearly demarcated from normal skin.

■ FOLLICULITIS

DESCRIPTION

- *Folliculitis* means an inflammation of the hair follicle.
- There are several types; common types include mechanical folliculitis from persistent trauma and tight clothing and bacterial folliculitis.
- Bacterial folliculitis includes follicular impetigo, a superficial form, and sycosis barbae, a deep form occurring in the beard area.

HISTORY

- Usually, there is an abrupt eruption.
- Lesions spread by trauma, scratching, or shaving.
- The distribution is variable; often, the scalp, arms, legs, axillae, and trunk are involved.

SKIN FINDINGS

- Dome-shaped pustules with small erythematous halos arise in the center of a follicle.
- In sycosis barbae, the inflammation is intense and deep; there is marked tenderness.

LABORATORY

- Culture is not routinely necessary. *Staphylococcus aureus* is most common infecting organism.
- Potassium hydroxide examination of the hair and surrounding scaling is performed to exclude an infection by a dermatophyte.

COURSE AND PROGNOSIS

- Folliculitis is responsive to antibiotic and hygienic measures.

DISCUSSION

- In a dermatophyte infection (Majocchi's granuloma), hair follicle infection is caused by a dermatophyte fungus. There are inflammatory papules and pustules with surrounding scaling. The results of a potassium hydroxide examination of the hair are positive.
- In eosinophilic folliculitis, pruritic, extensive follicular papules suddenly appear on the face, neck, and chest. Testing for the human immunodeficiency virus is performed.
- In gram-negative folliculitis, an acneiform eruption suddenly worsens and becomes pustular. Superficial gram-negative bacterial overgrowth occurs in patients on chronic antibiotics, often for acne.

- In hot tub folliculitis, erythematous papules and pustules appear, primarily on the trunk. *Pseudomonas* follicular infection is acquired from improperly sanitized hot tubs.
- Mechanical folliculitis results from chronic frictional exposure.
- Occlusion folliculitis results from occlusion, such as that which can occur after exposure to oil and greases.
- *Pityrosporum* folliculitis often appears on the back and chest. The results of potassium hydroxide testing are positive. There are short hyphae and round spores.
- In steroid folliculitis, multiple, small pustules and red papules appear within 2 weeks of systemic corticosteroid use; a neutrophilic inflammation of the hair follicles occurs.

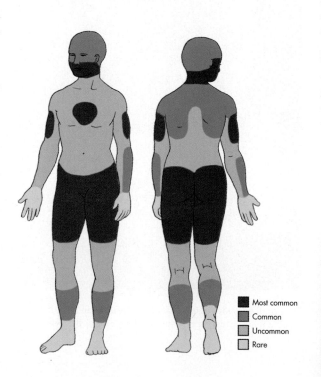

Most common
Common
Uncommon
Rare

TREATMENT

- Heat, friction, and occlusion should be minimized.
- Antibacterial soap, warm compresses, and topical antibiotics are used.
- Mupirocin (Bactroban) is effective in limited, superficial involvement.
- Oral antistaphylococcal antibiotics (oxacillin, dicloxacillin, cefuroxime) are indicated for extensive or spreading disease or deep involvement of sycosis barbae.

- *Pityrosporum* folliculitis can be treated with topical or oral antiyeast antibiotics.

CAVEAT

- Potassium hydroxide examination of the hair and any surrounding scaling should be performed to exclude a dermatophyte infection.

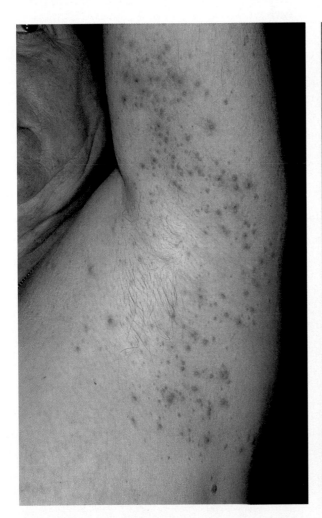

Folliculitis is inflammation of the hair follicle caused by infection, chemical irritation, or physical injury.

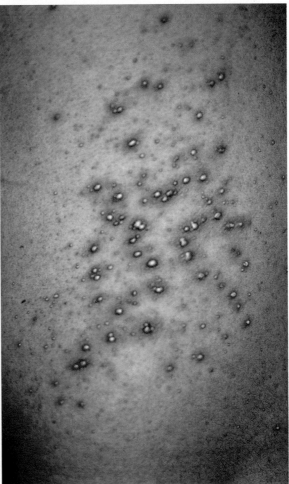

Staphylococcal folliculitis is the most common form of infectious folliculitis. A group of pustules may appear, usually without fever or other systemic symptoms, on any body surface. It may be a complication of occlusive topical steroid therapy, as occurred in this case.

■ PSEUDOFOLLICULITIS BARBAE (RAZOR BUMPS, INGROWN HAIRS)

DESCRIPTION

- Pseudofolliculitis barbae is a papular and pustular, foreign-body, inflammatory reaction that can affect any individual who has curly hair and who shaves closely on a regular basis. This condition is a particular nuisance to African-Americans.

HISTORY

- Pseudofolliculitis barbae is a significant problem in predisposed individuals required to shave closely.
- It is found in 50% to 75% of African-Americans and 3% to 5% of Caucasians who shave.
- The more severely affected site is the neck area.
- This is a chronic problem unless close shaving is avoided.

SKIN FINDINGS

- Pseudofolliculitis barbae affects people with curly hair or those with hair follicles oriented at oblique angle to the skin surface.
- A sharp, shaved, tapered, hair reenters the skin as it grows from below the skin surface and incites a foreign-body reaction, producing a microabscess.
- Red papules or pustules appear in the beard area.
- This condition occurs anywhere the hair is shaved (scalp, posterior neck, groin, legs).
- It results in scarring and hyperpigmentation.

LABORATORY

- The pustule is cultured. (Normal flora may be replaced by pathogenic organisms.)

DIFFERENTIAL DIAGNOSIS

- Acne
- Folliculitis

TREATMENT

- The imbedded hair shaft must be dislodged. A needle is inserted under the hair loop, and the hair is firmly elevated.
- A Buff Puff or toothbrush can be used to gently massage in a circular fashion and thus dislodge any ingrown hair.

- Shaving should be discontinued until inflammation is under control.
- A short course of antistaphylococcal antibiotics may hasten the resolution.
- Intralesional triamcinolone acetonide, 2.5 to 10 mg/ml, is used for persistent papules.
- Once lesions resolve, shaving may be resumed.
- Depilatories (Nair, Neet) with barium sulfide or calcium thioglycolate are effective alternatives to shaving. They are applied to the skin for 3 to 10 minutes and then wiped off. These products are irritating and can be tolerated only once or twice each week.
- If all measures fail, shaving must be discontinued indefinitely.
- Laser-assisted hair removal may provide a safe, effective means of treating recalcitrant cases.

Shaving Instructions

- The goal is to avoid close shaves and the production of sharply angled hair tips.
- The patient should hydrate the beard before shaving. The patient should shower before shaving and keep the beard hair in contact with warm water for at least 2 minutes.
- The patient should dislodge any hair tips that are beginning to pierce the skin. A soft-bristled toothbrush in a circular motion or a needle cleaned with rubbing alcohol should be used. This is done before shaving and at bedtime.
- A lather with thick shaving gels (Aveeno Therapeutic Shave Gel, Edge Gel for Tough Beards) should be used.
- The Bump Fighter razor (American Safety Razor Company, Verona, Va.) cuts the hair slightly above the skin surface.
- Alternatively, an electric razor can be used, avoiding the "closest" shave setting.
- The patient should shave in the direction of hair growth. The skin should not be stretched.
- Multiple razor strokes should be avoided.
- A moisturizing lotion should be used after shaving. Lacticare-HC (1% or 2.5%) intermittently can be used to reduce inflammation.

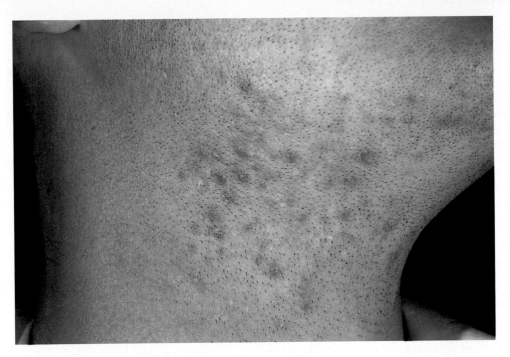

Pseudofolliculitis is a foreign body reaction to hair. The disease occurs only in men who have commenced shaving. It begins with the appearance of small follicular papules or pustules and rapidly becomes more diffuse as shaving continues.

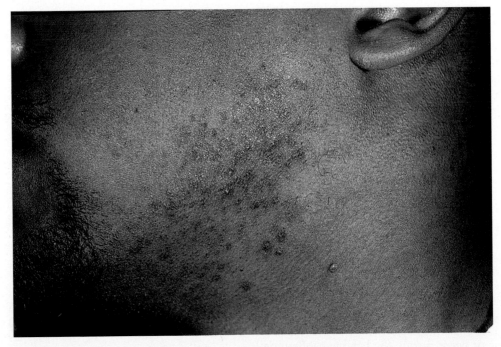

The problem is more severe in the neck areas, where hair follicles are more likely to be oriented at low angles to the skin surface, making repenetration of the skin more likely.

■ FURUNCLES AND CARBUNCLES

DESCRIPTION

- A furuncle (boil) is a walled-off, deep, painful, firm or fluctuant mass enclosing a collection of pus; often, it evolves from a superficial folliculitis.
- *Staphylococcus aureus* is the most commonly associated organism, but other organisms *(Escherichia coli, Pseudomonas aeruginosa, Streptococcus faecalis)* and anaerobes *(Peptostreptococcus, Peptococcus,* and *Lactobacillus* species) may cause lesions. Usually, a bacteriologic study of the abscess identifies the local flora.
- A carbuncle is an extremely painful, deep, interconnected aggregate of infected, abscessed follicles.

HISTORY

- Furuncles and carbuncles are uncommon in children.
- Occlusion and hyperhidrosis promote bacterial colonization.
- Most affected patients have normal immune systems, although certain conditions and immune defects (e.g., hyperimmunoglobulin E syndrome, chronic granulomatous disease, Wiskott-Aldrich syndrome, Chediak-Higashi syndrome, diabetes, leukemia, therapeutic immunosuppression, malnutrition, obesity) may predispose the patient to furuncles and carbuncles.

SKIN FINDINGS

- Any hair-bearing site can be affected. Sites of high friction and sweating are most typically affected; these include the areas under the belt, the anterior thighs, the buttocks, the groin, the axillae, and the waist.
- With a furuncle, a deep dermal or subcutaneous, red, swollen, painful mass later points and drains through multiple openings.
- With a carbuncle, deep, tender, firm subcutaneous erythematous papules enlarge to deep-seated nodules that can be stable or become fluctuant within several days.
- Favored sites for carbuncles are the back of the neck, the upper back, and the lateral thighs.

NONSKIN FINDINGS

- With a furuncle, the patient remains afebrile.
- With a carbuncle, malaise, chills, and fever may precede or occur during the height of inflammation.

LABORATORY

- Gram stain and culture are indicated if lesions recur or if they fail to respond to conventional therapy.

DIFFERENTIAL DIAGNOSIS

- Ruptured pilar or epidermal cyst
- Cystic acne
- Hidradenitis suppurativa

COURSE AND PROGNOSIS

- The abscess either remains deep and is reabsorbed or points toward the surface and ruptures.
- Ruptured lesions heal with a depressed, violaceous scar.
- Infection can spread to other sites.
- Recurrent furunculosis can be difficult to eradicate.

TREATMENT

- Furuncles
  - Warm, moist compresses are applied 15 to 30 minutes several times a day.
  - Drainage is the primary management for pointing, fluctuant lesions.

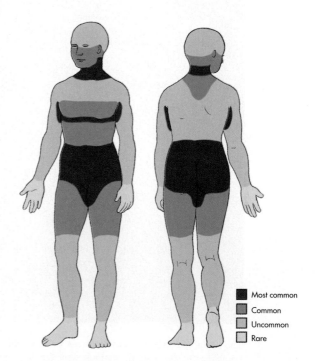

Most common
Common
Uncommon
Rare

- For fluctuant, localized lesions, incision and drainage with or without packing is performed. Local anesthesia is required. Iodoform gauze is used for packing large abscesses; it is removed or replaced when saturated.
- Recurrent furunculosis
  - Nasal carriage of *S. aureus* is eradicated by mupirocin 2% ointment applied to the anterior nares twice a day for 5 days; application to the nasal vestibule for 5 consecutive days of each month for 1 year should be considered.
  - If topical treatment fails, oral semisynthetic penicillin, 0.5 to 1.0 gm twice a day for 10 to 14 days, can be prescribed. Alternatively, for persistent colonization, combination therapy with rifampin, 600 mg once a day, and cloxacillin, 500 mg four times a day, for 7 to 10 days can eradicate nasal *S. aureus* carriage.
  - Other measures include washing the entire body and fingernails each day for 1 to 3 weeks with Betadine and changing and washing the towels, washcloths, and bed sheets daily. The patient should change the wound dressings frequently, clean or replace shaving tools daily, and avoid nose picking.
  - Applicable predisposing factors, including friction, tight clothing, industrial chemical exposure, obesity, poor hygiene, and diabetes, must be addressed.

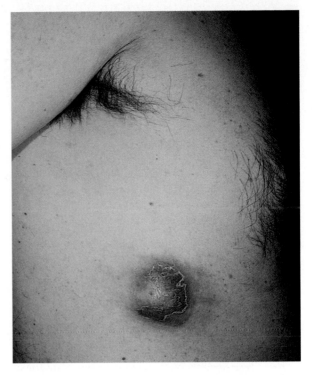

A furuncle (abscess or boil) is a walled-off collection of pus that is a painful, firm, or fluctuant mass. An abscess is not a hollow sphere but a cavity formed by fingerlike loculations of granulation tissue and pus that extends outward along planes of least resistance.

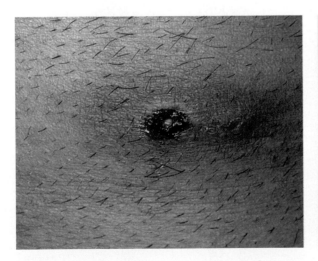

The abscess either remains deep and reabsorbs or points and ruptures through the surface.

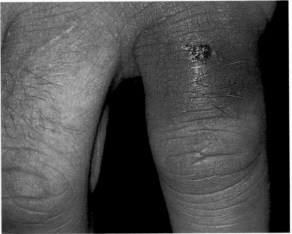

A single lesion on the finger.

■ *PSEUDOMONAS* FOLLICULITIS

- *Pseudomonas* folliculitis is an acute skin infection that follows exposure to contaminated water. The urticarial, red plaque with a central papule or pustule is highly distinctive.

HISTORY

- The attack rate is significantly higher in children than in adults, possibly because children tend to spend more time in the water.
- *Pseudomonas* folliculitis occurs from 8 hours to 5 days or longer after using a contaminated whirlpool, home hot tub, water slide, physiotherapy pool, or contaminated loofah sponge; 7% to 100% of those exposed to *Pseudomonas* species develop the disease.
- The spread of infection from person to person is unlikely.
- Prolonged exposure to the water, excessive numbers of bathers, and inadequate pool care predispose to infection.
- Desquamated skin cells in the water provide a rich, organic nutrient source for bacteria.
- In most cases, the eruption clears in 7 to 10 days, but recurrent crops of lesions may occur for as long as 3 months.

SKIN FINDINGS

- Few to more than 50 (0.5- to 3-cm), red, pruritic, round, urticarial plaques with a central papule or pustule appear.
- The rash is most severe in areas occluded by a snug bathing suit.
- Occlusion and superhydration of the stratum corneum favors colonization of the skin with *P. aeruginosa.*
- Women who wear one-piece bathing suits are at an increased risk.
- The rash resolves, leaving round spots of red-brown, postinflammatory hyperpigmentation.

NONSKIN FINDINGS

- Malaise and fatigue may occur during the initial few days of the eruption. Fever is uncommon and is low grade when it appears.

LABORATORY

- *P. aeruginosa* serotypes 0:9 and 0:11 are most commonly isolated from skin lesions, but other serotypes have been reported.

DIFFERENTIAL DIAGNOSIS

- Staphylococcal folliculitis
- Hives
- Insect bites

TREATMENT

- The infection is self-limited; treatment is usually not required.
- A wet compress of acetic acid 5% (white vinegar) is applied for 20 minutes two to four times a day; silver sulfadiazine cream (Silvadene) might help.
- Cases resistant to topical therapy can be treated orally with ciprofloxacin (Cipro), 500 or 750 mg twice each day for 5 to 10 days.

PREVENTATIVE MEASURES

- Continuous water filtration eliminates desquamated skin.
- Adequate chlorine levels should be maintained.
- The water in private hot tubs should be changed every 4 to 8 weeks.
- Public hot tubs should be drained daily.
- Showering after using the contaminated facility offers no protection.

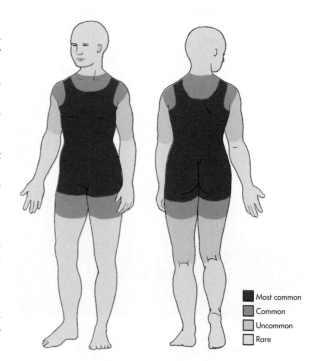

Most common
Common
Uncommon
Rare

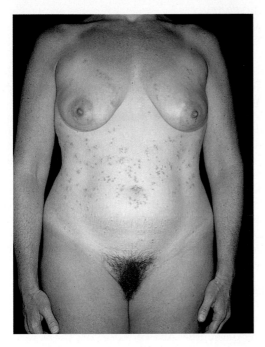

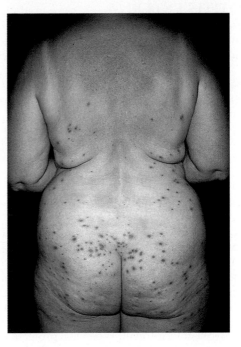

Occlusion and superhydration of the stratum corneum favors colonization of the skin with *Pseudomonas aeruginosa*. This may explain why the rash is most severe in areas occluded by a snug bathing suit. Women who wear one-piece bathing suits are at an increased risk.

About 48 hours after the patient uses a contaminated whirlpool, pruritic, round, urticarial plaques with a central papule or pustule appear.

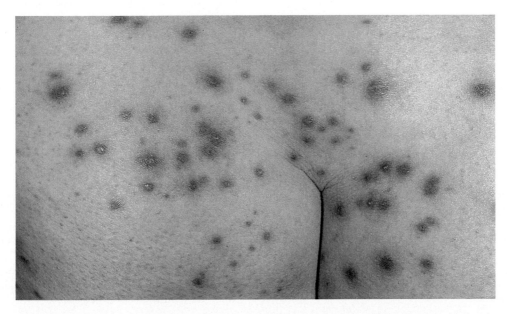

The rash may be a follicular, maculopapular, vesicular, pustular, or polymorphous eruption that includes all of these types of lesions.

■ OTITIS EXTERNA

DESCRIPTION

- Otitis externa is an inflammation of the external auditory canal, usually with secondary infection.

HISTORY

- Otitis externa is equally common among male and female patients.
- A mild, self-limited form known as *swimmer's ear* is especially common in children and during the summer.
- No racial or genetic predisposition has been reported.
- Symptoms range from itch and irritation to severe pain.
- Mechanical cleansing of the external canal and medicaments used to relieve symptoms can mask or exacerbate the condition.
- Cerumen is produced by modified apocrine glands of the external auditory canal. It forms a water-resistant barrier for the thin skin lining the canal. It inhibits bacterial growth by maintaining a low-pH environment. When this protective barrier is disrupted, bacterial overgrowth can occur.
- The usual pathogen is *Pseudomonas.*
- Mixed infections with *Staphylococcus* and *Pseudomonas* species are common.
- Secondary infections with *Candida* organisms also occur.

SKIN FINDINGS

- Dull pain is localized to the external auditory canal.
- The external auditory canal is inflamed with erythema and edema.
- Keratin and inflammatory cell debris accumulate within the canal. Most cases do not progress beyond this point.
- With progression, the pinna becomes red, hot, and edematous.
- Cellulitis involves the entire pinna and often extends to the preauricular skin. At this point, pain becomes sharp and constant.
- Purulent drainage exudes from the external auditory canal.

NONSKIN FINDINGS

- The regional lymph nodes are usually palpable and tender.

LABORATORY

- A skin biopsy is not recommended.
- The external canal should be cultured.

COURSE AND PROGNOSIS

- The protective cerumen barrier may be compromised by any number of mechanisms.
- Mechanical disruption (i.e., vigorous cleansing of the canal), inflammatory conditions (e.g., psoriasis, seborrheic dermatitis), and contact dermatitis (irritant and allergic) may all lead to disruption of the barrier.
- A rare severe form of otitis referred to as *malignant external otitis* may develop in patients who have diabetes or who have had ear surgery. Cellulitis extends from the external auditory canal into the bone at the base of the skull. The ipsilateral facial nerve becomes involved.

DISCUSSION

- Early in the course, the differential diagnosis includes psoriasis, seborrheic dermatitis, and contact dermatitis. Any of these conditions can lead to compromise of the natural barrier and ultimately to otitis externa.
- Both herpes zoster involving the geniculate ganglion and Ramsay Hunt syndrome can mimic early otitis externa with localized pain and inflammation. Careful examination reveals vesicles within the external auditory canal. Usually, ipsilateral Bell's palsy is present or develops soon after onset.
- When cellulitis involves the ear, the differential diagnosis includes relapsing polychondritis, a recurrent phenomenon presumably of autoimmune origin. Purulent discharge is not seen in this condition.

TREATMENT

- Treatment involves reestablishing the natural protective barrier.
- Cellular debris is flushed from the external canal with gentle irrigation.
- An acetic acid solution (VōSol otic solution or VōSol HC otic solution) helps lower the pH and inhibits bacterial and fungal growth.
- Ofloxacin otic solution 0.3% (Floxinotic solution) or ciprofloxacin and hydrocortisone (Cipro HC otic) are instilled two times a day.

- Topical steroids, wet dressings, and oral antibiotics (ciprofloxacin [Cipro]) are of value when cellulitis involves the pinna.
- Malignant external otitis requires hospitalization, the administration of intravenous antibiotics, and débridement.
- An otolaryngology consultation is recommended.

CAVEAT

- Lymphatic drainage from the pinna may be damaged by cellulitis. Such patients may be predisposed to future episodes of streptococcal erysipelas of the pinna.

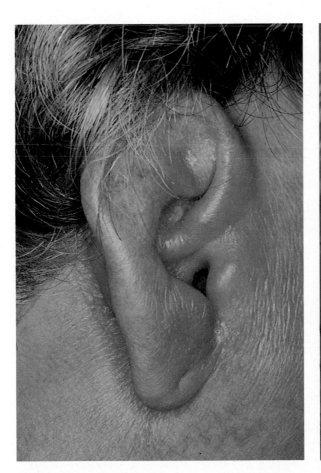

Pseudomonas cellulitis. The entire pinna and surrounding skin have become inflamed after an episode of external otitis.

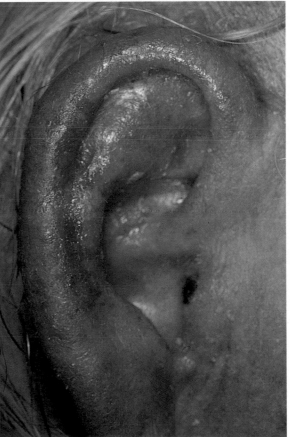

Malignant external otitis. Patients have a history of nonresolving otitis externa of many weeks' duration. Most patients are diabetic. *Pseudomonas* organisms invade underlying soft tissues. There is severe ear pain, purulent exudate, and granulation tissue. Nuclear scanning studies and CT scanning may reveal osteomyelitis of the skull base.

7

Sexually Transmitted Infections

More information can be found on the Internet by going to www.cdc.gov, clicking on *MMWR* and then *search*. Type, without commas, "Guidelines for Treatment of Sexually Transmitted Diseases" for all the latest disease descriptions and treatments for sexually transmitted diseases.

■ SYPHILIS

DESCRIPTION

- Syphilis is due to infection with *Treponema pallidum.*
- Untreated, syphilis may pass through three stages: primary infectious, secondary, and latent or progression to a rare tertiary stage.

HISTORY

- Syphilis is more common in men.
- The greatest age range is among 20 to 40 year olds.
- It was more common in male homosexuals before the epidemic of the acquired immunodeficiency syndrome.

Primary Syphilis

- A cutaneous ulcer (chancre) is acquired by direct contact with an infectious lesion.
- The chancre appears 10 to 90 days (average, 21 days) after exposure. It develops at the site of initial contact.
- Chancres are usually solitary, but multiple lesions can occur.
- Untreated disease resolves in 75% of cases.

Secondary Syphilis

- The secondary stage begins approximately 6 weeks after the chancre appears.
- Mucocutaneous lesions, an influenza-like syndrome, hepatosplenomegaly, and generalized adenopathy occur.
- This stage lasts 2 to 10 weeks.
- The distribution and morphologic characteristics of the lesions vary.
- Syphilis in this stage is easily confused with numerous other skin diseases.

Latent Syphilis

- The results of serologic tests are positive (not false positive) without evidence of active disease.
- The early latent period begins 1 year or less from the onset of primary disease; late latent syphilis lasts more than 4 years.
- Some 25% of untreated cases in the secondary stage relapse during the first year, a small percentage relapse in the second year, and no cases relapse after the fourth year.

Tertiary Syphilis

- Systemic disease develops in about 25% of untreated or inadequately treated cases. Cardiovascular disease, central nervous system lesions, and systemic granulomas (gummas) can occur.

Congenital Syphilis

- *T. pallidum* can be transmitted from an infected mother to her fetus.
- In untreated cases, 25% of neonates are stillborn, 25% of neonates die shortly after birth, 12% have no symptoms, and 40% will have late symptomatic congenital syphilis.
- In early congenital syphilis, symptoms (e.g., rash, hepatosplenomegaly, bone and joint changes) occur before age 2.
- In late congenital syphilis, symptoms (e.g., bone and joint changes, neural deafness, interstitial keratitis) occur after age 5.
- Therapy before the sixteenth week of gestation prevents infection of the fetus.
- A fetus is at greatest risk when the mother has syphilis no more than 2 years.

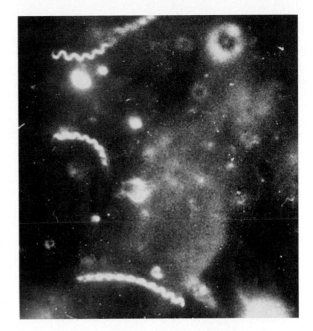

Treponema pallidum. Organism responsible for syphilis is seen here photographed through a dark-field microscope.

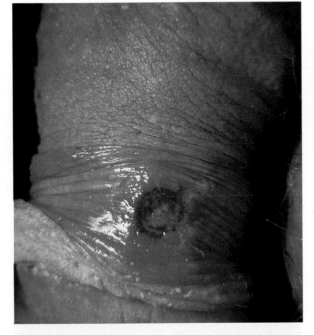

Primary syphilis. The lesion begins as a papule that undergoes ischemic necrosis and erodes, forming a 0.3- to 2.0-cm, painless to tender, hard, indurated ulcer; the base is clean, with a scant, yellow, serous discharge.

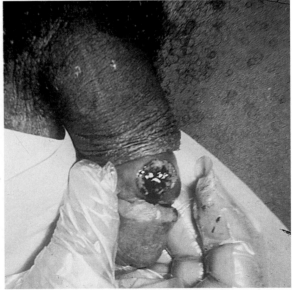

Primary syphilis. The borders of the ulcer are raised, smooth, and sharply defined.

SKIN FINDINGS

Primary Syphilis

- The lesion begins as a papule, undergoes ischemic necrosis, and erodes.
- A 0.3- to 2.0-cm, painless-to-tender, hard, indurated ulcer (chancre) forms.
- The borders are raised, smooth, and sharply defined.
- Painless, hard, discrete, nonsuppurative regional lymphadenopathy develops in 1 to 2 weeks.
- The chancre heals with scarring in 3 to 6 weeks.

Secondary Syphilis

- Lesions develop slowly and persist for weeks or months.
- Pain and itching are minimal or absent.
- There is a marked tendency for polymorphism; various lesions present simultaneously.
- The color of the lesion is characteristic: a coppery tint.
- The lesion appears in a variety of shapes, including round, elliptic, and annular.
- It may be limited and discrete, profuse, generalized, or more or less confluent.
- Lesions appear on the palms or soles in most patients.
- Lesions are isolated, oval, slightly raised, erythematous, and scaly.
- Irregular ("moth eaten") alopecia of beard, scalp, or eyelashes occurs.
- Moist, anal, wartlike papules (condylomata lata) are highly infectious.
- Classic split papules appear at the angle of the mouth.
- All secondary lesions are infectious.

LABORATORY

- Corkscrew-rotation motility of a small, spiral spirochete is observed via dark-field microscopy.
- Screening tests (rapid plasma reagin [RPR] or Venereal Disease Research Laboratory [VDRL]) are reactive by day 7 of the chancre.
- Positive results from RPR or VDRL tests should be confirmed with a fluorescent treponemal antibody absorption test.
- False-positive results are possible with all serologic tests.

DIFFERENTIAL DIAGNOSIS

Primary Syphilis

- Chancroid
- Herpes progenitalis
- Aphthae (Behçet's syndrome)
- Fixed drug eruption
- Traumatic ulcers

Secondary Syphilis

- Pityriasis rosea
- Guttate psoriasis
- Lichen planus
- Tinea versicolor
- Exanthematous drug eruption
- Viral eruptions

TREATMENT

- In early disease (primary, secondary, latent less than 1 year), the drug of choice is benzathine penicillin G, 2.4 million U intramuscularly once.
- In late disease (that lasting more than 1 year), the drug of choice is benzathine penicillin G, 2.4 million U intramuscularly once a week for 3 weeks.
- For patients allergic to penicillin, doxycycline, 100 mg twice a day for 2 weeks, or tetracycline, 500 mg four times a day for 2 weeks, is given.
- Successful therapy is indicated by a falling RPR titer.
- RPR testing should be repeated 3, 6, and 12 months after treatment is complete.
- Treatment is repeated when there is a sustained fourfold increase in the RPR titer.
- Therapy is repeated when a high titer does not show a fourfold decrease within a year.
- In most patients infected with the human immunodeficiency virus, syphilis responds to standard penicillin treatment.

Secondary syphilis. Temporary irregular ("moth eaten") alopecia of the beard, scalp, or eyelashes may occur.

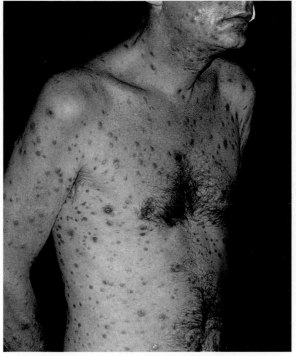

The lesions of secondary syphilis have marked tendency to polymorphism, with various types of lesions presenting simultaneously. They have a coppery tint and assume a variety of shapes. Eruptions may be limited and discrete, or profuse and generalized.

Secondary syphilis. A few oval lesions are present on the trunk. The initial diagnosis was pityriasis rosea.

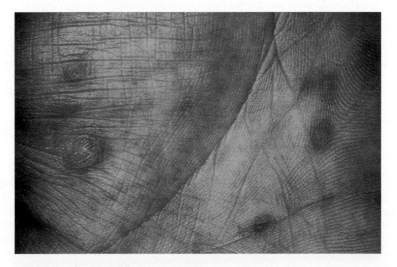

Secondary syphilis. Lesions on the palms and soles occur in the majority of patients with secondary syphilis. A coppery color resembling that of clean-cut ham is characteristic of secondary syphilis.

■ CHANCROID

DESCRIPTION

- Chancroid is an uncommon sexually transmitted disease caused by *Haemophilus ducreyi*.
- Painful genital ulceration and suppurative regional adenopathy occur.

HISTORY

- The male-to-female ratio is 10:1.
- Chancroid predominantly affects heterosexual men. Most cases originate from prostitutes, who are often asymptomatic carriers.
- It is uncommon in the United States and occurs in epidemics.
- It is common and endemic in many parts of the Third World.
- There is a high rate of infection with the human immunodeficiency virus (HIV) among patients with chancroid.

SKIN FINDINGS

- A painful, red papule appears at the contact site, becomes pustular, and ruptures to form a ragged ulcer with a red halo.
- The ulcer is deep, bleeds easily, and spreads laterally, burrowing under the skin.
- It has an undermined edge and a base covered by yellow-gray exudate.
- Ulcers are highly infectious, multiple lesions appearing on the genitals from autoinoculation.
- Autoinoculation results in lesions on the thighs, buttocks, and anal area.

SYSTEMIC SYMPTOMS

- Anorexia, malaise, and low-grade fever are occasionally present.
- Female carriers may have no detectable lesions and may have no symptoms.
- Unilateral or bilateral inguinal lymphadenopathy develops in about 50% of untreated patients, beginning 1 week after the onset.
- Nodes resolve spontaneously, or they suppurate and break down.
- Untreated cases resolve spontaneously or become chronic and require long periods to heal.

LABORATORY

- *H. ducreyi* cannot be cultured on routine medium. All the newly formulated transport media can maintain the viability of this organism.
- Exudate is obtained with a cotton swab from the base of a new ulcer. The swab is rolled in one direction over the slide to preserve the "school-of-fish" pattern (clumping of organisms). Gram-negative coccobacilli are seen in parallel arrays.
- There is a high rate of HIV infection among patients with chancroid. The patient should be tested for HIV infection and 3 months later tested for syphilis and HIV infection if the initial results were negative.

DIFFERENTIAL DIAGNOSIS

- Genital ulcerative diseases, including herpes simplex, primary syphilis, lymphogranuloma venereum, and granuloma inguinale
- Deep and painful chancroid ulcer, unlike in herpes (shallow ulcer) or in syphilis (painless ulcer)

TREATMENT

- Drug regimens are azithromycin, 1 gm orally in a single dose; ceftriaxone, 250 mg intramuscularly in a single dose; ciprofloxacin, 500 mg orally two times a day for 3 days; or erythromycin, 500 mg orally three times a day for 7 days.
- Asymptomatic carriage of *H. ducreyi* occurs; therefore aggressive tracing and treatment of sex partners is essential.

DISCUSSION

- The combination of a painful ulcer accompanied by suppurative inguinal adenopathy is almost pathognomonic.
- Chancroid is often misdiagnosed as a primary herpes simplex infection.
- Chancroid is the sexually transmitted disease most strongly associated with an increased risk of HIV transmission.
- Without proper treatment, ulcers require long periods to heal, thereby prolonging the patient's susceptibility to or risk for HIV transmission or acquisition. The treatment should not be delayed for the results of a culture; a clinical diagnosis should be made and the condition treated.

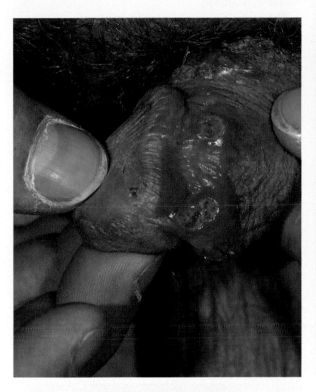

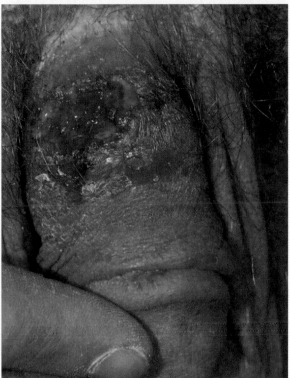

Several small, painful ulcers are usually present. The base is purulent, in contrast to the chancre of syphilis.

The ulcers have coalesced during a 4-week period without treatment.

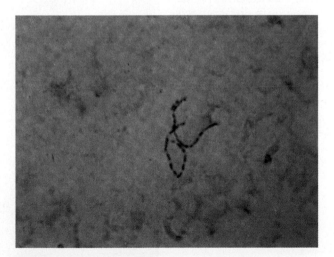

Wright's stain of purulent material of the base of the ulcer shows a chain of coccobacilli in the "school-of-fish" pattern.

■ GENITAL WARTS (CONDYLOMA ACUMINATA OR VENEREAL WARTS)

DESCRIPTION

- Infection of genital or anal skin by the human papilloma virus (HPV) results in epidermal proliferation.

HISTORY

- Warts spread rapidly over moist areas and may therefore be symmetric on opposing surfaces of the labia or rectum.
- Common warts can be the source of genital warts, although they are usually caused by different antigenic types of virus.
- Genital warts frequently recur after treatment.
- Latent virus exists beyond the treatment areas in clinically normal skin.
- Half of patients who have multiple and widespread infection with genital (HPV) and who practice orogenital sex have oral condylomata. The lesions are asymptomatic. Magnification is necessary to detect oral lesions.
- Half of cases of condyloma acuminata in children are the result of sexual abuse. Warts in the genital area can be acquired without sexual abuse. A child with warts on the hands can transfer the warts to the mouth, genitals, and anal area. A mother with hand warts can transfer warts to the child. Sexual play among children is another possible mode of transmission. The incubation period for warts is often many months in duration; this makes it difficult to associate past events.
- There is strong evidence that HPV types 16 and 18 are most strongly associated with genital cancers.
- The course is highly variable; spontaneous resolution may occur with time.

SKIN FINDINGS

- The skin is pale pink with numerous, discrete, narrow-to-wide projections on a broad base.
- The surface is smooth or velvety and moist and lacks the hyperkeratosis of warts found elsewhere.
- The lesions may coalesce in the rectal or perineal area to form a large, cauliflower-like mass.
- Warts may extend into the vaginal tract, urethra, and rectum, in which case a speculum or sigmoidoscope is required for visualization and treatment.

DIFFERENTIAL DIAGNOSIS

- Pearly penile papules, which are dome-shaped or hairlike projections that appear on the corona of the penis and sometimes on the shaft just proximal to the corona in up to 10% of male patients (These small angiofibromas are normal variants but are sometimes mistaken for warts. No treatment is required [see p. 138].)
- Molluscum contagiosum, which consists of dome-shaped, firm, white papules that usually have a central depression

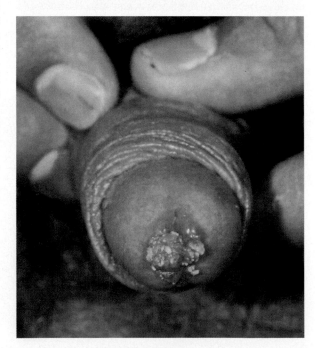

Wart at the urethral meatus.

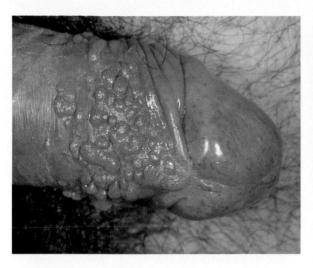

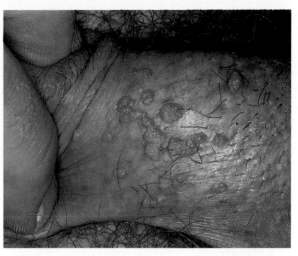

Warts spread rapidly over moist areas such as under the fore-skin and the vulva and tend to be more numerous than on skin in other areas.

These warts are similar in appearance to common warts.

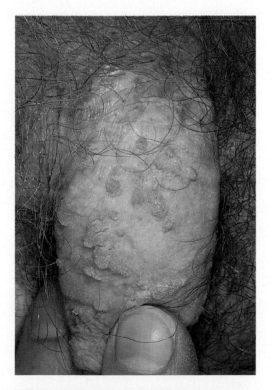

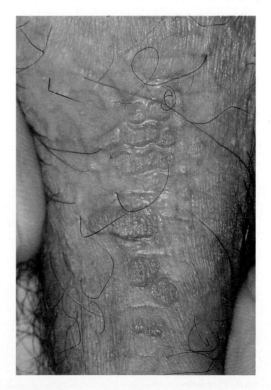

Multiple discrete warts on the shaft of the penis.

Genital warts are pale pink with numerous, discrete, narrow to wide projections on a broad base.

TREATMENT

- Warts that are flat and inconspicuous, especially on the penile shaft and urethral meatus, escape treatment; these can be visualized after the application of gauze soaked in acetic acid (vinegar) for 5 to 10 minutes.
- Treatment can be difficult, and multiple visits and treatments are often necessary for success.
- When liquid nitrogen cryotherapy is performed, the wart is frozen until a 1-mm rim appears around it. Another treatment is done in 2 to 3 weeks. The treatment is painful, and blisters may form.
- When electrocautery and curettage are used, a light touch with monopolar electrocautery is effective for treating a few isolated lesions. Scarring is possible.
- Patients are instructed to apply podofilox (Condylox gel) to the external genital warts twice each day for 3 consecutive days, followed by 4 days without treatment. This cycle is repeated at weekly intervals for a maximum of 4 weeks. Local adverse effects of the drug, such as pain, burning, inflammation, and erosion, have occurred in more than 50% of patients.
- Imiquimod (Aldara cream 5%) is an immune response stimulator. It is applied every other night at bedtime, left on the wart for 6 to 10 hours, and removed by washing with mild soap and water. This regimen is continued until the warts have resolved or 16 weeks maximum have passed. Treatment may have to be temporarily interrupted if irritation occurs.
- Examination of sexual partners is unnecessary for the management of genital warts because the role of reinfection is probably minimal. The majority of partners are probably already subclinically infected with HPV, even if they have no visible warts.
- The use of condoms may reduce transmission to partners likely to be uninfected, such as new partners.

CAVEAT

- Individual variations in cell-mediated immunity may explain differences in severity and duration.
- Warts occur more frequently, last longer, and appear in greater numbers in patients with acquired immunodeficiency syndrome and lymphomas and in patients who are taking immunosuppressive medications.

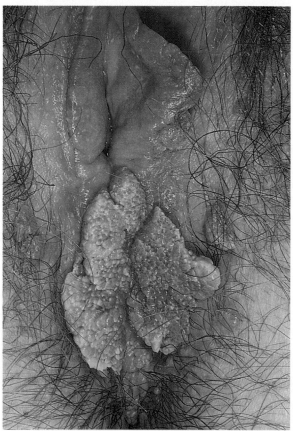

A large cauliflower-like wart projects from the vagina.

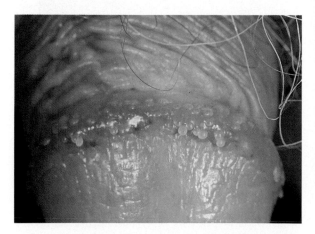

Pearly penile papules. An anatomic variant of normal, most commonly found on the corona of the penis. They are sometimes mistaken for warts. No treatment is required.

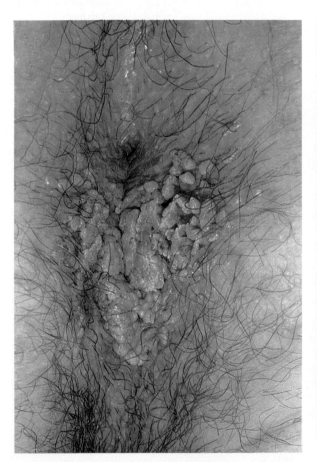

Warts spread rapidly over moist areas and may coalesce in the rectal area to form a large, cauliflower-like mass.

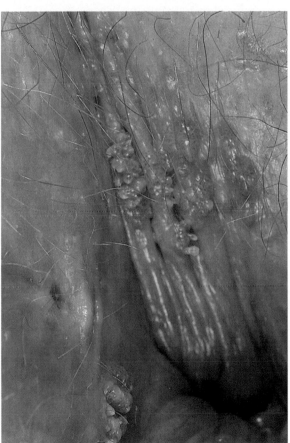

Many small warts may be found in the anal area.

■ GENITAL HERPES SIMPLEX

DESCRIPTION

- Genital herpes simplex is a sexually transmitted disease caused by the herpes simplex virus (HSV).
- The primary infection is followed by recurrent outbreaks of grouped vesicles on a red base.
- Many cases are transmitted by people who are unaware that they have the infection or are asymptomatic when transmission occurs.

HISTORY

Primary Infection

- A total of 2 to 20 days after exposure, influenza-like systemic complaints (e.g., fever, headache, malaise, myalgia) begin; the complaints peak 3 to 4 days after viral vesicles develop.
- Tender lymphadenopathy occurs in the second and third weeks.

Recurrent Infection

- Influenza-like symptoms are less intense or most often are absent.
- The prodrome is burning or itching.
- Chronic disease with recurrence is common.

SKIN FINDINGS

- A primary infection is more severe (greater number of lesions) and extensive than a secondary infection.
- The lesions in a recurrent infection occur in same sequence but on a lesser scale.
- This condition presents with a red plaque followed by grouped vesicles that evolve into pustules.
- Umbilication (a central depression) is a characteristic feature of herpetic vesicles.
- The pustules rupture or break, may crust, and form shallow, painful erosions.
- Large confluent erosions and ulcers can occur.
- The lesions heal in 2 to 4 weeks; recurrent lesion may heal in 1 to 2 weeks.
- Hypopigmentation or hyperpigmentation and sometimes scars may be left.
- In women, primary infection is often the most extensive and severe; lesions are seen on the labia majora and minora, perineum, and inner thighs. Secondary infections occur on the labia and buttocks.
- Regional lymphadenopathy (painful) occurs with primary infection.

LABORATORY

- The most definitive method is viral culture.
- Lesions must be sampled in the vesicular or early ulcerative stage.
- A rapid test is the Tzanck smear. The best results are obtained from intact vesicles. Giant cells with 2 to 15 nuclei are the characteristic finding.
- A Papanicolaou (Pap) smear is useful for detecting HSV in women without symptoms.
- An intact vesicle can be biopsied.
- A rapid immunofluorescent test is available at some centers.

DIFFERENTIAL DIAGNOSIS

- Syphilis
- Chancroid

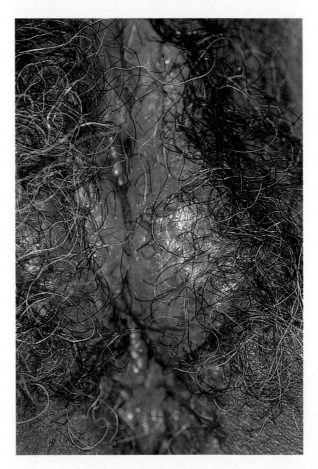

Primary herpes simplex. Numerous lesions form on moist surfaces.

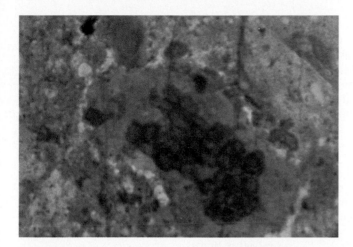

Tzanck smear. Multinucleated giant cell.

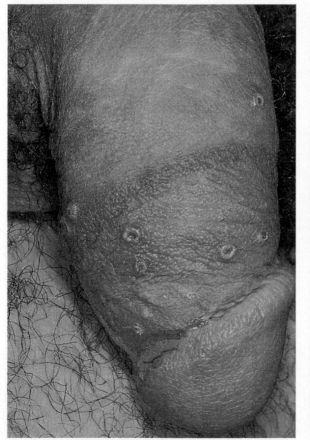

Primary herpes simplex. Lesions spread over a wide area.

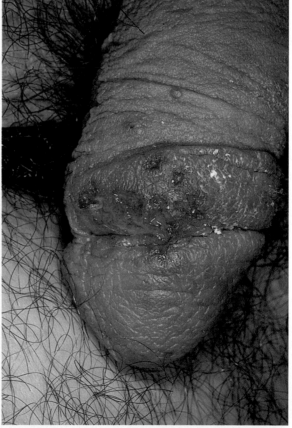

Primary herpes simplex. Vesicles became confluent and then eroded.

TREATMENT
Counseling

- The natural history of the disease, the potential for recurrent episodes, asymptomatic viral shedding, and sexual transmission should be explained.
- The patient should be instructed to use condoms during all sexual exposures with new or unaffected sex partners.

Systemic Therapy

- Systemic antiviral drugs partially control the symptoms and signs of herpes episodes.
- These drugs neither eradicate latent virus nor affect the risk, frequency, or severity of recurrences after the drug is discontinued.

Primary Infection

- Treatment is initiated within 72 hours of the onset of signs and symptoms.
- Valacyclovir (Valtrex), 1 gm every 12 hours for 10 days, can be prescribed.
- Famciclovir (Famvir), 250 mg, can be administered every 8 hours for 10 days.
- Cool, wet water compresses suppress inflammation.
- Acyclovir (Zovirax), 200 mg every 4 hours 5 times a day, 400 mg every 8 hours, or 800 mg orally every 12 hours for 10 days, can be administered.
- Severe primary infections are treated intravenously (5 mg/kg every 8 hours for 7 days). This regimen should be considered in immunocompromised patients.

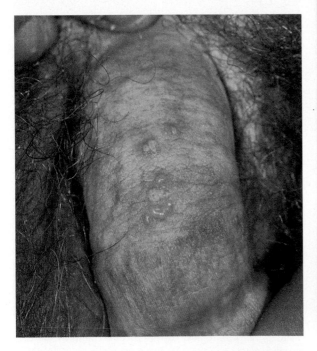

Recurrent herpes simplex with vesicles on a red base.

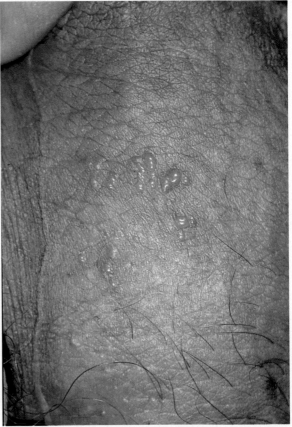

Recurrent herpes simplex. A group of vesicles on a red base.

Recurrent Infection

- Treatment is initiated within 24 to 48 hours of the onset of signs and symptoms.
- Valacyclovir (Valtrex), 500 mg every 12 hours for 5 days, can be prescribed.
- Famciclovir (Famvir), 125 mg every 12 hours for 5 days, can be administered.
- Acyclovir (Zovirax), 400 mg every 8 hours for 5 days, can be given.
- Patients should be provided with a prescription for the medication so that treatment can be started at the first sign of prodrome or genital lesion.

Long-Term Suppressive Therapy

- Valacyclovir (Valtrex), 1 gm every day or 500 mg every day, can be prescribed for fewer than 9 recurrences a year.
- Famciclovir (Famvir), 250 mg every 12 hours, can be administered.
- Acyclovir (Zovirax), 400 mg every 12 hours, may be given. (The dosage may need to be adjusted.)
- Treatment is continued for at least 6 to 12 months.
- If treatment is successful, a trial without medication may be considered.
- Daily suppressive therapy reduces the frequency of genital herpes recurrences by at least 75% among patients who have frequent recurrences (i.e., six or more occurrences per year). Suppressive treatment reduces but does not eliminate asymptomatic viral shedding.

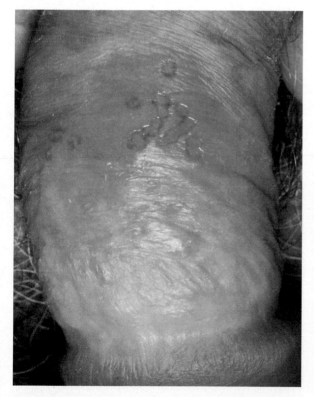

Recurrent herpes simplex under the foreskin. A group of discrete erosions is present. Crusts do not form on this moist surface.

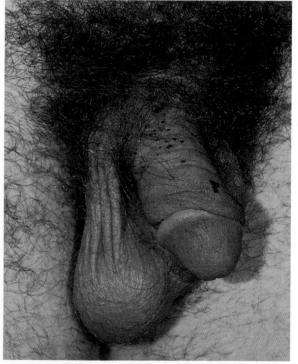

Recurrent herpes simplex with scattered small crusts and lack of vesicles.

■ PUBIC LICE (PEDICULOSIS PUBIS)

DESCRIPTION

- Pubic lice are the most contagious sexually transmitted problem known.
- The chance of acquiring pubic lice from one sexual exposure with an infested partner is more than 90%.
- Up to 30% of patients infested with pubic lice have at least one other sexually transmitted disease.
- Direct contact is the primary source of transmission.
- Eggs (nits) are cemented to the shaft 1 cm from the skin surface.
- Nits hatch in 8 to 10 days.
- Infested adults may spread pubic lice to the eyelashes of children.
- Additional information can be obtained from the National Pediculosis Association (www.head-lice.org).

HISTORY

- Fomite transmission is common (e.g., from hats, brushes, earphones).
- The majority of patients complain of pruritus.
- Many patients are aware that something is crawling on the groin but are not familiar with the disease and have never seen lice.

SKIN FINDINGS

- Nits are firmly cemented to the hair.
- The pubic hair is the most common site of infestation, but lice frequently spread to the hair around the anus.
- On hairy persons, lice may spread to the upper thighs, abdominal area, axillae, chest, and beard.
- Occasionally, gray-blue macules (maculae ceruleae) varying in size from 1 to 2 cm are seen in the groin and at sites distant from the infestation. Their cause is not known, but they may represent altered blood pigment.
- Approximately 50% of patients have little inflammation, but those who delay seeking help may develop widespread inflammation and infection of the groin with regional adenopathy.

TREATMENT

- All agents attack the louse's nervous system; young nits are not affected.
- The use of all agents should be repeated in 1 week.
- Strains resistant to synergized pyrethrins, permethrin 1% (Nix) and 5% (Elimite), have emerged.

STANDARD THERAPIES

- An over-the-counter (OTC) permethrin rinse 1% (Nix creme rinse) is often the drug of first choice. It is applied and washed off after 10 minutes.
- OTC synergized pyrethrin shampoos (RID, A-200, R & C) are also used.
- Permethrin 5% (Elimite cream) is prescribed when OTC treatment fails. It is left on the hair overnight.
- Lindane (Kwell) shampoo is left in for 5 minutes and then washed out; treatment is repeated in 1 week. It is used if OTC treatment fails. Lindane-resistant lice have emerged.
- Malathion lotion (Ovide) is highly effective. It is applied to dry hair and shampooed out after 8 to 12 hours.

Oral Medication

- Ivermectin, 200 μg/kg, is given in a single oral dose that is repeated in 10 days. It attacks invertebrate nerve and muscle cells in the louse and causes paralysis and death. It has selective activity against parasites but no systemic effects on mammals.

Nit Removal

- It is important to remove nits.
- Shaving the pubic and abdominal hair may be helpful.
- Fomite control is essential.

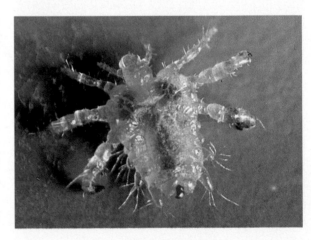

Phthirus pubis (pubic or crab louse). The crab louse is the smallest louse, with a short, oval body and prominent claws resembling those of sea crabs.

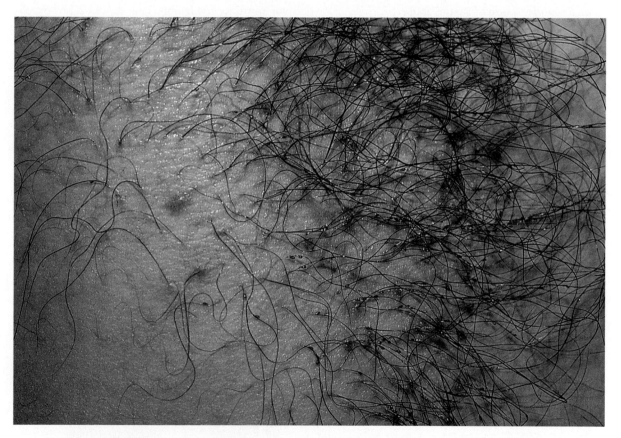

Pediculosis pubis. Lice become rust colored from the ingestion of blood; their color is an identifying characteristic. Lice feces can be seen on the skin as small, rust-colored flecks.

■ MOLLUSCUM CONTAGIOSUM

DESCRIPTION

- Molluscum contagiosum is a viral infection of the skin characterized by discrete papules.

HISTORY

- Molluscum contagiosum spreads by autoinoculation, by scratching, or by touching a lesion.
- Genital molluscum contagiosum in children may be a manifestation of sexual abuse.
- Molluscum contagiosum is a common and at times a severely disfiguring eruption in patients with infection of the human immunodeficiency virus. It is often a marker of late-stage disease.

SKIN FINDINGS

- Discrete, 2- to 5-mm, slightly umbilicated, flesh-colored, and dome-shaped lesions appear.
- The pubic and genital areas are most commonly involved in adults.
- The lesions are frequently grouped. There may be a few or many covering a wide area.
- Erythema and scaling at the periphery of a single or several lesions may occur. This may be the result of inflammation from scratching, or it may be a hypersensitivity reaction.
- Papules are often camouflaged by pubic hair. Most patients have just a few lesions that can be easily overlooked.
- The focus of examination is the pubic hair, genitals, anal area, thighs, and trunk. Lesions may appear anywhere except the palms and soles.

DIFFERENTIAL DIAGNOSIS

- Warts
- Herpes simplex

TREATMENT

- Genital lesions should be treated to prevent spread through sexual contact.
- New lesions too small to be detected at the first examination may appear after treatment and require attention at a subsequent visit.
- Small papules can be quickly removed with a curette with or without local anesthesia. Bleeding is controlled with gauze pressure or Monsel's solution. Curettage is useful when there are a few lesions because it provides the quickest, most reliable treatment. A small scar may form; therefore this technique should be avoided in cosmetically important areas.

- Lidocaine/prilocaine (EMLA Cream) applied 30 to 60 minutes before treatment effectively prevents the pain of curettage for children.
- Cryosurgery is the treatment of choice for patients who do not object to the pain. The papule is sprayed or touched lightly with a nitrogen-bathed cotton swab until the advancing, white, frozen border has progressed down the side of the papule to form a 1-mm halo on the normal skin surrounding the lesion. This should take approximately 5 seconds. A conservative approach is necessary because excessive freezing produces hypopigmentation or hyperpigmentation.
- A small drop of cantharidin 0.7% (Cantharone) is applied over the surface of the lesion, and contamination of normal skin is avoided. Lesions blister and may resolve without scarring. New lesions occasionally appear at the site of the blister created by cantharidin. Hypopigmentation or hyperpigmentation may occur.
- Potassium hydroxide 10% is be prepared by the pharmacist. A drop is applied with a cotton-tipped applicator once each day, taking care to avoid the surrounding normal skin. This medication is caustic and must be kept away from children.

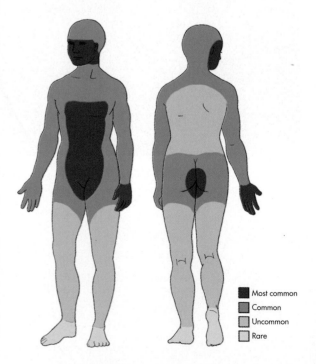

Most common
Common
Uncommon
Rare

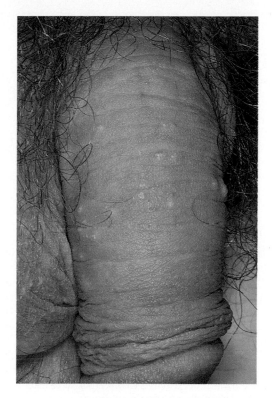

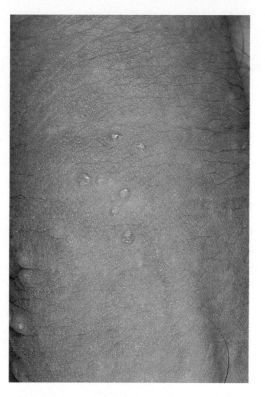

Lesions are usually discrete, white, and dome shaped. They lack the many small projections found on the surface of warts.

Close observation of individual lesions is necessary to confirm the diagnosis. Lesions are often misdiagnosed as warts.

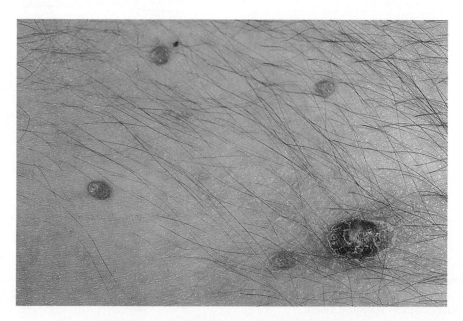

A single lesion became inflamed and disappeared 10 days later.

■ WARTS (VERRUCA VULGARIS)

DESCRIPTION

- Warts are benign epidermal proliferations caused by human papillomavirus infection.
- There are over 70 different types of HPV, many associated with a particular clinical and pathologic entity.
- Transmission is by simple contact, often at sites with small skin breaks, abrasions, or other trauma.
- Local spread is often by autoinoculation.

HISTORY

- The estimated incidence of infection is 10% in children and young adults.
- The peak incidence is age 12 to 16.
- The incubation period is variable: 1 to 6 months.

SKIN FINDINGS

- Flesh-colored papules evolve to dome-shaped, gray-brown, hyperkeratotic growths with black dots on the surface.
- The black dots are thrombosed capillaries.
- They are usually few in number but may be numerous.
- Common sites are the hands, periungual skin, elbows, knees, and plantar surfaces.
- Filiform warts are growths with fingerlike, flesh-colored projections on a narrow or broad base; they often occur on the face.

COURSE AND PROGNOSIS

- The course is highly variable; spontaneous resolution with time is the rule.
- In children, approximately two thirds of all warts spontaneously regress within 2 years.

TREATMENT

- Treatment can be difficult, and multiple visits and treatments are often necessary for success.
- Over-the-counter topical salicylic acid preparations are applied once a day. The preparations may be occluded to increase penetration. The duration of treatment is often lengthy; soreness and irritation are side effects.
- With liquid nitrogen cryotherapy, the 15-second freeze time is repeated once. A follow-up visit for retreatment occurs in 2 to 3 weeks. Side effects are pain and a blister after treatment.

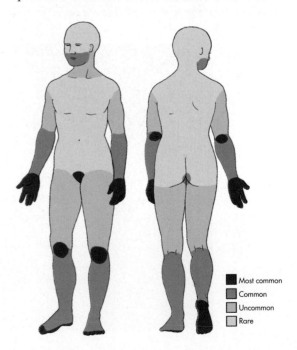

■ Most common
■ Common
■ Uncommon
□ Rare

- The limitations of electrocautery and curettage are pain, secondary infection, and scarring.
- The limitations of laser surgery are pain and potential scarring.
- Filiform warts are easiest to treat. Local anesthesia can be used and the lesion removed with a snip or a curette. Light electrocautery and cryotherapy are other alternatives.

CAVEAT

- Individual variations in cell-mediated immunity may explain differences in severity and duration.
- Warts occur more frequently, last longer, and appear in greater numbers in patients with acquired immunodeficiency syndrome and lymphomas and in patients on immunosuppressive medications.

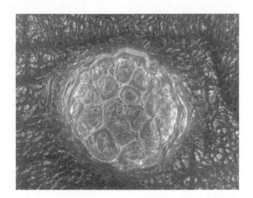

Warts form cylindric projections. The projections become fused in common warts on thicker skin and form a highly organized mosaic pattern on the surface.

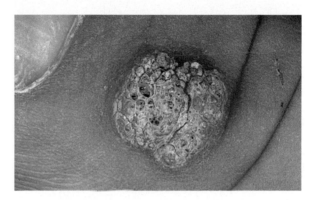

The surface projections are long and have a large surface area. Liquid salicylic acid should be effective for this type of wart because it can penetrate between the projections.

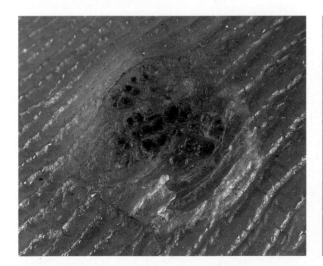

Warts remain confined to the epidermis and interrupt normal skin lines. The wart is gone when normal skin lines reappear.

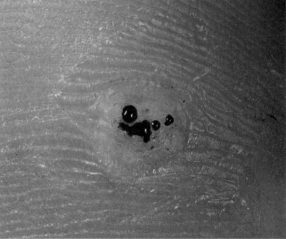

Thrombosed black vessels become trapped in the projections and are seen as black dots on the surface. They bleed when pared with a blade.

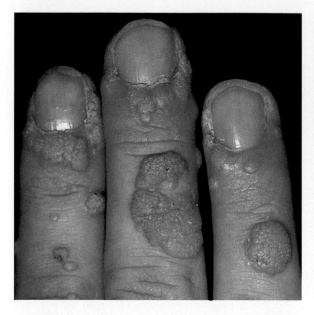

The hands are the most commonly involved area. Warts become confluent and obscure large areas of normal skin. Biting or picking the skin around the nails can spread warts.

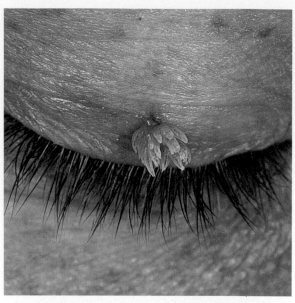

Filiform and digitate warts consist of a few or several finger-like, flesh-colored projections emanating from a narrow or broad base. They are most commonly observed about the mouth, beard, eyes, and nose.

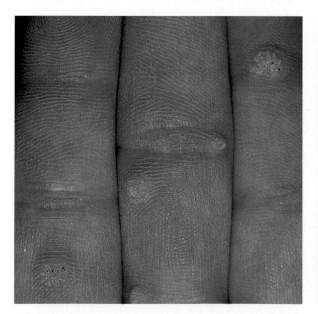

Warts on the palms have a similar appearance to those on the soles. The skin is thick, and the warts are more difficult to treat with liquid nitrogen and salicylic acid.

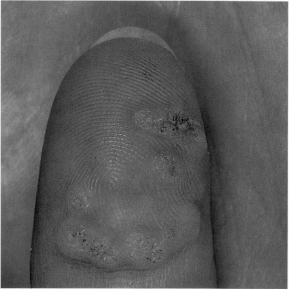

These warts have become confluent. Freezing a wide area of the fingertip is very painful. Localized areas should be treated in two or three treatment sessions

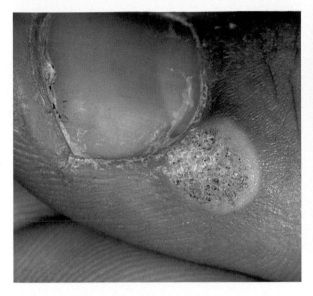

Warts are frozen until the "freeze front" extends for about 1 or 2 mm beyond the growth. Using two freeze-thaw cycles during one treatment session may increase the cure rate.

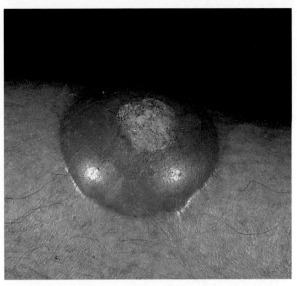

Warts blister a day or two after freezing with liquid nitrogen. The size of the blister varies depending on the location and the individual. Blisters are often filled with blood and are painful. These may be punctured and drained with an #11 surgical blade.

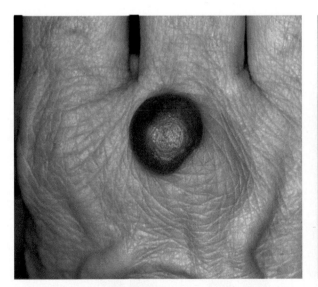

Large blisters commonly form on the backs of the hands after treatment with liquid nitrogen.

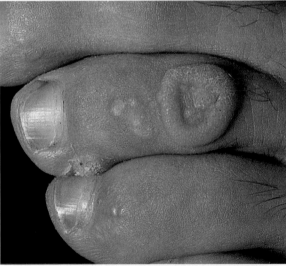

The wart virus spread to the edge of the blister and formed a wart larger than the lesion that was originally treated. This is one possible side effect of cryosurgery.

■ FLAT WARTS

DESCRIPTION

- Pink, light brown, or light yellow papules that are slightly elevated and flat-topped vary in size from 0.1 to 0.3 cm. They may be few or numerous and may occur in a line as a result of spread within a scratch or traumatized skin.

SKIN FINDINGS

- Typical sites are the forehead, back of the hands, chin, neck, and legs. Flat warts are easily spread within areas of shaving.

COURSE AND PROGNOSIS

- The duration may be lengthy; flat warts may be very resistant to treatment. They are generally located in cosmetically important areas where aggressive, scarring procedures must be avoided.
- Immunocompromised patients often have a protracted course.

TREATMENT

- Tretinoin cream, 0.025%, 0.05%, or 0.1%, is applied at bedtime over the entire involved area. The frequency of application is adjusted to produce fine scaling and mild erythema. Treatment may be required for weeks or months.
- Liquid nitrogen or a very light touch with an electrocautery needle may be performed for quick results. Flat warts may not respond to cryotherapy, even after many treatment sessions.
- Applied once or twice a day for 3 to 5 weeks, 5-fluorouracil cream (Efudex 5%) may produce dramatic clearing of flat warts. Persistent hyperpigmentation may follow the use of 5-fluorouracil and is minimized by applying it to individual lesions with a cotton-tipped applicator.

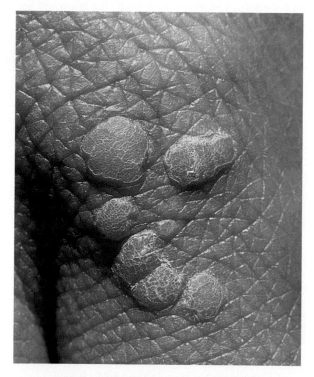

Warts are often grouped and are easily spread by scratching. The surface projections in these warts are very small and require magnification to be seen.

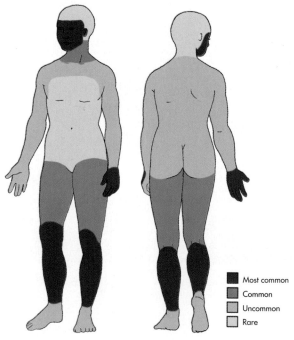

Most common
Common
Uncommon
Rare

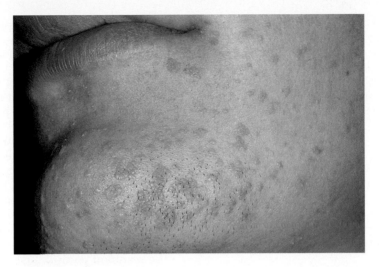

Flat warts are pink, light brown, or light yellow and are slightly elevated, flat-topped papules that vary in size from 0.1 to 0.3 cm. There may be only a few, but generally there are many.

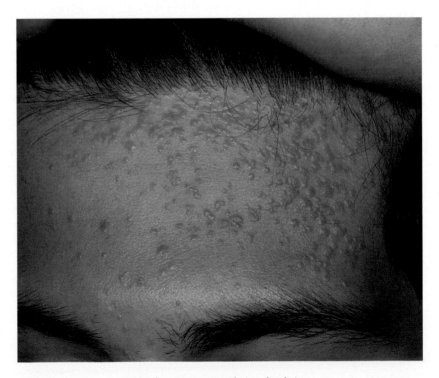

The face is a commonly involved site.

■ PLANTAR WARTS

DESCRIPTION

- Human papilloma virus (HPV) infection on the plantar foot surface frequently occurs at points of maximal pressure, such as over the heads of the metatarsal bones or the heels.
- A cluster of many warts is referred to as a *mosaic wart.*

SKIN FINDINGS

- The round, single or multiple, coalescing, flesh-colored, rough keratotic papules often look depressed.
- Punctate black dots within the wart, often seen on paring, are capillary loops.
- The papules may be tender with pressure.

LABORATORY

- Biopsy may be indicated in warts that are rapidly growing, ulcerated, atypical, or resistant to treatment; squamous cell carcinoma or melanoma may mimic a wart. HPV types 1, 2, and 4 are associated with plantar warts.

COURSE AND PROGNOSIS

- Treatment is often difficult; warts can be very refractory and recurrent. Often, multiple treatment sessions are required.
- Hyperhidrosis is associated with a more widespread distribution of warts that are often refractory to treatment.

TREATMENT

- There are multiple treatment options, indicating no single best option.
- Plantar warts do not require therapy as long as they are painless. Spontaneous resolution with time is the rule.
- Keratolytic therapy with salicylic acid (DuoPlant, Occlusal) is a conservative initial treatment. There is no scarring. The wart is pared, the affected part is soaked in warm water, and the salicylic acid preparation is applied to the wart surface. Limitations include irritation and soreness. Treatment may require 6 to 8 weeks.
- Plasters with salicylic acid 40% (Mediplast) are useful in treating mosaic warts covering large areas. It is left on for 24 to 48 hours and replaced. Treatment may require 6 to 8 weeks.
- Blunt dissection is a fast, effective surgical treatment (90% cure rate) and usually produces no scarring. It is superior to both electrodesiccation/curettage and excision because normal tissue is not disturbed. Many podiatrists are experienced at this procedure.
- In cryosurgery with liquid nitrogen, the nitrogen is applied for 15 to 30 seconds, twice to a wart. The resultant painful blister can interfere with mobility. Repeated light applications of liquid nitrogen are preferred.
- Carbon dioxide and pulsed dye laser treatment is also available but is expensive.
- Electrodesiccation/curettage can cause pain from the anesthesia, postoperative pain, and a risk of scarring.
- Bleomycin, 0.5 U/ml, is injected into the wart to achieve blanching. The size of the wart determines the injection quantity:

<5 mm	0.2 ml
5-10 mm	0.2-0.5 ml
≤1.0 ml	3 ml (1.5 U) maximum per visit

Responsive warts show hemorrhagic eschars that heal without scarring. Treatment is very painful; necrosis or severe vasospasm may occur. Pregnancy is a contraindication.

CAVEAT

- Calluses can be mistaken for warts.
- A wart lacks surface skin lines and has centrally located black dots that bleed with paring. Corns have a hard, painful, translucent central core.

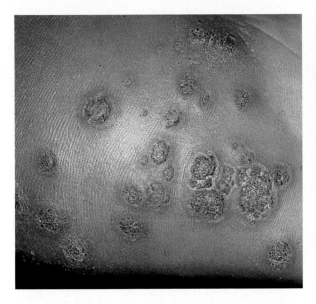

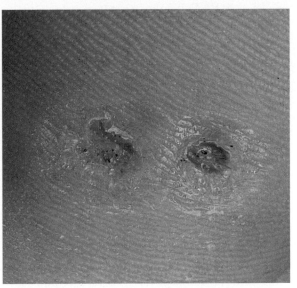

Plantar warts frequently occur at points of maximal pressure, such as over the heads of the metatarsal bones or on the heels. A cluster of many warts that appears to fuse is referred to as a *mosaic wart*.

A thick, painful callus forms in response to pressure, and the foot is repositioned while walking. This may result in distortion of posture and pain in other parts of the foot, leg, or back. This callus should be removed before treatment.

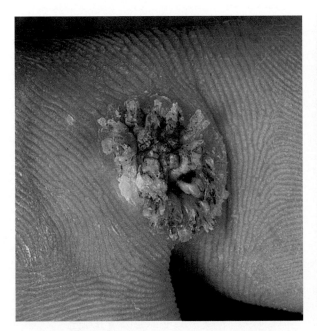

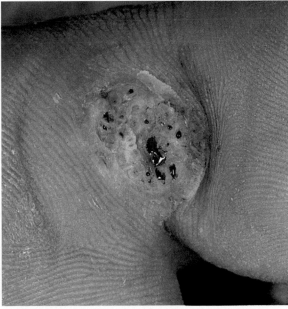

This wart has little callus on the surface and will bleed if pared with a blade.

Care should be used when removing the callus. Some warts have a thick surface callus, but others are fragile and bleed easily when pared.

■ MOLLUSCUM CONTAGIOSUM

DESCRIPTION

- Molluscum contagiosum is a localized, self-limited viral infection of the skin; it is spread on the skin by autoinoculation and is transmitted to others by skin-to-skin contact.
- The etiologic agent is a virus of the poxvirus family.

HISTORY

- Molluscum contagiosum may occur at any age.
- Peak ages affected are between ages 3 and 9 and again between ages 16 and 24.
- Lesions tend to occur in different areas of the body within different age groups.
- Most lesions are asymptomatic, although tenderness and itching do occur and are usually associated with mild local inflammation.
- Individual lesions often resolve spontaneously within 6 to 9 months but may persist for up to 24 months.
- The risk of transmission appears to be lower than that of herpesvirus and papillomavirus.

SKIN FINDINGS

- Molluscum contagiosum begins as a 1- to 2-mm shiny, white to flesh-colored, dome-shaped, firm papule.
- There is a small central punctum that is best seen when the epidermis is lightly frozen with ethyl chloride or liquid nitrogen.
- Over weeks, the lesion maintains its discrete dome shape, attaining its maximum size of 2 to 5 mm.
- Larger lesions occur in immunocompromised hosts.
- With time, the papule becomes softer and more pink in color, and the central umbilication becomes more obvious.
- Untreated lesions usually persist for 6 to 9 months before slowly involuting, at times leaving a minute pitted scar.
- Inflammation surrounding a lesion of molluscum contagiosum implies a host immune response and predicts resolution.
- Excoriations as well as crusting from secondary impetiginization may be present.
- The body area involved varies by age.

- Children tend to have lesions on the upper trunk, extremities, and especially on the face.
- Autoinoculation around the eyes is particularly common.
- The palms and soles are not involved.
- Molluscum contagiosum is primarily a sexually transmitted disease in young adults. Lesions tend to occur on the lower abdomen, pubic area (including the genitalia), and thighs. Lesions occurring solely in these areas in children should raise suspicion of sexual abuse.
- Individuals with atopic dermatitis are prone to developing numerous lesions within eczematous areas through inoculation of inflamed skin. Such lesions are notoriously difficult to clear until the eczema is brought under control.
- Molluscum contagiosum is similarly difficult to treat in immunocompromised hosts such as in the setting of the human immunodeficiency virus (HIV). In such cases, lesions are often more numerous and widespread, and individual lesions can become quite large and tend to persist.

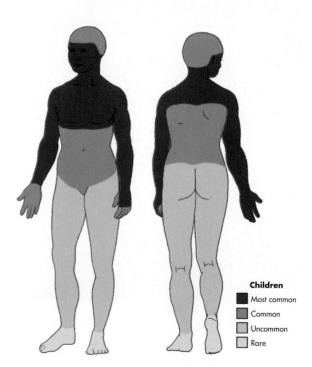

Children

■ Most common
■ Common
■ Uncommon
□ Rare

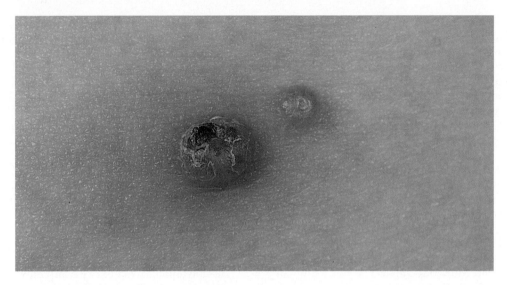

It is common to see erythema and scaling at the periphery of a single or several lesions. This may be the result of inflammation from scratching or may be a hypersensitivity reaction. Inflamed molluscum may spontaneously clear.

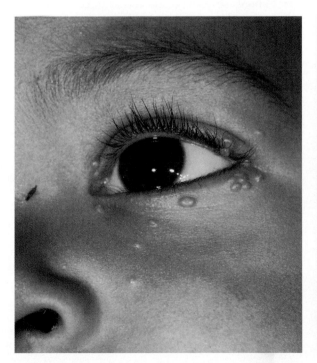

Inoculation around the eye, a typical presentation for children.

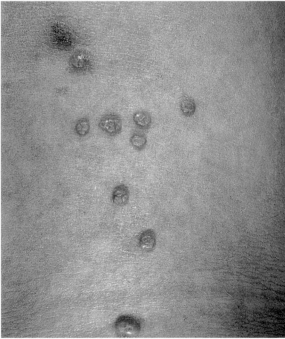

Molluscum contagiosum is characterized by discrete, 2- to 5-mm, slightly umbilicated, flesh-colored, dome-shaped papules. It spreads by autoinoculation, by scratching, or by touching a lesion.

LABORATORY

- Skin biopsy is rarely needed to establish the diagnosis in an immunocompetent host.
- Biopsy confirms the presence of large intracytoplasmic viral inclusions known as *molluscum bodies* within infected keratinocytes.
- Curettage of a lesion expresses a white, rubbery core of infected keratinocytes suitable for potassium hydroxide examination.
- Infected keratinocytes are strikingly round and separate easily from one another.
- Normal keratinocytes are flat and cohesive, forming a sheet of adherent cells.
- Lesions occurring in an immunocompromised host such as those with HIV disease should be biopsied to confirm the diagnosis. Other infections that also occur in such patients may mimic molluscum contagiosum.

DISCUSSION

- The differential diagnosis of molluscum lesions in immunocompetent hosts includes flat warts, genital warts, and herpes infection.
- Warts lack the central umbilication and may occur on the palms and soles.
- Herpes lesions are vesicles and are only transiently umbilicated.
- Herpes lesions are usually tender and have a more rapid onset and shorter clinical course.
- In HIV disease, other opportunistic fungal infections, including cryptococcosis and histoplasmosis, may produce lesions resembling those of molluscum contagiosum.
- Biopsy is recommended to confirm the diagnosis.

TREATMENT

- Skin-to-skin contact should be avoided to minimize transmission of the virus.
- In children, lesions should be kept covered by clothing if possible.
- Genital lesions in sexually active adults should be treated (see p. 146).
- Sexual partners of affected individuals should be checked for lesions.
- The use of condoms should be encouraged because lesions may be too small to detect during the initial examination.
- Depending on the location of lesions, the patient should be advised not to shave lesional areas because it can also lead to autoinoculation.
- Because lesions resolve spontaneously in healthy individuals and because there is some risk of scarring with treatment, the decision to treat must be made on an individual basis.
- Curettage is fairly painless and clears the lesions immediately.
  - Anesthesia may not be required but is recommended, especially in children.
  - Curettage is particularly useful for genital lesions.
  - There is some risk of scarring, and caution should be used, especially on the face.
- Cryosurgery with liquid nitrogen is effective and in trained hands, rarely produces scarring. Treatment can be painful, especially for genital lesions.
- Cantharidin 0.7% solution is painless, effective, and well tolerated, especially by children.
  - A drop of solution is applied to the molluscum lesion and allowed to dry completely before occlusion with Blenderm tape.
  - The tape is left in place for several hours and then removed, and the treated areas are carefully washed.
  - Patients should be advised to remove the tape sooner if any tenderness develops.
  - The lesion develops a small blister, which then resolves along with the lesion; scarring rarely occurs.
- Topical tretinoin applied daily to individual lesions may also hasten resolution.
  - A month or more of continuous treatment is usually required.
  - Significant local irritation from the tretinoin may develop.
- Hypoallergenic surgical adhesive tape may be used.
  - The tape is applied to each lesion.
  - The tape is changed each day after showering.
  - Treatment is continued until the lesion has ruptured, which may require several weeks.
- Potassium hydroxide 10% is best prepared by the pharmacist. A drop is applied with a cotton-tipped applicator once each day, taking care to avoid the surrounding normal skin. This medication is caustic and must be kept away from children.

CAVEAT

- Treatment should be individualized; lesions are self-limited.
- Significant scarring may result from overtreatment.

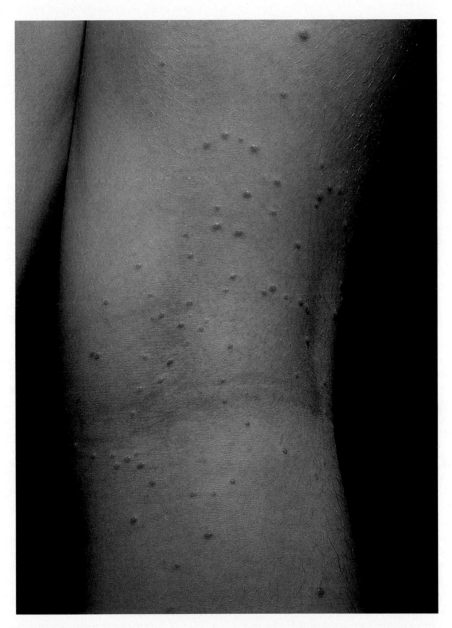

Lesions spread to inflamed skin, such as areas of atopic dermatitis. Most lesions are self-limiting and clear spontaneously in 6 to 9 months; however, they may last much longer.

■ HERPES SIMPLEX (COLD SORES, FEVER BLISTERS)

DESCRIPTION

- Herpes simplex virus (HSV) infections are caused by two different virus types (HSV-1 and HSV-2) that can be distinguished in the laboratory.
  - HSV-1 is generally associated with oral infections and HSV-2 with genital infections (see p. 140).
  - HSV-1 genital infections and HSV-2 oral infections are becoming more common, possibly as a result of oral-genital sexual contact.
- Both types produce identical patterns of infection.
- HSV infections have two phases: the primary infection, after which the virus becomes established in a nerve ganglion, and the secondary phase, characterized by recurrent disease at the same site.
- Infections can occur anywhere on the skin. Infection in one area does not protect the patient from subsequent infection at a different site.
- Herpes labialis (infection of the lips) is the most common presentation.

Primary Infection

- Nearly one third of primary infections are asymptomatic and can be detected only by an elevated immunoglobulin G antibody titer.
- The virus may be spread by respiratory droplets, direct contact with an active lesion, or contact with virus-containing fluid such as saliva or cervical secretions in patients with no evidence of active disease.
- Symptoms occur from 3 to 7 or more days after contact.
- Tenderness, pain, mild paresthesias, or burning occurs before the onset of lesions at the site of inoculation.
- Gingivostomatitis and pharyngitis are the most frequent manifestations of first-episode HSV-1 infection.
- Localized pain, tender lymphadenopathy, headache, generalized aching, and fever are characteristic prodromal symptoms.
- Grouped vesicles on an erythematous base appear and subsequently erode.
- The vesicles in primary herpes simplex are more numerous and scattered than in the recurrent infection.
- Lesions on the mucous membrane accumulate exudate, whereas lesions on the skin form a crust.
- Lesions last for 2 to 6 weeks and heal without scarring.

- During this primary infection, the virus enters the nerve endings in the skin directly below the lesions and ascends through peripheral nerves to the dorsal root ganglia, where it apparently remains in a latent stage.

Recurrent Infection

- Local skin trauma (e.g., ultraviolet light exposure, chapping, abrasion) or systemic changes (e.g., menses, fatigue, fever) reactivate the virus, which then travels down the peripheral nerves to the site of initial infection and causes the characteristic focal, recurrent infection.
- Recurrent infection is not inevitable. In many individuals, there is a rise in the antibody titer, and these people never experience recurrence.
- The prodromal symptoms, lasting 2 to 24 hours, resemble those of the primary infection. Tenderness, pain, mild paresthesias, or burning occurs before the onset of lesions at the site of inoculation.
- Within 12 hours, a group of lesions evolves rapidly from an erythematous base to form papules and then vesicles.
- The dome-shaped, tense vesicles rapidly umbilicate.
- In 2 to 4 days, the vesicles rupture, forming aphthae-like erosions in the mouth and vaginal area or erosions covered by crusts on the lips and skin.
- Crusts are shed in approximately 8 days to reveal a pink, reepithelialized surface.
- In contrast to the primary infection, systemic symptoms and lymphadenopathy are rare unless there is secondary infection.
- Many people experience a decrease in the frequency of recurrences with time, but others experience an increase.

CUTANEOUS HERPES SIMPLEX

- Herpes simplex may appear on any skin surface.
- Herpetic whitlow (herpes simplex of the fingertips) can resemble a group of warts or a bacterial infection. It is most often reported in pediatric patients with gingivostomatitis and in women with genital herpes.
- Herpes gladiatorum (cutaneous herpes in athletes involved in contact sports) is transmitted by direct skin-to-skin contact. This is a recognized health risk for wrestlers.

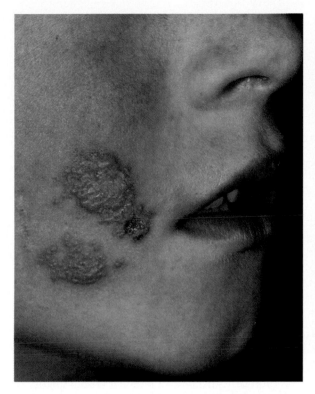

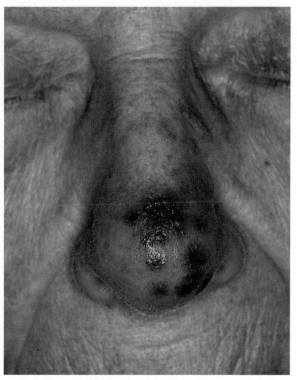

Primary herpes simplex infection. Primary infections in children typically begin in or about the oral cavity. Blisters are numerous.

Recurrent herpes. The diagnosis of herpes can be made at any stage in the evolution of lesions.

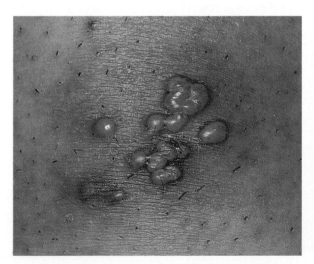

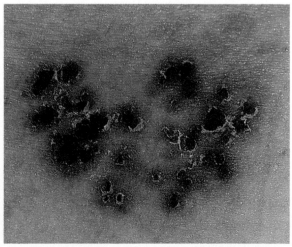

Recurrent infection. Tense, dome-shaped vesicles.

Recurrent infection. A group of crusts.

- Herpes simplex of the buttock area seems to be more common in women.
- Herpes simplex of the lumbosacral region or trunk may be very difficult to differentiate from herpes zoster; the diagnosis becomes apparent only at the time of recurrence.
- Eczema herpeticum (Kaposi's varicelliform eruption) is the association of two common conditions: atopic dermatitis and herpes simplex virus infection. The disease is most common in areas of active or recently healed atopic dermatitis, particularly the face, but normal skin can be involved. In most cases, the disease is a primary herpes simplex infection. In one third of the patients in a particular study, there was a history of herpes labialis in a parent in the previous week.

LABORATORY DIAGNOSIS

- In culture testing, the base of the vesicle is swabbed with the special viral culture kits provided by the laboratory. Results can be available in 24 hours.
- In Tzank smears, the base of the vesicle is swabbed with a cotton swab and smeared onto a glass slide. The sample can be stained directly or the slide submitted to the laboratory. The characteristic multinucleated giant cells help confirm the diagnosis.

TREATMENT

- Infections resolve without treatment. The need for treatment of first-episode infections, recurrent infections, and suppressive therapy is based on each patient's needs.
- Long-term suppressive therapy can greatly improve the quality of life for people with frequent and painful recurrences.
- The subsequent recurrence rate is not influenced by any topical or oral medication.

Topical Antiviral Agents

- Tetracaine cream 1.8% (Cepacol Viractin Cream [over the counter]), when applied frequently, reduces the healing time of recurrent herpes labialis lesions by about 2 days.
- Penciclovir cream (Denavir), when applied several times each day, reduces the duration of herpes labialis by about half a day. It is very expensive.

- Topical acyclovir is not approved for use on cold sores in the immunocompetent host because of its lack of efficacy.
- The lips should be protected from sun exposure with opaque creams such as zinc oxide or with sun-blocking agents incorporated into a lip balm.
- A compress with cool water decreases erythema and débrides crusts to promote healing.

Oral Antiviral Agents

- Therapy is initiated at the first sign or symptom.
- Therapy is most effective when administered within 48 hours of the onset of signs and symptoms.
- The frequency and severity of episodes of untreated herpes may change over time. After 1 year of suppressive therapy, the frequency and severity of the infection should be reevaluated to assess the need for continued therapy.

Valacyclovir (Valtrex)
- For initial episodes, 1 gm is given twice a day for 10 days.
- For recurrent episodes, 500 mg is administered twice a day for 5 days.
- Suppressive therapy requires the administration of 1 gm/day. In patients with a history of no more than nine recurrences a year, an alternative dose is 500 mg/day.

Famciclovir (Famvir)
- For recurrent episodes, 125 mg twice a day is given for 5 days.
- For suppressive therapy, 250 mg is administered twice a day for up to 1 year.

Acyclovir (Zovirax)
- For initial episodes, 200 mg is given every 4 hours five times a day for 10 days.
- For suppressive therapy, 400 mg is administered twice a day for up to 12 months. Then the case is reevaluated. Alternative regimens have included doses ranging from 200 mg three times a day to 200 mg five times a day.
- For recurrent episodes, 400 mg is administered every 8 hours three times a day for 5 days.

L-Lysine is ineffective.

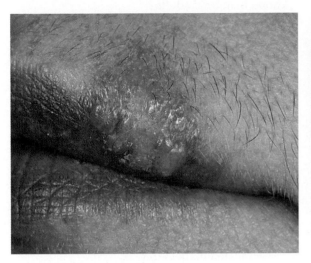

Recurrent herpes. Vesicles are confluent.

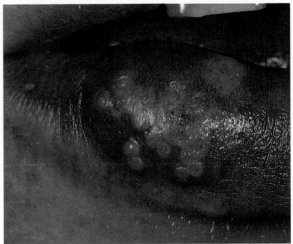

Recurrent herpes. Umbicated vesicles.

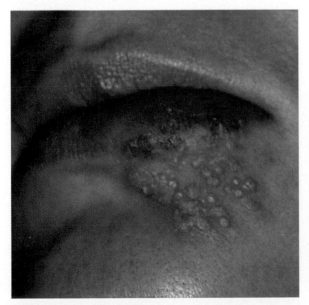

Recurrent herpes. A large group of vesicles followed sun exposure.

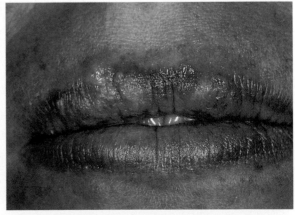

Recurrent herpes. Extensive infection after sun exposure.

■ VARICELLA (CHICKEN POX)

DESCRIPTION

- Varicella, a highly contagious condition, is caused by the varicella zoster virus, resulting in lifetime immunity.
- Transmission is via airborne droplets or vesicular fluid.
- Patients are contagious from 2 days before the onset of the rash until all lesions have crusted.

HISTORY

- The incubation period is approximately 14 to 16 days.
- In children, prodromal symptoms are absent or consist of low-grade fever, headache, and malaise; fever, malaise, and a generalized vesicular rash develop and last 4 to 7 days.
- Adolescents, adults, and immunocompromised persons have more severe disease.
- Moderate to intense pruritus is present during the vesicular stage.
- The patient's temperature varies from 101° to 105° F but returns to normal when the vesicles disappear.

SKIN FINDINGS

- There is a simultaneous presence of lesions (i.e., vesicles, pustules, crusts) in all stages.
- The rash begins on the trunk and spreads to the face and extremities. The extent of involvement varies considerably.
- A lesion starts as a 2- to 4-mm, red papule, and then a thin-walled, clear vesicle appears on the surface. The vesicle becomes umbilicated and cloudy and breaks in 8 to 12 hours to form a crust as the red base disappears. The formation of new lesions ceases by the fourth day.
- Crusts fall off in about 7 days and heal without scarring.
- Secondary infection or excoriation extends the process into the dermis.
- Vesicles often form in the oral cavity and vagina and rupture quickly to form multiple, aphthae-like ulcers.

NONSKIN FINDINGS

- Pneumonia is the most common serious complication in normal adults.
- Hepatitis is the most common complication in immunosuppressed patients.

LABORATORY

- Culture and a Tzanck smear are performed for questionable cases.

COMPLICATIONS

- Bacterial skin infections, pneumonia, dehydration, encephalitis, and hepatitis are complications.
- Since the association between Reye syndrome and aspirin use was identified, the incidence of Reye syndrome is now rare.

DIFFERENTIAL DIAGNOSIS

- Disseminated zoster
- Disseminated herpes simplex
- Eczema herpeticum
- Folliculitis
- Impetigo

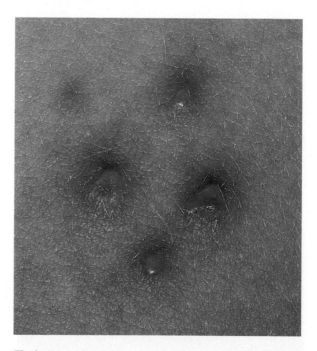

The lesion starts as a 2- to 4-mm red papule, which develops an irregular outline (rose petal) as a thin-walled clear vesicle appears on the surface (dew drop).

TREATMENT

- Symptomatic treatment consists of bland antipruritic lotions (e.g., Sarna). Antihistamines (hydroxyzine) may help control excoriation.

AMERICAN ACADEMY OF PEDIATRICS RECOMMENDATIONS FOR ACYCLOVIR THERAPY OF VARICELLA-ZOSTER INFECTIONS

Indications	Recommended therapy
• Nonpregnant, healthy adolescents ≥13 year of age who have varicella	Consider acyclovir: should be initiated within 24 hours of onset of rash
• Children >12 months of age who have chronic cutaneous or pulmonary disorder or are on long-term salicylate therapy	Dosage: 20 mg/kg (800 mg maximum) orally four times a day for 5 days
• Children receiving short, intermittent, or aerosolized courses of corticosteroids	
• Children infected from household contact	
• Healthy children and adults with complications of varicella	Intravenous acyclovir
• Immunocompromised children (including secondary to high-dose corticosteroids) with primary varicella	Dosage: 10 mg/kg intravenously every 8 hours for 7 days
• Immunocompromised children with recurrent zoster	
• Pregnant patients with complications of varicella	
• Healthy children with varicella	Routinely, no therapy
• Pregnant patients with uncomplicated varicella	
• Healthy children exposed to varicella	

Treatment of Adolescents and Adults

- Early therapy with oral acyclovir decreases the time to cutaneous healing of adult varicella, decreases the duration of fever, and reduces the severity symptoms but does not alter viral shedding. The initiation of therapy after the first day of illness is of no value in uncomplicated cases of adult varicella.
- There is a high morbidity rate even in normal patients with clinically evident varicella pneumonia; intravenous acyclovir (10 mg/kg intravenously every 8 hours for 7 days) may help.

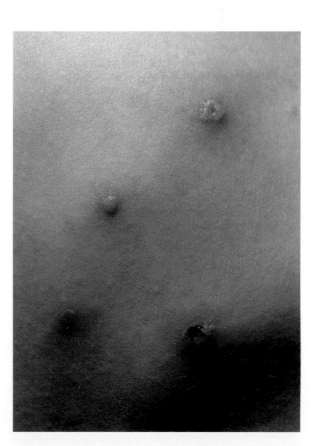

Vesicles become umbilicated and cloudy and break in 8 to 12 hours to form a crust as the red base disappears.

Immunocompromised Patients

- Immunosuppressed patients treated with acyclovir have decreased morbidity from visceral dissemination; there is a modest effect on cutaneous disease. The recommended schedule is acyclovir, 10 mg/kg intravenously every 8 hours for 7 to 10 days.
- The use of varicella zoster immune globulin (VZIG) is recommended for postexposure prophylaxis. VZIG may be administered within 96 hours after exposure.

RECOMMENDATION FOR THE USE OF VZIG FOR POSTEXPOSURE PROPHYLAXIS

Persons <13 years of age	Persons >13 years of age
Used for passive immunization of susceptible, immunocompromised children after substantial exposure to varicella or herpes zoster, including: • Children with primary and acquired immunodeficiency disorders • Children with neoplastic diseases who are receiving immunosuppressive treatment • Neonates whose mothers have signs and symptoms of varicella within 5 days before and 2 days after delivery • Premature infants who have substantial postnatal exposure and who should be evaluated on an individual basis	• A healthy, unvaccinated adolescent or adult who has had substantial exposure and is determined as being susceptible • VZIG should be considered for susceptible pregnant women who have been exposed in order to prevent complications of varicella in the mother, rather than to protect the fetus. NOTE: If varicella is prevented through the use of VZIG, vaccination should be offered later.

IMMUNIZATION: VARICELLA VACCINE RECOMMENDATIONS (VARIVAX [MERCK & CO., INC. WHITEHOUSE STATION, NJ])

Persons <13 years of age	Persons >13 years of age
A single, 0.5-ml subcutaneous dose is recommended for all healthy children 1-12 years old with no history of varicella. • Children with a reliable history are considered immune. • Those with an uncertain history are immunized. • Serologic testing is not warranted because the vaccine is well tolerated in seropositive persons.	Two 0.5-ml doses of varicella vaccine given 4 to 8 weeks apart are recommended for healthy adolescents and adults with no history of the disease. • Those with a reliable history of previous infection are considered immune. • Those who do not have such histories are considered susceptible and can be tested to determine immune status or can be vaccinated without testing.

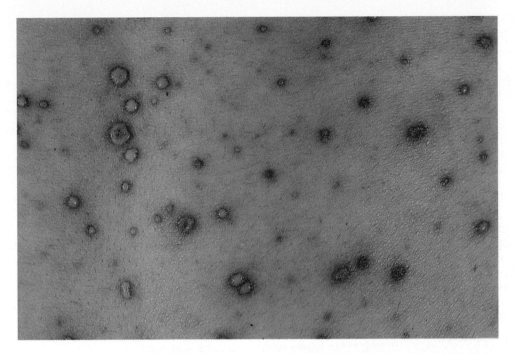

Lesions of different stages are present at the same time in any given body area.

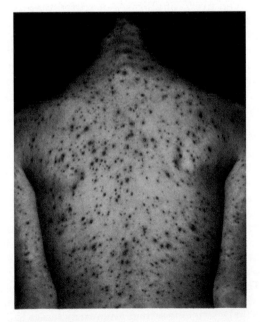

Numerous lesions on the trunk (centripetal distribution).

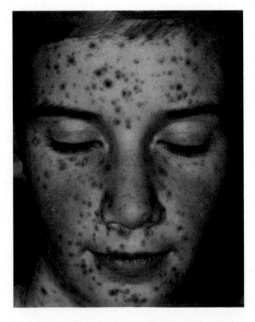

Lesions present in all stages of development.

■ HERPES ZOSTER (SHINGLES)

DESCRIPTION

- Herpes zoster is a cutaneous viral infection generally involving the skin of a single dermatome.
- Zoster results from the reactivation of varicella virus that entered the cutaneous nerves during an earlier episode of chicken pox.
- This condition occurs during the lifetime of 10% to 20% of all persons.
- People of all ages are afflicted; the incidence increases with age.
- Patients with zoster are not more likely to have an underlying malignancy.
- Zoster may be the earliest clinical sign of the development of the acquired immunodeficiency syndrome in high-risk individuals.
- Age, immunosuppressive drugs, lymphoma, fatigue, emotional upsets, and radiation therapy have been implicated in reactivating the virus.
- The elderly are at greater risk for developing segmental pain, which can continue for months after the skin lesions have healed.
- Patients with Hodgkin's disease are uniquely susceptible to herpes zoster.

HISTORY

- Preeruptive tenderness or hyperesthesia throughout the dermatome is a useful predictive sign.
- Preeruptive pain, itching, or burning, generally localized to the dermatome, may precede the eruption by 4 to 5 days.
- The pain may simulate pleurisy, myocardial infarction, abdominal disease, or migraine headache and may present a difficult diagnostic problem until the characteristic eruption provides the answer.
- The constitutional symptoms of fever, headache, and malaise may precede the eruption by several days. Regional lymphadenopathy may be present.
- An attack of herpes zoster does not confer lasting immunity, and it is not abnormal to have two or three episodes in a lifetime.

SKIN FINDINGS

- Although generally limited to the skin of a single dermatome, the eruption may involve one or two adjacent dermatomes.
- Occasionally, a few vesicles appear across the midline.

- Approximately 50% of patients with uncomplicated zoster have a viremia, with the appearance of 20 to 30 vesicles scattered over the skin surface outside the affected dermatome.
- The thoracic region is affected in two thirds of cases.
- The eruption begins with red, swollen plaques of various sizes and spreads to involve part or all of a dermatome.
- The vesicles arise in clusters from the erythematous base and become cloudy with purulent fluid by the third or fourth day.
- The vesicles vary in size, in contrast to the cluster of uniformly sized vesicles noted in herpes simplex.
- Vesicles either umbilicate or rupture before forming crusts, which fall off in 2 to 3 weeks.
- Elderly or debilitated patients may have a prolonged and difficult course. For them, the eruption is typically more extensive and inflammatory, occasionally resulting in hemorrhagic blisters, skin necrosis, secondary bacterial infection, or extensive scarring.

Ophthalmic Zoster

- Involvement of any branch of the ophthalmic nerve is called *herpes zoster ophthalmicus*. It is involved in 7% of all cases of zoster, with 20% to 72% of patients developing ocular complications.
- With ophthalmic zoster, the rash extends from eye level to the vertex of the skull but does not cross the midline.
- Vesicles on the side or tip of the nose (Hutchinson's sign) are associated with the most serious ocular complications.

Postherpetic Neuralgia

- Pain is the major cause of morbidity in zoster.
- The incidence and duration of pain increase with age.
- Pain can persist in a dermatome for months or years after lesions have disappeared.
- The pain is often severe, intractable, and exhausting. The patient protects areas of hyperesthesia to avoid the slightest pressure, which activates another wave of pain.
- The majority of patients under 30 years of age experience no pain. By age 40, the risk of prolonged pain lasting longer than 1 month increases to 33%. By age 70, the risk increases to 74%.

- The degree of pain is related neither to the extent of involvement nor to the number of vesicles or degree of inflammation or fibrosis in peripheral nerves.

LABORATORY

- Culture is specific, but the virus is labile and not easily isolated.
- Complement fixation tests can be used for retrospective diagnosis.
- Direct immunofluorescence of cellular material from skin lesions can be performed.
- In a Tzanck smear, the base of a vesicle is scraped with a cotton swab, and the material is smeared onto a glass slide. It is submitted to the laboratory or stained directly to see multinucleated giant cells.

TREATMENT
Suppression of Inflammation, Pain, and Infection

- Topical therapy is tried. Cool tap water can be used in a wet compress. The compresses, applied for 20 minutes several times a day, macerate the vesicles, remove serum and crust, and discourage bacterial growth.
- With oral steroids, there is a decrease of acute pain and a quicker rash resolution but no effect on postherpetic neuralgia. There is no difference in pain at 6 months when acyclovir and prednisone are used together compared with acyclovir alone or prednisone alone. There are no significant differences between steroid-treated and non–steroid-treated patients in the time to a first or a complete cessation of pain. The incidence of adverse effects is higher in patients treated with corticosteroids.
- Sympathetic blocks (stellate ganglion or epidural) with bupivacaine 0.25% may terminate the pain of acute herpes zoster and prevent or relieve postherpetic neuralgia.

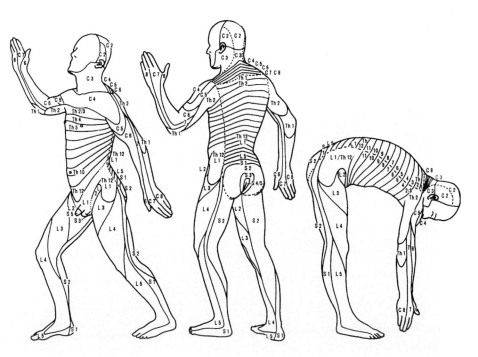

Dermatome areas.

Attenuation of the Acute Phase

- Oral antiviral drugs decrease acute pain, inflammation, vesicle formation, and viral shedding.
- The duration and severity of postherpetic neuralgia may be reduced by treating acute herpes zoster with valacyclovir or famciclovir.
- Treatment is most effective when started within the first 48 hours of infection.
- It is reasonable to use antiviral therapy in the patient seeking medical treatment more than 48 hours after the vesicles appear if the lesions are not completely crusted.
- The recommended oral dosage for adults is a 7- to 10-day course of acyclovir (Zovirax), 800 mg five times a day; valacyclovir (Valtrex), 1000 mg three time a day; or famciclovir (Famvir), 500 mg three times a day.
- The drugs are given empirically to patients who are older than 50 years of age, are immunocompromised, or have trigeminal zoster.

Prevention of Postherpetic Neuralgia

- Famciclovir and valacyclovir may decrease the duration of postherpetic neuralgia.
- Oral steroids used to prevent postherpetic neuralgia have not proved effective.
- Some authors recommend starting amitriptyline at low doses (10 to 25 mg) and gradually increasing this to doses of 50 to 75 mg over 2 to 3 weeks in all patients older than 60 years of age as soon as shingles is diagnosed. A 50% decrease in the incidence of postherpetic neuralgia has been reported.

Treatment of Postherpetic Neuralgia

- There is no reliable treatment for postherpetic neuralgia.
- Tricyclic antidepressants, such as amitriptyline (75 mg/day), nortriptyline (25 to 75 mg/day), and desipramine, and the anticonvulsants carbamazepine (400 to 1200 mg/day) and phenytoin (300 to 400 mg/day) relieve pain in some patients.
- Some clinicians advocate a short course of steroids (e.g., prednisone, 40 to 60 mg/day for 3 to 5 days or longer).
- Narcotics and analgesics are effective in many patients.
- Topical capsaicin cream (Zostrix, Zostrix HP) acts by enhancing the release or inhibiting the reaccumulation of substance P from cell bodies and nerve terminals. Patients experience some pain relief but may not be able to tolerate the burning. Applying EMLA or topical lidocaine (Lignocaine) before capsaicin use may make the treatment more tolerable. Capsaicin should not be applied to unhealed skin lesions.

EVOLUTION OF LESIONS

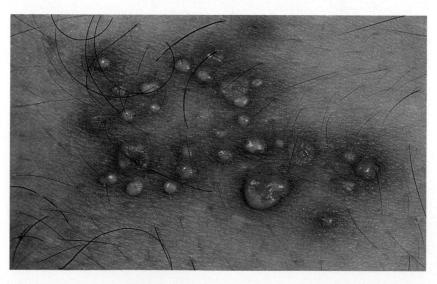

The vesicles vary in size, in contrast to the cluster of uniformly sized vesicles noted in herpes simplex.

HERPES ZOSTER EVOLUTION OF LESIONS—CONT'D

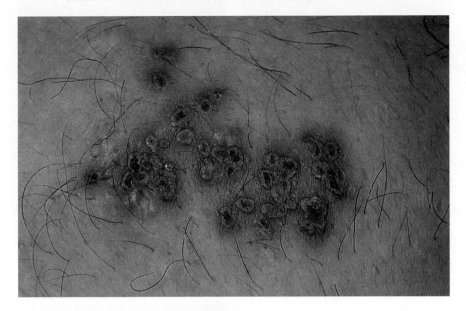

Vesicles either umbilicate or rupture.

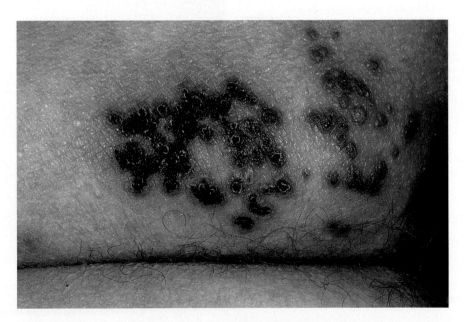

A crust forms; it falls off in 2 to 3 weeks.

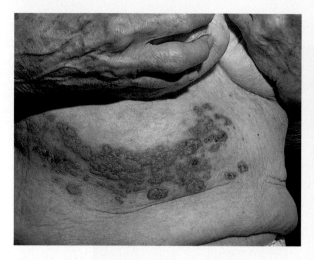

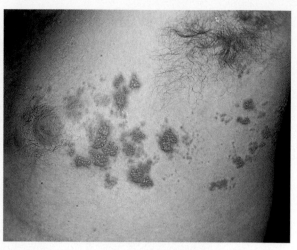

The eruption begins with red, swollen plaques of various sizes and spreads to involve part or all of a dermatome. Elderly or debilitated patients may have a prolonged and difficult course. For them, the eruption is typically more extensive and inflammatory.

Vesicles arise in clusters from the red base. Lesions often involve more than one dermatome.

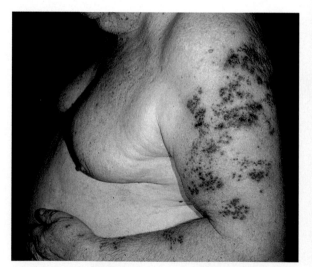

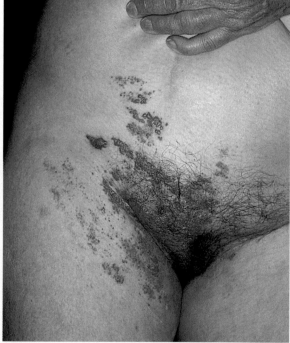

Herpes zoster may involve any dermatome. Many patients think that "shingles" involves only the trunk.

Sacral zoster. A neurogenic bladder with urinary hesitancy or urinary retention can be associated with zoster of the sacral dermatome S2, S3, or S4. Migration of virus to the adjacent autonomic nerves is responsible for these symptoms.

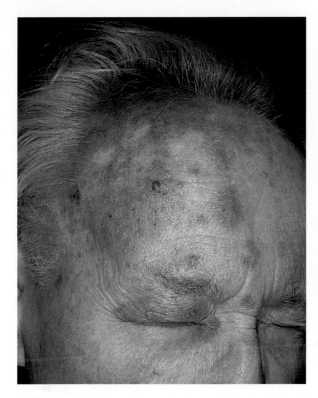

Ophthalmic zoster. Involvement of any branch of the ophthalmic nerve is called *herpes zoster ophthalmicus*. The rash extends from eye level to the vertex of the skull but does not cross the midline. This is the initial vesicular stage.

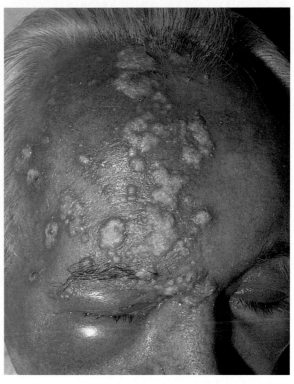

Ophthalmic zoster. Vesicles on the side or tip of the nose (Hutchinson's sign) that occur during an episode of zoster are associated with the most serious ocular complications, including conjunctival, corneal, scleral, and other ocular diseases, although this is not invariable.

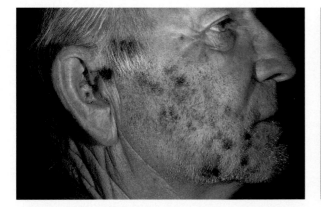

Varicella zoster of the geniculate ganglion is called *Ramsay Hunt syndrome*. There is involvement of the sensory and motor portions of the seventh cranial nerve. There may be unilateral loss of taste on the anterior two thirds of the tongue and vesicles on the tympanic membrane, external auditory meatus, concha, and pinna.

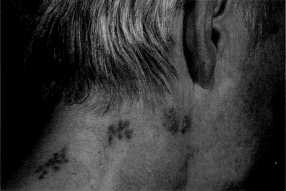

A classic presentation of grouped vesicles and crusts involving a cervical dermatome.

■ HAND, FOOT, AND MOUTH DISEASE

DESCRIPTION

- Hand, foot, and mouth disease is a highly contagious virus infection that causes aphthae-like oral erosions and a vesicular eruption on the hands and feet.
- It is caused by the coxsackie A16 virus, but A5, A10 and other enteroviruses have been implicated.

HISTORY

- The incubation period is 4 to 6 days.
- Hand, foot, and mouth disease usually presents with acute stomatitis and a mild fever.
- There may be mild symptoms of sore throat and malaise or abdominal pain for 1 or 2 days.
- Some 20% of patients develop submandibular lymphadenopathy, cervical lymphadenopathy, or both conditions.
- Epidemics usually occur in the summer and autumn but may appear at any time.
- Children younger than 5 years of age are most commonly affected, but the rate of infection among close household contacts is high.

SKIN FINDINGS

- The number of aphthae-like erosions (3 to 6 mm) varies from a few to 10 or more. They are irregularly distributed anywhere in the oral cavity. They are more painful in younger children. Each erosion lasts 3 to 5 days.
- Cutaneous lesions occur in two thirds of patients and appear less than 24 hours after the oral lesions. They begin as 3- to 7-mm, red macules that rapidly become pale, white, oval vesicles with red areolae. The vesicles have a unique rhomboidal shape of "square blisters." There may be a few inconspicuous lesions, or there may be dozens. The vesicles occur on the palms, soles, dorsal aspects of the fingers and toes, and occasionally on the face, buttocks, and legs. They heal in approximately 7 days, usually without crusting or scarring.

COURSE

- Hand, foot, and mouth disease is usually mild and self-limited. It resolves without treatment in about 10 days.
- Oral ulcerations are painful in infants and interfere with feeding.

LABORATORY

- The diagnosis is usually made clinically.
- Laboratory studies are usually unnecessary.
- Virus can be cultured from the vesicles, throat, and stool.
- Convalescent sera show elevated titers of specific complement-fixing viral antibodies.
- Both varicella and herpes have multinucleated, giant cells in smears taken from the moist skin exposed when a vesicle is removed (Tzanck smear). Giant cells are not present in the lesions of hand, foot, and mouth disease.

Differential Diagnosis

- Herpangina, in which lesions are limited to the posterior oral cavity, tonsils, and soft palate and the disease is associated with a higher temperature
- Aphthous stomatitis, in which patients are afebrile and tend to have recurrences (Herpetic gingivostomatitis is the most common cause of stomatitis in children younger than 5 years of age. Gingival involvement is severe and associated with lymphadenopathy and a high fever. The oral erosions of hand, foot, and mouth disease are usually small and uniform.)

TREATMENT

- Children may be isolated during the most contagious period, usually for 3 to 7 days. Some may be carriers up to 3 months after the infection. Symptomatic relief is important in infants to prevent dehydration. Fever and pain are controlled with acetaminophen. Cool fluids are best tolerated; acidic foods are avoided.
- Acyclovir suspension, 200 to 300 mg five times a day for 5 days, was reported to provide rapid relief of signs and symptoms in children age 9 months to 5 years.

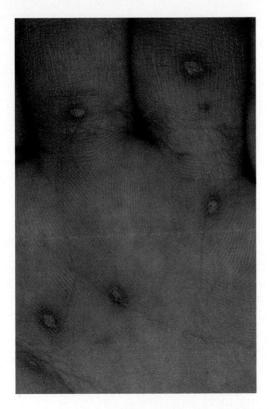

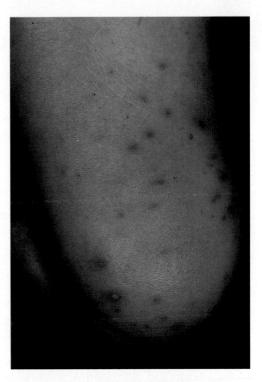

Cloudy vesicles with red halos are highly characteristic of this disease.

Cloudy vesicles with red halos in hand, foot, and mouth disease.

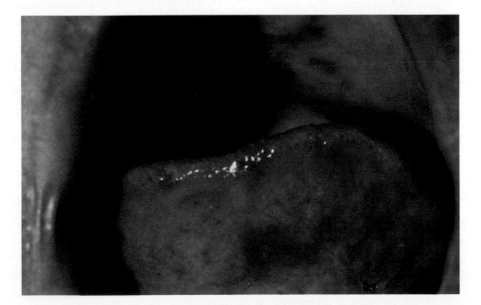

Pale, white oval vesicles with red areolae in hand, foot, and mouth disease.

9 Fungal Infections

■ CANDIDIASIS

DESCRIPTION

- *Candida albicans* and a few other *Candida* species are capable of producing skin and mucous membrane infections.
- The organism lives with the normal flora of the mouth, vaginal tract, and gut, and it reproduces through the budding of oval yeast forms.
- Pregnancy, oral contraception, antibiotic therapy, diabetes, skin maceration, topical steroid therapy, certain endocrinopathies, and factors related to the depression of cell-mediated immunity may allow the yeast to become pathogenic and produce budding spores and elongated cells (pseudohyphae) or true hyphae with septate walls.

CLINICAL PRESENTATION

- The yeast infects only the outer layers of the epithelium of the mucous membrane and skin (stratum corneum).
- The primary lesion is a pustule, the contents of which dissect horizontally under the stratum corneum and peel it away. This process results in a red, denuded, glistening surface with a long, cigarette paper–like, scaling, advancing border.
- Yeast grows best in a warm, moist environment; therefore infection is usually confined to the mucous membranes and intertriginous areas.
- The advancing infected border usually stops when it reaches dry skin.

LABORATORY

- The pseudohyphae and hyphae are indistinguishable from dermatophytes in potassium hydroxide preparations (see p. 199).
- Culture must be interpreted carefully because the yeast is part of the normal flora in many areas.

■ CANDIDAL BALANITIS

DESCRIPTION

- Yeast invades the superficial epidermis, producing pustules and exudate.
- The uncircumcised penis provides a warm, moist environment ideally suited for yeast infection, but the circumcised male patient is also at risk.
- Diabetics are at greater risk.

HISTORY

- In men infection can occur after intercourse with an infected woman but may occur and persist without sexual exposure.
- Tenderness, pain, edema, and swelling from intense inflammation may prevent retraction of the foreskin.
- Candidal balanitis is persistent and recurrent if not treated.

SKIN FINDINGS

- Red, pinpoint papules and pustules become umbilicated.
- Pustules rupture under the foreskin and leave 1- to 2-mm, white, doughnut-shaped, possibly confluent rings.
- Erosions, ulceration, and fissures may follow.

LABORATORY

- In potassium hydroxide examination, the exudate is gently sampled with a cotton swab. Pseudohyphae and spores are often numerous.
- Samples from the pustules and exudate are taken with cotton swabs. Yeast survives in the commonly available transportable bacterial culture tube kits. Bacterial superinfection may be identified by culture.

DIFFERENTIAL DIAGNOSIS

- Molluscum contagiosum, which forms umbilicated papules
- Genital warts
- Psoriasis
- Eczema
- Umbilicated pustules, which occur with herpes simplex and acute candidal infection. (These pustules may be clinically indistinguishable.)

TREATMENT

Topical Therapy

- The eruption responds quickly with the application of miconazole, clotrimazole, ketoconazole, or econazole (Spectazole), twice a day for 10 days.
- Relief is almost immediate, but treatment should be continued for 10 days.
- Preparations containing topical steroids (betamethasone 0.5% and clotrimazole 1% [Lotrisone]) give temporary relief by suppressing inflammation, but the eruption rebounds and worsens, sometimes even before the cortisone cream is discontinued.

Systemic Therapy

- Resistant cases may respond to itraconazole (Sporanox), 200 mg/day for 3 to 7 days, or fluconazole, 150 mg/day for 1 to 3 days.

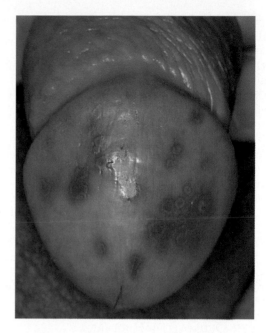

Candida balanitis. Tender, pinpoint, red papules and pustules appear on the glans and shaft of the penis.

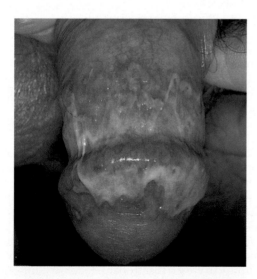

White exudate similar to that seen in candidal vaginal infections may be present. The infection may occur and persist without sexual exposure.

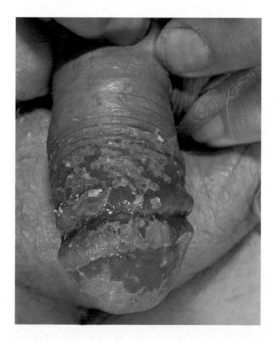

The uncircumcised penis provides the warm, moist environment ideally suited for yeast infection. Here, the inflammation is intense, causing superficial erosions.

■ CANDIDIASIS (DIAPER DERMATITIS)

DESCRIPTION

- There are several causes of inflammation in the diaper area.
- Diaper candidiasis is an acute candidal infection of the superficial layers of the skin.

HISTORY

- An artificial intertriginous area is created under a wet diaper, predisposing the area to infection and inflammation.
- Diaper dermatitis is often treated with steroid or steroid-combination creams that contain antibiotics. Although these creams (e.g., betamethasone 0.5% and clotrimazole 1% [Lotrisone]) may contain the antifungal agent, clotrimazole, its concentration may not be sufficient to control the yeast infection. The cortisone component may alter the clinical presentation and prolong the disease.

DIAPER DERMATITIS PATTERNS

Contact irritant diaper dermatitis
- This is the most common diaper dermatitis.
- It is most prominent on the convex skin surfaces (hill areas) that are in contact with the diaper.
- Rash is usually absent in the skin creases.
- Erosions occur if the rash persists.

Candidiasis
- The 1- to 2- mm pustules erode and form collarette scales.
- Satellite pustules occur outside the plaque area.
- Eruption may occur as a superinfection secondary to seborrheic dermatitis, atopic dermatitis, or psoriasis.
- A nodular, granulomatous form of candidiasis occurs in the diaper area, appearing as dull, red, irregularly shaped nodules, sometimes on a red base. This may represent an unusual reaction to *Candida* organisms or to a *Candida* infection modified by steroids.

Atopic dermatitis
- Erythema and scaling occur.
- Areas of lichenification (thickening) cause persistent scratching.
- This form is relatively uncommon.
- The diaper makes groin scratching difficult.

Psoriasiform napkin dermatitis
- Dull to bright red plaques appear.
- This form may be indistinguishable from seborrheic dermatitis.
- There may be no other signs of psoriasis.

Seborrheic dermatitis
- Erythema and macerated scaling are present in the creases and relatively absent on the convex surfaces.
- This form is associated with seborrheic dermatitis on the scalp and face.
- This is an uncommon eruption.

LABORATORY

- In a potassium hydroxide examination, the pustules or advancing border is sampled with a cotton swab, and the material is applied to a slide. Pseudohyphae and spores are often numerous.
- The pustules or moist areas of the plaque are sampled with a cotton swab. Yeast survive in the commonly available transportable bacterial culture tube kits. Bacterial superinfection may be identified by culture.

DIFFERENTIAL DIAGNOSIS

- Streptococcal anal cellulitis
- Staphylococcal impetigo

TREATMENT

- Minimizing wetness is most important. Diapers should be changed frequently or left off for short periods.
- Barrier ointments such as petrolatum or zinc oxide are useful for prophylaxis.
- Overzealous cleaning with irritating baby wipes should be avoided.
- Initially, hydrocortisone cream 1% is applied twice a day until the inflammation is controlled.
- Betamethasone 0.5% and clotrimazole 1% (Lotrisone) is avoided in the diaper area because the steroid component is too potent.
- Candidal infection is treated with miconazole, clotrimazole, ketoconazole, or econazole (Spectazole) applied twice a week for 1 or 2 weeks. It is applied about 2 hours after the hydrocortisone.
- Localized bacterial infection can be treated with mupirocin cream (Bactroban). Extensive infection requires systemic therapy.

- Pampers Rash Guard diapers (Procter & Gamble) may be recommended. These diapers reduce the severity and frequency of diaper rash by delivering petrolatum to the diaper area. Stripes of petrolatum transferred to the baby's skin provide a moisture barrier, and breathable fabric between the stripes absorbs the moisture.

CAVEAT

- Psoriasis should be considered when diaper dermatitis fails to respond to antifungal topical medication.

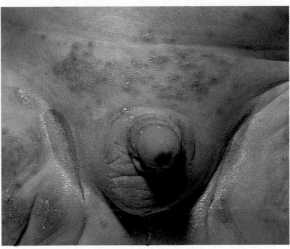

Diaper dermatitis is often treated with steroid combination creams. The cortisone component may alter the clinical presentation and prolong the disease.

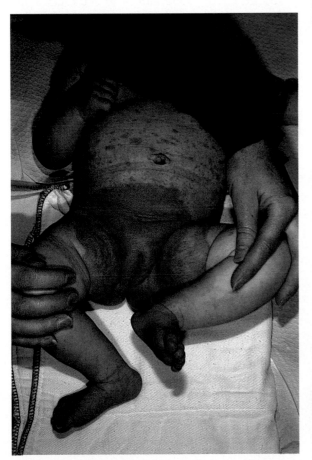

Intense erythema occurring under the entire diaper area. Disease may progress to this extent if topical steroids are the only treatment. Psoriasis would be the differential diagnosis for this patient.

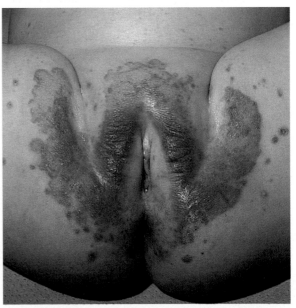

An artificial intertriginous area is created under a wet diaper, predisposing the area to a yeast infection with the characteristic red base and satellite pustules.

CANDIDIASIS OF LARGE SKINFOLDS (CANDIDAL INTERTRIGO)

DESCRIPTION

- Yeasts thrive in intertriginous areas where skin touches skin.
- Large skinfolds retain heat and moisture, providing the environment suited for yeast infection.

HISTORY

- Predisposed individuals include older women with pendulous breasts and obese men and women with overhanging abdominal folds; other common areas of involvement include the groin, rectal area, and axillae.
- Predisposing factors include hot, humid weather; tight or abrasive underclothing; poor hygiene; and inflammatory diseases occurring in the skinfolds, such as psoriasis. The use of topical steroids make a yeast infection more likely.

SKIN FINDINGS

- Pustules form but become macerated under apposing skin surfaces and develop into red papules with fringes of moist scaling at the border. Intact pustules may be found outside the opposing skin surfaces.
- Red, moist, glistening plaques extend to or just beyond the limits of the opposing skinfolds. The advancing border is long, is sharply defined, and has an ocean wave-shaped fringe of macerated scale.
- There is a tendency for painful fissuring in the skin creases.

LABORATORY

- In potassium hydroxide examination, the pustules or advancing border is sampled with a cotton swab, or material is gently collected with a #15 surgical blade. Pseudohyphae and spores are often numerous.
- A cotton swab is used to obtain a culture specimen from the pustules or moist areas of the plaque. Yeast survive in the commonly available transportable bacterial culture tube kits. Bacterial superinfection may be identified by culture.

COURSE AND PROGNOSIS

- Candidal intertrigo may persist or may recur after treatment.

DIFFERENTIAL DIAGNOSIS

- Psoriasis
- Seborrheic dermatitis
- Intertrigo
- Erythrasma
- Eczema
- Bacterial folliculitis

TREATMENT

- A compress with cool water or Burow's solution is applied for 20 to 30 minutes several times a day to promote dryness. The application of compresses should be continued until the skin remains dry.
- An antifungal cream (miconazole, clotrimazole, ketoconazole, or econazole [Spectazole] is applied in a thin layer twice a day until the rash clears.
- An absorbent powder, not necessarily medicated, such as Zeasorb, may be applied after the inflammation is gone. The powder absorbs a small amount of moisture and acts as a dry lubricant, allowing skin surfaces to slide freely and thus preventing moisture accumulation in a potentially stagnant area.

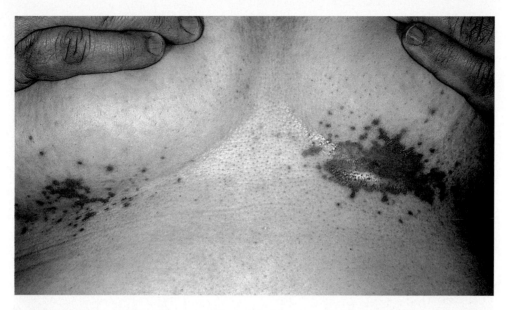

Skinfolds contain heat and moisture, providing an environment suited for yeast infection. Hot, humid weather; tight or abrasive underclothing; poor hygiene; and inflammatory diseases occurring in the skinfolds, such as psoriasis, make a yeast infection more likely.

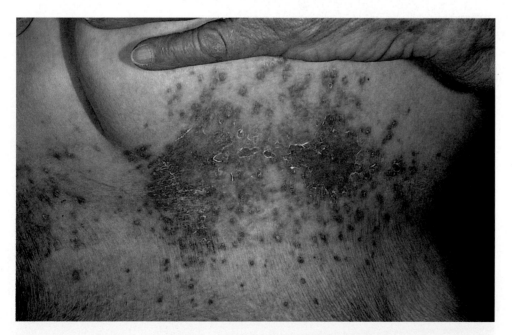

Pustules form but become macerated under apposing skin surfaces and develop into red papules with a fringe of moist scale at the border. Intact pustules may be found outside the apposing skin surfaces.

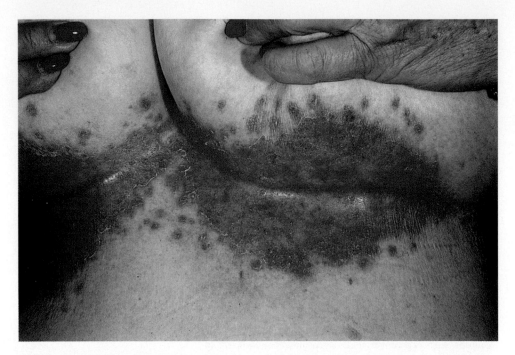

Red, moist, glistening plaques extend to or just beyond the limits of the apposing skinfolds. Pinpoint pustules appear outside the advancing border. There is a tendency for painful fissuring in the skin creases.

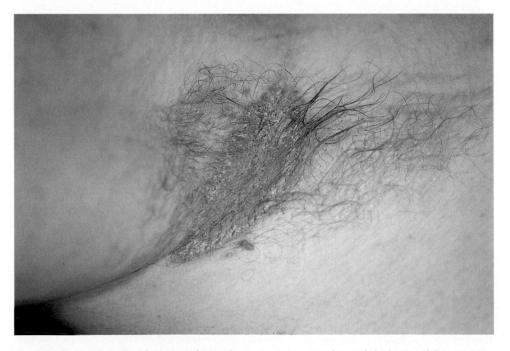

Candidiasis. A red, moist, glistening plaque that extends to or just beyond the limits of the apposing skinfolds.

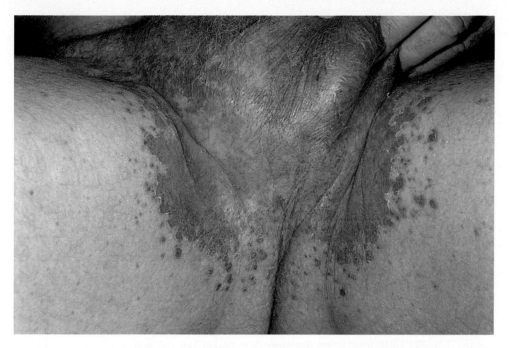

Candidiasis. A fringe of moist scale is present at the border. A red, moist, glistening plaque extends to the limits of the opposing thigh and scrotum. Compare this to tinea of the groin (see p. 205).

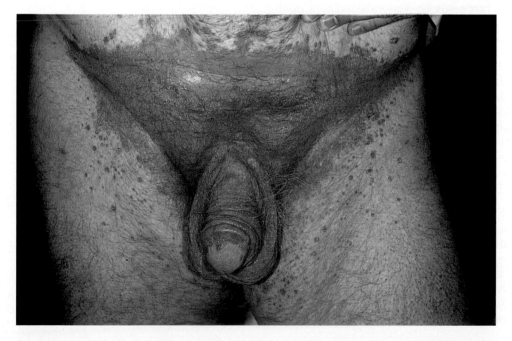

Candidiasis. Papules and pustules are found outside the opposing skin surfaces. A red plaque extends to the border of all apposing skinfolds.

■ TINEA VERSICOLOR

DESCRIPTION

- Tinea versicolor (TV) is a common infection caused by the lipophilic yeast *Pityrosporum orbiculare*. The organism is part of the normal skin flora.
- TV may be contagious. Individuals with oily skin may be more susceptible.
- Excess heat and humidity predispose to infection.

HISTORY

- TV is more common during the years of higher sebaceous activity (i.e., adolescence, young adulthood).
- It is very common especially in tropical and semitropical regions.
- It varies in activity for years and diminishes or disappears with advancing age.
- It may itch, but TV is usually asymptomatic. Appearance is often the patient's major concern.

SKIN FINDINGS

- The common presentation involves multiple small, circular, white, scaling macules on the upper trunk.
- Powdery scaling that may not be obvious on inspection can easily be demonstrated by scraping lightly with a #15 surgical blade.
- Lesions are white in tanned skin and pink or brown in untanned skin, They are hyperpigmented in African-Americans.
- The color is uniform in each patient. Lesions may be inconspicuous in fair-complexioned individuals during the winter.
- The upper trunk is most commonly affected; TV may spread to the upper arms, neck, and abdomen. Involvement of the face, back of the hands, and legs is rare. Facial lesions (forehead) are more common in children.

NONSKIN FINDINGS

- Adrenalectomy, Cushing's disease, pregnancy, malnutrition, burns, corticosteroid therapy, immunosuppression, and oral contraceptives may lower the patient's resistance, allowing this normally nonpathogenic resident yeast to proliferate in the upper layers of the stratum corneum.

LABORATORY

- In potassium hydroxide examination, the scale is scraped with a #15 surgical blade onto a slide, a drop of 10% to 20% potassium hydroxide is added, and the sample is covered with a coverslip and gently heated.
- Examination at the microscope's 10× ocular power shows numerous hyphae that tend to break into short, rod-shaped fragments intermixed with round spores in grapelike clusters, giving the so-called spaghetti-and-meatballs pattern.
- Wood's light examination reveals an irregular, pale, yellow-to-white fluorescence that fades with improvement. Some lesions do not fluoresce. Vitiligo is white and does not scale.
- Culture is possible but is rarely necessary.

DIFFERENTIAL DIAGNOSIS

- Vitiligo
- Pityriasis alba
- Seborrheic dermatitis
- Secondary syphilis
- Pityriasis rosea
- Nummular eczema
- Guttate psoriasis

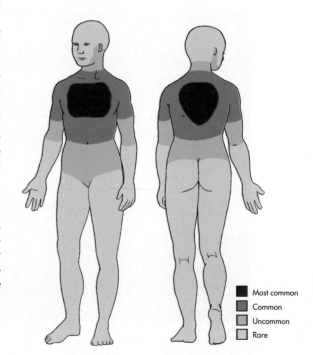

Most common
Common
Uncommon
Rare

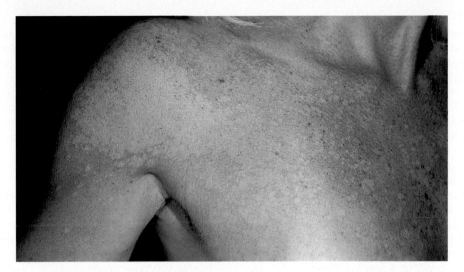

Tinea versicolor infections produce a spectrum of clinical presentations and colors.

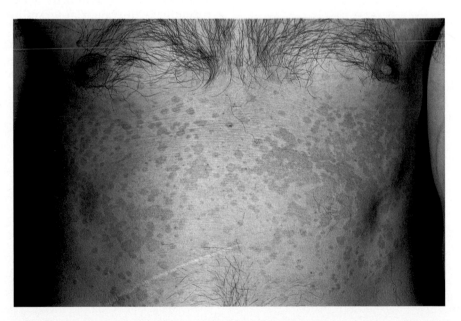

Lesions begin as multiple small, circular macules of various colors (white, pink, brown) that enlarge radially. The lesions may be inconspicuous in fair-complexioned individuals during the winter.

TREATMENT

- Topical treatment is indicated for limited disease.
- A variety of medicines eliminate the fungus, but relief is usually temporary, and recurrences are common (40% to 60%).
- Selenium sulfide lotion 2.5% is applied and washed off in 10 minutes; this regimen is repeated every day for 7 consecutive days. The suspension is applied to the entire skin surface from the lower posterior scalp area down to the thighs.
- Ketoconazole 2% shampoo is applied to dampened skin, lathered and left on for 5 minutes, and then it is rinsed. The clinical response rate is about 70 % when this medication is used as a single application or is used daily for 3 days.
- Miconazole, clotrimazole, econazole, or ketoconazole is applied to the entire affected area once or twice a day for 2 to 4 weeks. These creams are odorless and are not greasy, but they are expensive.
- Salicylic acid soap (from Stiefel Laboratories, Inc.) may be useful for preventing recurrences in patients who can tolerate the drying effect.
- Terbinafine spray (Lamisil) is also effective. It is available in both over-the-counter and prescription forms.

Oral Treatment

- Oral treatment is used in patients who have extensive disease, whose condition does not respond to topical treatment, or who have frequent recurrences. Cure rates may be greater than 90%.
- Itraconazole, 200 mg/day for 5 to 7 days, is administered. Food enhances absorption.
- Ketoconazole, 400 mg in a single dose or 200 mg a day for 5 to 10 days, can be prescribed. Efficacy can be enhanced by refraining from antacids and taking the drug at breakfast with fruit juice.
- Fluconazole, 150 mg (two capsules/wk for 4 weeks or two capsules as an initial dose to be repeated after 2 weeks), is given.
- Sweating may improve transfer of ketoconazole and fluconazole to the skin surface. The patient should not bathe for at least 12 hours after treatment. Refraining from bathing allows the medication to accumulate in the skin.

Response to Treatment

- Hypopigmented areas do not disappear immediately after treatment.
- Sunlight accelerates repigmentation.
- The inability to produce powdery scales by scraping with a #15 surgical blade indicates that the fungus has been eradicated.

General Measures

- Fungal elements may be retained in frequently worn garments that are in contact with the skin; discarding or boiling such clothing might decrease the chance of recurrence.
- Patients without obvious involvement who have a history of multiple recurrences might consider repeating a treatment program just before the summer to avoid uneven tanning.

CAVEAT

- The diagnosis of TV is often made in any patient with white spots on the trunk. A potassium hydroxide examination can quickly establish the correct diagnosis.

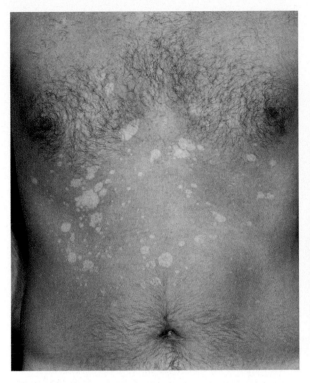

Classic presentation of tinea versicolor with white, oval or circular patches on tan skin.

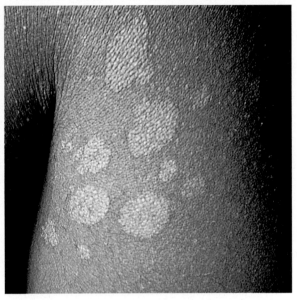

Lesions may be hyperpigmented or hypopigmented in African-Americans. The color is uniform in each individual. The lesions may be inconspicuous in fair-complexioned individuals during the winter.

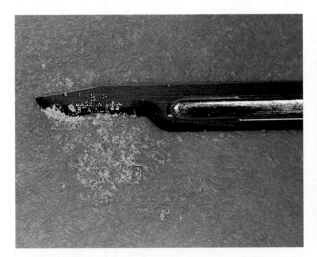

A powdery scale that may not be obvious on inspection can easily be demonstrated by scraping lightly with a #15 surgical blade.

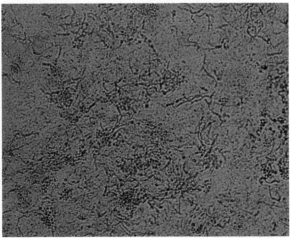

Tinea versicolor. A potassium hydroxide wet mount. A low-power view showing numerous, short, broad hyphae and clusters of budding cells, which have been described as having the appearance of "spaghetti and meatballs."

■ *PITYROSPORUM* FOLLICULITIS

DESCRIPTION

- *Pityrosporum* folliculitis is an infection of the hair follicle caused by the yeast *Pityrosporum orbiculare*, the same organism that causes tinea versicolor.
- A discrete, often itchy, papulopustular eruption, localized mainly to the upper portion of the trunk and shoulders, appears.

HISTORY

- *Pityrosporum* folliculitis occurs in young and middle-aged adults.
- The male/female ratio is 1:3.
- Follicular occlusion may be a primary event, with yeast overgrowth as a secondary occurrence.
- Diabetes mellitus and broad-spectrum antibiotics or corticosteroids are predisposing factors.

SKIN FINDINGS

- Asymptomatic or slightly itchy, dome-shaped follicular papules and pustules, 2 to 4 mm in diameter, appear.
- *Pityrosporum* folliculitis occurs on the upper back, chest, and upper arms.
- It is very common in the tropics, where it presents with follicular papules, pustules, nodules, and cysts. The face is often affected. Lesions are localized to the mandible, chin, and sides of the face.
- Steroid acne is a folliculitis that can result from treatment with systemic steroids. It presents with discrete follicular papules localized to the upper trunk or face. Over 85% of these patients have large numbers of *P. orbiculare* in the lesional follicle.

LABORATORY

- In potassium hydroxide examination, there are abundant round, budding yeast cells and sometimes hyphae.
- Biopsy reveals abundant round, budding yeast cells and occasionally hyphae in a dilated follicle. Methenamine silver is used to stain the hyphae.
- Cultures are usually necessary.

DIFFERENTIAL DIAGNOSIS

- Acne
- Bacterial folliculitis
- Scabies

DISCUSSION

- Patients may have associated tinea versicolor, seborrheic dermatitis, or acne. Their active sebaceous glands presumably provide the lipid-rich environment required by the yeast.
- Occlusion and greasy skin may be important predisposing factors.
- The lack of comedones differentiates *Pityrosporum* folliculitis from acne.

TREATMENT

- Selenium sulfide shampoo (Selsun) is applied for 30 minutes in the shower. This regimen is repeated for another 2 days and once each week for maintenance treatment.
- Topical antifungal agents (e.g., econazole cream [Spectazole]) are applied every night for 1 week, followed by application once a week for several weeks or months.
- Itraconazole (Sporanox), 200 mg for 5 days, is prescribed.
- Predisposed individuals should avoid the use of heavy emollients.
- The itch is relieved in the first week of treatment; the papules remain for up to 3 to 4 weeks.
- Recurrence is seen in most cases if topical treatment is not maintained intermittently.

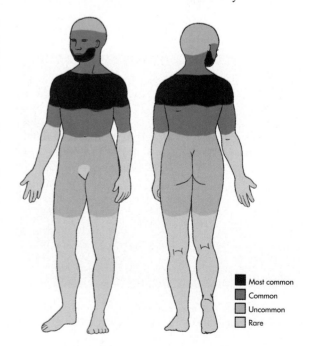

Most common
Common
Uncommon
Rare

CAVEAT

- Patients who appear to have acne may instead have *Pityrosporum* folliculitis.

- This condition should be considered in young and middle-aged adults with itching and follicular lesions on the trunk.

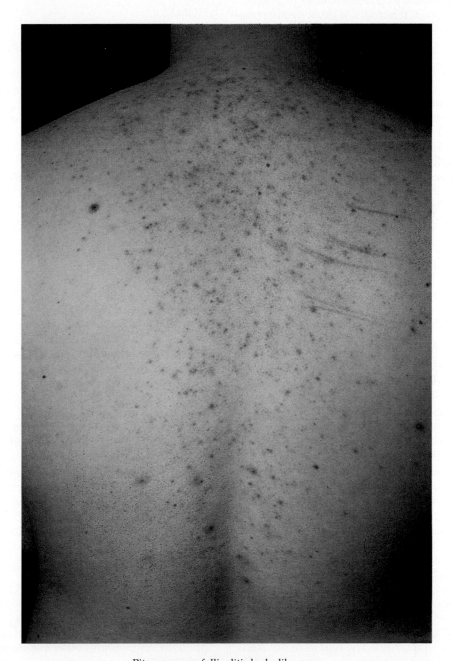

Pityrosporum folliculitis looks like acne.

■ FUNGAL NAIL INFECTIONS

DESCRIPTION

- Tinea of the nails is a fungal infection of the finger or toe nail plate.
- It is caused by many different species of fungus.
- Once established, it persists. It causes embarrassment and pain if the nail plate is distorted.

HISTORY

- The incidence of fungal nail infections increases with age.
- These infections occur in 15% to 20% of the population between 40 and 60 years of age.
- They are life long; there is no spontaneous remission.
- Trauma predisposes to infection.
- A large mass composed of a thick nail plate and underlying debris may cause discomfort with footwear.

SKIN FINDINGS

There are four distinct patterns of nail infection. Several patterns may occur simultaneously in the nail plate.

- Distal subungual onychomycosis is the most common pattern. Fungi invade the distal area of the nailbed. The distal plate turns yellow or white as an accumulation of hyperkeratotic debris causes the nail to rise and separate from the underlying bed.
- White superficial onychomycosis is caused by surface invasion of the nail plate, most often by *Trichophyton mentagrophytes.* The nail surface is soft, dry, and powdery and can easily be scraped away. The nail plate is not thickened and remains adherent to the nailbed.
- In proximal subungual onychomycosis, microorganisms enter the posterior nailfold-cuticle area and invade the nail plate from below. The surface remains intact. Hyperkeratotic debris causes the nail to separate. *Trichophyton rubrum* is the most common cause. This is the most common pattern seen in patients with infection of the human immunodeficiency virus.
- In candidal onychomycosis, nail-plate infection caused by *Candida albicans* is seen almost exclusively in chronic mucocutaneous candidiasis, a rare disease. It generally involves all of the fingernails. The nail plate thickens and turns yellow-brown.

- Nail infection may occur with hand or foot tinea or may occur as an isolated phenomenon.
- All nails and the skin are examined to rule out other diseases that mimic onychomycosis.

ETIOLOGY

- The dermatophytes *T. rubrum* and *T. mentagrophytes* are responsible for most fingernail and toenail infections.
- *Aspergillus, Cephalosporium, Fusarium,* and *Scopulariopsis* species, considered contaminants or nonpathogens, can also infect the nail plate.
- Multiple pathogens may be present in a single nail.

LABORATORY

- There is a tendency to label any process involving the nail plate as a fungal infection, but many other cutaneous diseases can change the structure of the nail. Some 50% of thick nails are not infected with fungus.
- In a potassium hydroxide wet mount, the subungual debris and nail plate are examined for hyphae.
- The species of fungus is identified before oral antifungal treatment is started. A culture is performed to establish the presence of dermatophytes (organisms susceptible to itraconazole [Sporanox], terbinafine [Lamisil], and fluconazole [Diflucan]).
- There are no clear guidelines for monitoring patients treated with terbinafine, itraconazole, or fluconazole. A prudent approach would be to order a complete blood count and liver function tests before and 6 weeks into treatment. Laboratory monitoring is not required in patients treated with itraconazole (Sporanox) pulse dosing.
- Histologic study of a nail clipping is performed if the results of the potassium hydroxide examination and culture are negative but clinical suspicion is high. The results of the histologic tests and periodic acid–Schiff staining are highly reliable for establishing the diagnosis.

DIFFERENTIAL DIAGNOSIS

- Psoriasis, which is most commonly confused with onychomycosis (The two diseases may coexist. Psoriatic nail disease may present as an isolated phenomenon without other cutaneous signs. The single distinguishing feature of psoriasis, pitting of the nail-plate surface, is not a feature of fungal infection [see p. 91].)

- Leukonychia, which is the occurrence of white spots or bands that appear proximally and proceed outward with the nail, probably caused by minor trauma
- Eczema or habitual picking of the proximal nail-fold, which causes the nail plate to be wavy and ridged
- Onycholysis, a very common finding in women with long fingernails (It is caused by separation of the nail plate from the nailbed. The yellow or opaque separated nail looks like tinea.)

TREATMENT

- Topical antifungal creams are of little value.
- Oral therapy has the highest success rate in fingernail and nail infections in young individuals.
- Prolonged use of a topical antifungal agent, after clinical response of onychomycosis to an oral agent, may prevent nail reinfection.
- Systemic therapy is 50% to over 80% effective. The relapse rate is approximately 15% to 20% in 1 year.
- Indications for treatment include pain with thick nails, functional limitations, secondary bacterial infection, and appearance.
- Terbinafine (Lamisil), 250 mg/day, is administered 6 weeks for infection of the fingernails and 12 weeks for infection of the toenails. Terbinafine may provide the highest cure rates and longest remission. It is not effective for some candidal species.
- Itraconazole (Sporanox), 200 mg/day, is prescribed 6 weeks for fingernail infection and 12 weeks for toenail infection. Pulse dosing, 200 mg twice a day, 1 week on and then 3 weeks off, is also an option. Fingernail infection requires two or three pulses; toenail infection requires three or four pulses.
- Fluconazole, 300 mg once a week for 6 to 9 months or until the nail is normal, is administered. This treatment has not been approved by the Food and Drug Administration.
- Griseofulvin may be effective at very high doses if used for many months but the other drugs are clearly superior.
- Patients are monitored at 6 weeks and at the end of oral therapy. The infected nail plate is débrided at each visit.

- In most cases, nails do not appear clear at 12 weeks. Patients are reassured that the drug remains in the nail plate for months and will continue to kill fungus.
- Ciclopirox topical solution 0.8% (Penlac Nail Lacquer) has been approved for topical treatment of nail infections. It is applied every day for 1 year.
- A nail clipper with pliers handles may be used to remove substantial amounts of hard, thick debris. The pointed tip of the instrument is inserted as far down as possible between the diseased nail and the nailbed.
- Removing the infected nail plate provides higher cure rates and longer remissions.

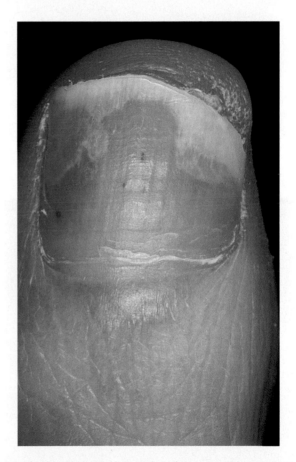

Distal subungual onychomycosis is the most common pattern of nail invasion. Fungi invade the distal area of the nailbed. The distal nail plate turns yellow or white as an accumulation of hyperkeratotic debris causes the nail to rise and separate from the underlying bed.

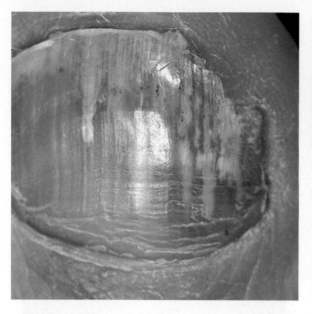

Distal subungual onychomycosis. Various patterns are produced as the fungi grow proximally. Yellow longitudinal channels are highly characteristic of tinea.

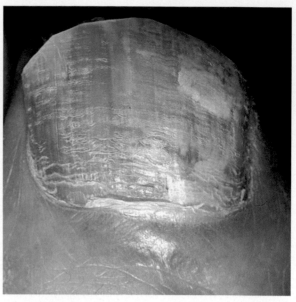

Distal subungual onychomycosis. Fungus has invaded the entire nail plate.

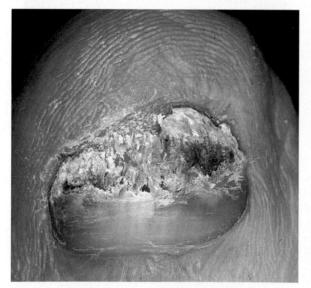

Distal subungual onychomycosis. Fungus grows in the substance of the plate, causing it to crumble and fragment.

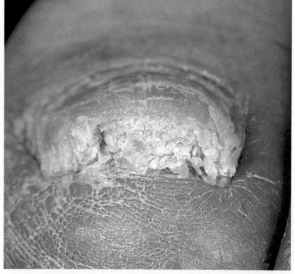

Distal subungual onychomycosis. A large mass composed of thick nail plate and underlying debris may cause discomfort with footwear.

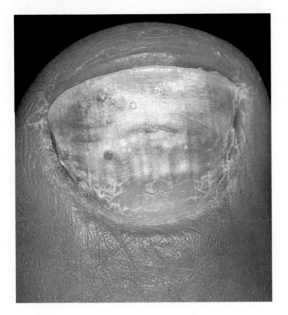

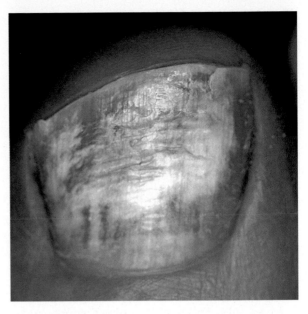

White superficial onychomycosis. The surface of the nail is soft, dry, and powdery and can easily be scraped away. The nail plate is not thickened and remains adherent to the nail bed.

White superficial onychomycosis. The nail-plate surface has been invaded and is crumbling away.

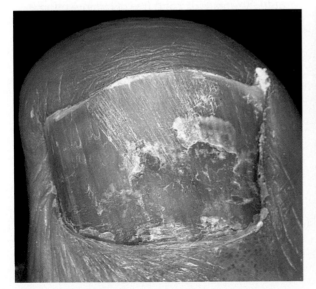

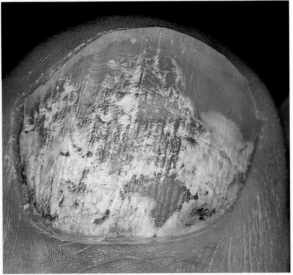

Proximal subungual onychomycosis. Microorganisms enter the posterior nailfold-cuticle area, migrate to the underlying matrix, and finally invade the nail plate from below.

Proximal subungual onychomycosis. Hyperkeratotic debris accumulates and causes the nail to separate.

■ ANGULAR CHEILITIS

DESCRIPTION

- Angular cheilitis is an inflammation at the angles of the mouth. Saliva macerates and irritates this small intertriginous area and may lead to fissuring, bacterial and yeast infections, and eczema.

HISTORY

- Angular cheilitis occurs more commonly in the elderly.
- It occurs frequently in patients treated with isotretinoin (Accutane).
- It may be long standing; recurrence is common.
- The patient experiences soreness, pain, and itching.

ETIOLOGY

- The presence of saliva at the angles of the mouth is the most important factor.
- Excess saliva occurs as a result of mouth-breathing secondary to nasal congestion, of malocclusion resulting from poorly fitting dentures, and of compulsive lip licking.
- Aggressive use of dental floss may cause mechanical trauma to mouth angles.
- In young patients, lip licking, biting the corners of the mouth, or thumb sucking causes perlèche. Continued irritation may lead to eczematous inflammation.
- In older patients, a moist, intertriginous space forms in skinfolds at the angles of the mouth as a result of advancing age, congenital excessive-angle skinfolds, sagging that occurs with weight loss, or abnormal vertical shortening of the lower third of the face from loss of teeth and resultant resorption of the alveolar bone.
- Also in older patients, capillary action draws fluid from the mouth into the fold, creating maceration, chapping, fissures, erythema, exudation, and secondary infection with candidal organisms, staphylococci, or both species.

SKIN FINDINGS

- In the primary lesion, papules and pustules surround a fissure.
- In secondary lesions, erythema, fissures, erosions, and ulceration occur with persistent inflammation.

LABORATORY

- Culture reveals mixed bacterial infection and yeast.

COURSE AND PROGNOSIS

- The inflammation starts as a sore fissure in the depth of the skinfold.
- Erythema, scales, and crust form at the sides of the fold.
- Patients lick and moisten the area in an attempt to prevent further cracking.
- This attempt at relief aggravates the problem and may lead to eczematous inflammation, staphylococcal infection, or hypertrophy of the skinfold.

TREATMENT

- Antifungal creams (e.g., clotrimazole, miconazole) are applied twice a day. Application is followed in a few hours by a group VI steroid cream or lotion with a nongreasy base (alclometasone 0.05% cream [Aclovate] or desonide 0.05% lotion [DesOwen]) until the area is dry and free of inflammation.
- Topical steroids are discontinued when inflammation has resolved. Thereafter, a thick, protective lip balm (e.g., ChapStick) or ointment (Aquaphor or Eucerin) is applied frequently.
- Secondary bacterial infection requires topical antibiotics (e.g., mupirocin [Bactroban]) or systemic antibiotics active against staphylococci.

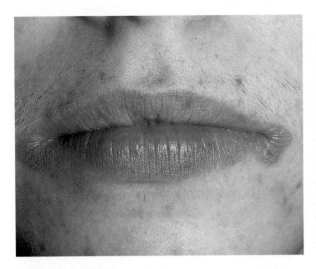

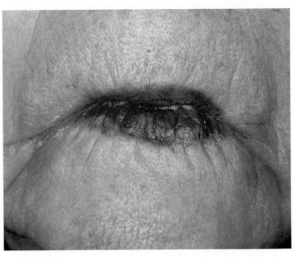

Patients lick and moisten the area in an attempt to prevent cracking. This only aggravates the problem and may lead to eczematous inflammation, staphylococcal infection, or hypertrophy of the skinfold.

Angular cheilitis or perlèche. A moist, intertriginous space forms in skinfolds at the angles of the mouth as a result of advancing age. Capillary action draws fluid from the mouth into the fold, creating maceration, chapping, fissures, and erythema.

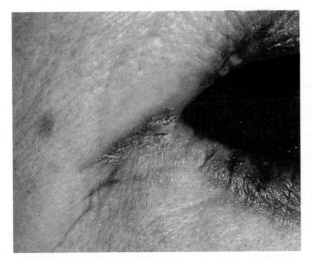

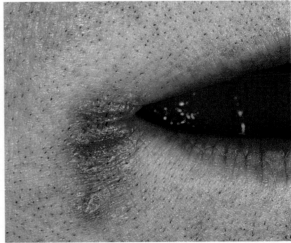

This elderly patient experiences recurrent inflammation from saliva flowing into the deep skinfold at the angle of the mouth.

Eczematous inflammation and a staphylococcal infection have developed in this chronically inflamed area.

■ CUTANEOUS FUNGAL INFECTIONS

Dermatophytes

- Dermatophytes can infect and survive only on dead keratin (the top layer of the skin [stratum corneum or keratin layer]), the hair, and the nails.
- They cannot survive in the mouth or vagina, where the keratin layer does not form.
- They are responsible for the majority of skin, nail, and hair fungal infections.
- Genetic susceptibility may predispose a patient to infection.
- *Tinea* is the clinical term for infection.

Biologic Classification

- There are three genera: *Microsporum, Trichophyton,* and *Epidermophyton.*
- There are several species of *Microsporum* and *Trichophyton* and one species of *Epidermophyton.*

Origin

- Anthropophilic dermatophytes grow only on human skin, hair, or nails.
- Zoophilic varieties originate from animals but may infect humans.
- Geophilic dermatophytes live in soil but may infect humans.

Type of Inflammation

- Zoophilic and geophilic dermatophytes elicit a brisk inflammatory response.
- Anthropophilic fungi elicit a mild response.

Type of Hair Invasion

- Some species are able to infect the hair shaft.
- In the endothrix pattern, fungal hyphae are inside the hair shaft.
- In the ectothrix pattern, fungal hyphae are inside and on the hair shaft surface.
- Spores of fungi are either large or small.
- The type of hair invasion is further classified as large- or small-spore ectothrix and large-spore endothrix.

Body Region Classification

- Dermatophytes produce a variety of disease patterns that vary with location.
- It is important to know the general patterns of inflammation in different body regions.

DESCRIPTION

- The greatest number of hyphae are located in the active border.
- This is the best area to get a sample for a potassium hydroxide examination.
- The active border is scaly, red, and slightly elevated.
- Vesicles appear at the active border when inflammation is intense.
- This pattern is present in all locations except the palms and soles.

LABORATORY

Potassium Hydroxide Wet-Mount Preparation

- The most important test for diagnosis is direct visualization of the branching hyphae in keratinized material under the microscope.
- A #15 surgical blade is held perpendicular to the skin surface and smoothly but firmly drawn against the scale with several short strokes. If an active border is present, the blade is drawn along the border at right angles to the fringe of the scale.
- The scale is placed on a microscope slide and gently separated, and a coverslip is applied. Potassium hydroxide (10% or 20% solution) is applied with a toothpick or eyedropper to the edge of the coverslip and allowed to run under by capillary action.
- The preparation is gently heated under a low flame and then pressed to facilitate separation of the epithelial cells and fungal hyphae.
- Lowering the condenser of the microscope and dimming the light enhances contrast, making hyphae easier to identify.
- Nail-plate keratin can be softened by leaving the fragments along with several drops of potassium hydroxide in a watch glass covered with a Petri dish for 24 hours. A nail micronizer can be used to pulverize nails for microscopy and culture.
- Hair specimens require no special preparation and can be examined immediately.

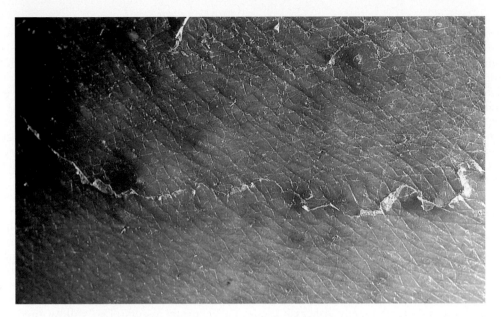

A very characteristic pattern of inflammation is the active border of infection. The highest numbers of hyphae is located in the active border, and this is the best area to get a sample for a potassium hydroxide examination. This pattern is present in all locations except the palms and soles.

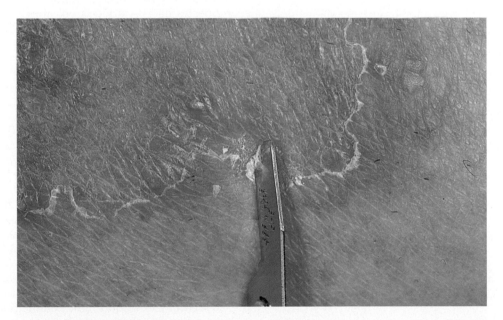

Scale is obtained by holding a #15 surgical blade perpendicular to the skin surface and smoothly but firmly drawing the blade with several short strokes against the scale.

Microscopy

- The entire area is scanned under the coverslip at low power. The presence of hyphae is confirmed by examination at 40× objective power. Slight back-and-forth rotation of the focusing knob aids visualization of the entire segment of the hyphae.
- Dermatophytes appear as translucent, branching, rod-shaped filaments (hyphae) of uniform width, with lines of separation (septa) spanning the width and appearing at irregular intervals.
- The uniform width and branching distinguish hyphae from hair and other debris. Hair tapers at the tip.
- A mosaic artifact produced by lipid droplets appearing in a single-file line between cells, especially from specimens taken from the palms and soles, may cause confusion. These disappear when the cells are separated further by additional heating and pressure.
- Longitudinal, rod-shaped potassium hydroxide crystals that simulate hyphae may appear if the wet mount is heated excessively.
- A drop of Parker's blue ink added to the wet mount clearly stains hyphae, rendering them visible under low power.

Culture

- It is usually not necessary to know the species of dermatophyte infecting skin in most cases because the same oral and topical agents are active against all of them.
- Fungal culture is helpful for hair and nail fungal infections.
- A sterile cotton swab moistened with sterile water or agar from an agar plate is rubbed vigorously over the active part of the lesion and then rubbed onto the surface of the agar plate.

Culture Media

- Dermatophytes are aerobic and grow on the surface of media.
- Cultures usually become positive in 1 to 2 weeks.

There are three types of culture media for tinea.
- Mycosel agar is Sabouraud dextrose medium that contains cycloheximide and chloramphenicol to prevent the growth of bacteria and saprophytic fungi. It is best for the evaluation of hair tinea because only dermatophytes cause hair tinea.
- Sabouraud dextrose medium does not contain antibiotics and allows the growth of most fungi, including nondermatophytes. It is useful for nail infections because the detection of nondermatophytes is desirable in such infections.
- Dermatophyte test medium (DTM) culture can be performed in the physician's office; it is supplied in vials. It produces fast but slightly less accurate results. The yellow medium turns pink in the presence of dermatophytes in 6 or 7 days but remains yellow in the presence of nonpathogenic fungi. It must be discarded after 2 weeks because saprophytes can induce a similar color change from this time on.
- Species identification is possible but is more accurately determined with Mycosel agar and Sabouraud dextrose medium.

Culture media for yeast
- Initial isolation can occur on Sabouraud's agar.
- Other techniques are used for the isolation and identification of *Candida* species.

Wood's light examination
- Hair, but not the skin of the scalp, fluoresces with a blue-green color if infected with *Microsporum canis* or *Microsporum audouinii*.
- No other dermatophytes that infect hair produce fluorescence.
- Fungal infections of the skin do not fluoresce. The exception is tinea versicolor, which produces a pale white-yellow fluorescence.
- Erythrasma, a noninflammatory, pale brown, scaly eruption of the toe webs, groin, and axillae caused by the bacteria *Corynebacterium minutissimum*, shows a brilliant coral-red fluorescence with Wood's light examination.
- Wood's light examination should be performed in a dark room with a high-intensity instrument.

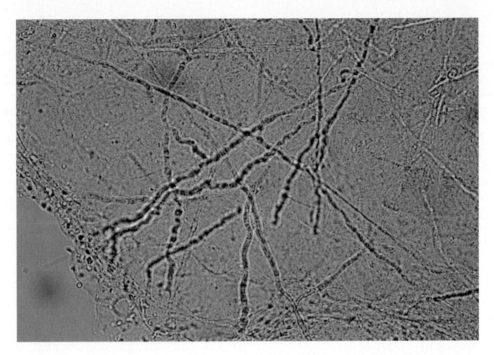

Dermatophytes appear as translucent, branching, rod-shaped filaments (hyphae) of uniform width, with lines of separation (septa) spanning the width and appearing at irregular intervals.

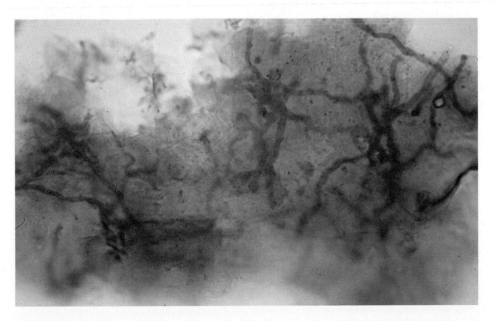

Hyphae may be difficult to find in a potassium hydroxide wet mount. Parker's blue ink and other stains easily stain hyphae, rendering them visible under low power.

■ TINEA OF THE FOOT (TINEA PEDIS)

DESCRIPTION

- The feet are the most common area infected by dermatophytes (tinea pedis, "athlete's foot").
- There are many different clinical presentations.

HISTORY

- Tinea of the foot is common in young and middle-aged adults. It is uncommon in prepubertal children.
- It is common in men and less common in women.
- This infection is probably inevitable in immunologically predisposed individuals regardless of any elaborate precautions taken to avoid the infecting organism.

PREDISPOSING FACTORS

- Shoes promote warmth and sweating, thus encouraging fungal growth.
- Locker-room floors contain fungal elements; communal baths may create an ideal condition for repeated exposure to infected material.

SKIN FINDINGS

- Tinea of the feet may present with the classic ringworm pattern, but most infections are found in the toe webs or on the soles.

Interdigital Tinea Pedis (Toe Web Infection)

- The web between the fourth and fifth toes is most commonly involved, but all webs may be infected.
- Tight-fitting shoes compress the toes, creating a warm, moist environment.
- The webs become dry, scaly, and fissured or white, macerated, and soggy. Itching is most intense when the shoes and socks are removed.
- Overgrowth of the bacterial population determines the severity of infection.
- Extension out of the web space onto the plantar surface or the dorsum of the foot is common and occurs with the typical, chronic, ringworm type of scaly, advancing border or with an acute, vesicular eruption.

Chronic Scaly Infection of the Plantar Surface

- Plantar hyperkeratotic or moccasin-type tinea pedis is a chronic form of tinea that is resistant to treatment.
- The entire sole is usually infected and covered with fine, silvery white scales.
- The skin is pink, tender, pruritic, or a combination thereof.
- The hands may be similarly infected. It is rare to see both palms and soles infected simultaneously; rather, the pattern is infection of two feet and one hand or of two hands and one foot.
- *Trichophyton rubrum* is the usual pathogen.

Acute Vesicular Tinea Pedis

- A highly inflammatory infection may originate from a more chronic web infection.
- Vesicles evolve rapidly on the sole or on the dorsum. Vesicles may fuse into bullae or remain as collections of fluid under the thick scale of the sole and never rupture through the surface.
- Secondary bacterial infection occurs.
- A second wave of vesicles may follow in the same areas or at distant sites such as the arms, chest, and along the sides of the fingers. These itchy, sterile vesicles represent an allergic response to the fungus and are termed a *dermatophytid* or *id reaction*. At times, the id reaction is the only clinical manifestation of a fungal infection. Examination of these patients may show an asymptomatic fissure or area of maceration in the toe webs.

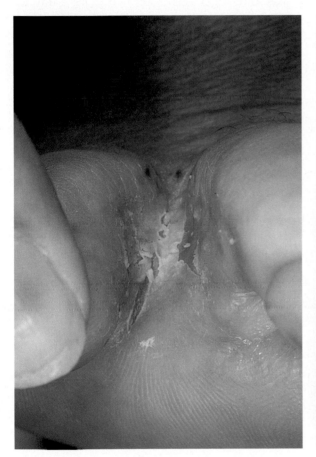

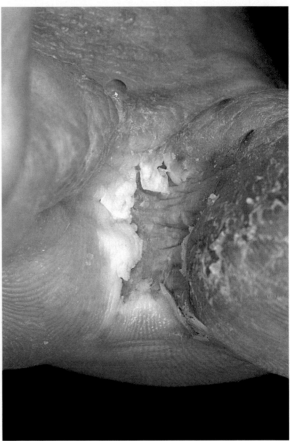

Interdigital tinea pedis (toe web infection). Tight-fitting shoes compress the toes, creating a warm, moist environment in the toe webs; this environment is suited to fungal growth.

Interdigital tinea pedis (toe web infection). The web can become dry, scaly, and fissured or white, macerated, and soggy.

LABORATORY

- Identification of fungal hyphae in the macerated skin of the toe webs may be difficult using potassium hydroxide examination.
- Fungal hyphae are difficult to identify in severely inflamed skin.
- A culture is obtained if the potassium hydroxide examination is negative and clinical suspicion exists.

COURSE AND PROGNOSIS

- Once the infection is established, the individual becomes a carrier and is more susceptible to recurrences.

DIFFERENTIAL DIAGNOSIS

- Psoriasis
- Eczema
- Chapped, fissured feet

TREATMENT
Topical Therapy

- Allylamines and related compounds (e.g., butenafine [Mentax], terbinafine [Lamisil], naftifine [Naftin]) may produce higher cure rates than imidazoles (clotrimazole, miconazole, econazole [Spectazole]) when applied twice a day for 2 to 4 weeks. These agents produce higher cure rates and have a lower relapse rate than a combination of an antifungal and a corticosteroid (betamethasone 0.5% and clotrimazole 1% [Lotrisone]).
- Econazole nitrate (Spectazole) has activity against several bacterial species associated with severely macerated interdigital interspaces.
- Acute vesicular tinea pedis responds to compresses with wet Burow's solution applied for 30 minutes several times a day in combination with topical antifungal creams applied twice a day.

Oral Therapy

- The following may be administered: terbinafine (Lamisil), 250 mg/day for 2 weeks; itraconazole (Sporanox Pulse Pack), 200 mg twice a day for 1 week; or fluconazole (Diflucan), 150 mg once a week for weeks. Griseofulvin may be less effective.
- An oral antifungal agent may be started and topical antifungal agents applied twice a day for acute or extensive infection.
- Secondary bacterial infection is treated with oral antibiotics.
- A vesicular id reaction sometimes occurs at distant sites during an inflammatory foot infection. Cool and wet dressings, group V topical steroids, and occasionally, prednisone, 20 mg twice a day for 8 to 10 days, are required to control such reactions.

General Measures

- Recurrence is prevented by wearing wider shoes and expanding the web space with a small strand of lamb's wool (Dr. Scholl's Lamb's Wool).
- Powders, not necessarily medicated, absorb moisture. The powders should be applied to the feet rather than to the shoes. Wet socks should be changed.

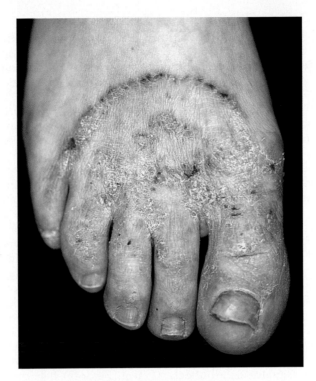

Classic ringworm pattern of fungal infection.

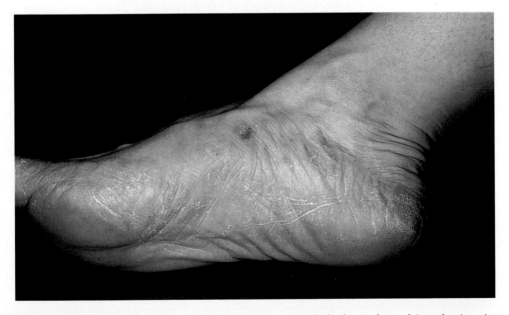

Plantar hyperkeratotic or moccasin-type tinea pedis is a particularly chronic form of tinea that is resistant to treatment. The entire sole is usually infected and covered with a fine, silvery white scale.

■ TINEA OF THE GROIN (TINEA CRURIS, JOCK ITCH)

DESCRIPTION

- Tinea of the groin is a dermatophyte infection of the crural fold.

HISTORY

- Tinea of the groin occurs almost exclusively in postpubertal male patients.
- It occurs in the summer after sweating or in the winter after wearing layers of clothing.
- Many patients are unaware of the infection.
- Itching becomes worse as moisture accumulates.

SKIN FINDINGS

- Often bilateral, tinea of the groin begins in the crural fold.
- A half moon–shaped plaque forms as well-defined scaling, and sometimes a vesicular border advances out of the crural fold onto the thigh.
- Skin within the border turns red-brown, is less scaly, and may develop red papules.
- Acute inflammation may appear after wearing occlusive clothing.
- The infection occasionally migrates to the buttock and gluteal cleft area.

LABORATORY

- Specimens for potassium hydroxide examination should be taken from the advancing scaling border.
- Culture can be taken if results from the wet-mount study are negative.

COURSE AND PROGNOSIS

- The infection may improve or resolve if the moist environment is eliminated.
- Involvement of the scrotum is unusual in tinea of the groin, unlike in candidal infections, in which it is common.

DIFFERENTIAL DIAGNOSIS

- Intertrigo
- Psoriasis
- Erythrasma

TREATMENT

- Antifungal creams with activity against *Candida* species and dermatophytes (e.g., econazole [Spectazole], miconazole [Micatin], clotrimazole [Lotrimin]) applied twice a day for 10 to 14 days are effective.
- Moist lesions may be treated with a compress with cool, water or Burow's solution for 20 to 30 minutes two to six times a day until the skin has dried.
- Resistant infections respond to griseofulvin ultra-microsize 333 to 500 mg/day for 2 weeks; itraconazole, 200 mg/day for 1 to 2 weeks; terbinafine, 250 mg/day for 2 weeks; or fluconazole, 150 mg once a week for 2 to 4 weeks.
- Betamethasone 0.5% and clotrimazole 1% (Lotrisone) cream, a steroid (betamethasone dipropionate), and an antifungal (clotrimazole) mixture may be used initially for inflamed lesions. A pure antifungal cream should be used once symptoms are controlled. Prolonged use of steroid-antifungal cream may not cure the infection and may cause striae in this intertriginous area.
- Absorbent powders, not necessarily medicated (e.g., Zeasorb), help control moisture and prevent infection. They are applied after the infection is gone.

CAVEAT

- Steroid creams are frequently prescribed for inflammatory disease of the groin and can modify the typical clinical presentation of tinea. This modified form, called *tinea incognito,* may not be immediately recognized as tinea.
- Intertrigo is commonly misinterpreted as tinea. The rash in intertrigo is symmetric and involves an equal area on the scrotum and thigh. It responds to weak topical steroids and measures to enhance dryness (powder and cool, wet compresses).

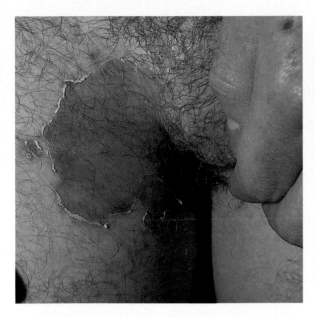

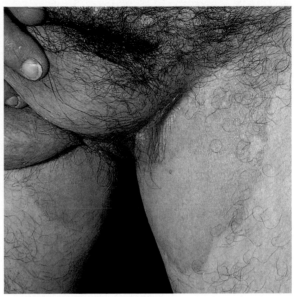

A half moon–shaped plaque forms as a well-defined scaling, and sometimes a vesicular border advances out of the crural fold onto the thigh. The skin within the border turns red-brown, is less scaly, and may develop red papules.

The entire surface of this lesion is dry and scaling. Involvement of the scrotum is unusual–unlike candidal reactions, in which it is common.

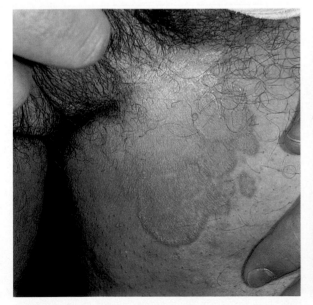

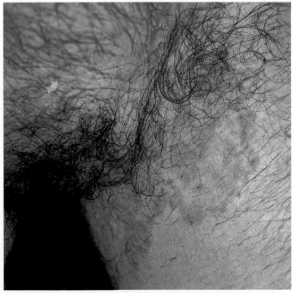

The ringworm pattern of infection may also appear in the groin.

The advancing border may sometimes be vesicular.

■ TINEA OF THE BODY (CORPUS) AND FACE (FACIEI)

DESCRIPTION

- Tinea of the face (excluding the beard area in men), trunk, and limbs is called tinea corporis (ringworm of the body).

HISTORY

- Tinea corporis is more common in warm climates.
- Epidemics can occur in wrestlers.

SKIN FINDINGS

- There is a broad range of clinical presentations, with lesions varying in size, degree of inflammation, and depth of involvement.

Round Annular Lesions (Classic Ringworm)

- Lesions begin as flat, scaly spots and then develop a raised border that extends out at variable rates in all directions.
- An advancing, scaly border may have red, raised papules or vesicles.
- The central area becomes brown or hypopigmented and less scaly as the active border progresses outward.
- Red papules may occur in the central area.
- Several annular lesions may enlarge to cover large areas of the body surface.
- Larger lesions tend to be mildly itchy or asymptomatic.
- Lesions may reach a certain size and remain for years with no tendency to resolve.

Deep Inflammatory Lesions

- Fungi from animals such as *Trichophyton verrucosum* from cattle may produce a very inflammatory skin infection.
- The round, intensely inflamed lesions have uniformly elevated, red, boggy, pustular surfaces.
- The pustules are follicular and represent deep penetration of the fungus into the hair follicle.
- Secondary bacterial infection can occur.
- The process ends with brown hyperpigmentation and scarring.

LABORATORY

- Potassium hydroxide examinations usually show abundant hyphae.
- Deep inflammatory lesions are cultured to identify an animal source of infection.

DIFFERENTIAL DIAGNOSIS

- Nummular eczema, psoriasis, pityriasis alba
- Pityriasis rosea (The appearance of the lesions of pityriasis rosea and the multiple small, annular lesions of ringworm may be similar. The scaly ring of pityriasis rosea does not reach the edge of the red border, as it does in tinea.)

TREATMENT

- Superficial lesions respond to antifungal creams (e.g., clotrimazole, miconazole, econazole [Spectazole], oxiconazole [Oxistat], terbinafine [Lamisil], butenafine [Mentax]) applied twice each day for a minimum of 2 weeks. Treatment is continued for at least 1 week after resolution of the infection.
- Extensive lesions or those with red papules require oral therapy, including griseofulvin ultramicrosize, 333 mg/day or 250 mg twice a day for adults and 5 to 7 mg/kg/day for 2 to 6 weeks for children; itraconazole, (Sporanox), 200 mg/day for 2 weeks; terbinafine (Lamisil), 250 mg/day for 2 weeks; or fluconazole (Diflucan), 150 mg once a week for 3 to 4 weeks.
- Secondary bacterial infection is treated with oral antibiotics.
- A short course of prednisone may be considered for highly inflamed lesions.

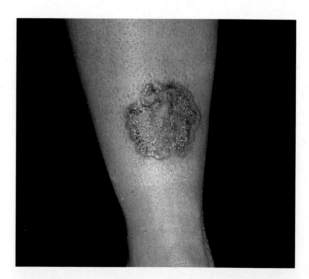

Inflammatory lesions. In classic ringworm, lesions begin as flat, scaly spots that then develop a raised border that extends out at variable rates in all directions. The advancing, scaly border may have red, raised papules or vesicles.

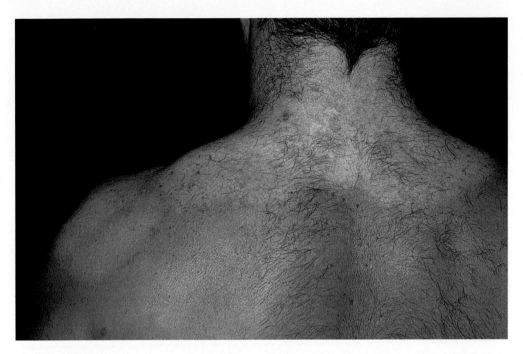

Round annular lesions. Larger lesions tend to be mildly itchy or asymptomatic. They may reach a certain size and remain for years with no tendency to resolve.

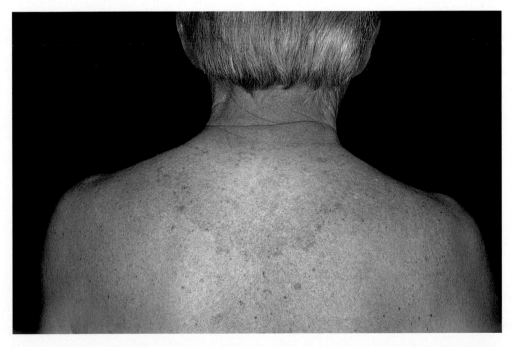

Round annular lesions. The border areas are fairly distinct. The central area is uniform and scaling. There are no papules.

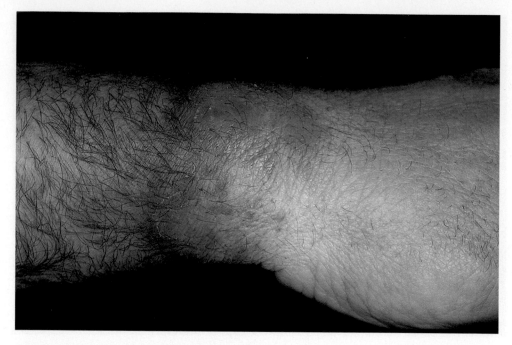

Round annular lesions. This highly inflamed lesion was initially diagnosed as bacterial cellulitis. The potassium hydroxide examination showed fungal hyphae.

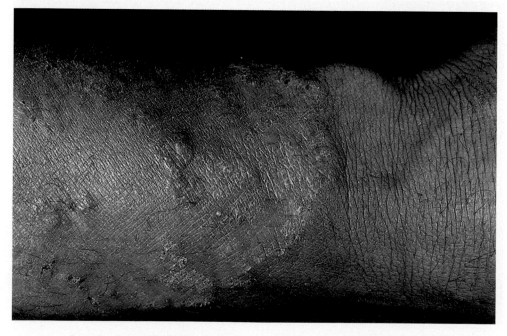

Round annular lesions. The border and central area are papular and vesicular.

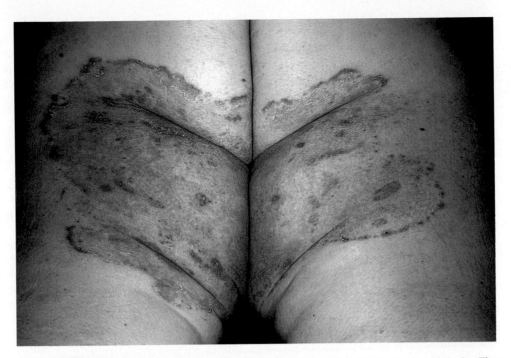

Clear, central areas of the larger lesions are yellow-brown and usually contain several red papules. The borders are serpiginous or annular and very irregular.

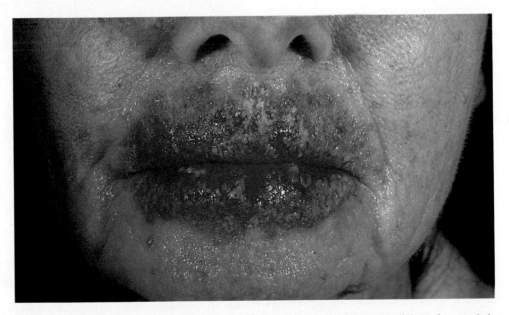

Tinea incognito. Fungal infections treated with topical steroids often lose some of their characteristic features. Diffuse erythema, diffuse scale, scattered pustules or papules, and brown hyperpigmentation may all result.

■ TINEA OF THE HAND (TINEA MANUUM)

HISTORY

- Children are rarely affected.
- Tinea of the hand may be insidious and progresses slowly over a period of weeks, months, or years.
- Itching is moderate, minimal, or absent.
- Pain occurs if there is secondary staphylococcal follicular infection of the dorsum.

SKIN FINDINGS

Ringworm Pattern of the Back of the Hand

- Tinea of the back of the hand has all the features of classic ringworm lesions of the body. There is a raised, red, scaly advancing border. Papules or vesicles may be present at the border or in the central area. A follicular infection with staphylococci or dermatophytes causes papules or pustules.

Chronic Scaling Infection of the Palms

- Tinea of the palm has the same appearance as the dry, diffuse, keratotic form of tinea on the soles. It is frequently seen in association with tinea pedis. The usual pattern of infection is involvement of one foot and two hands or of two feet and one hand. A fingernail fungal infection may accompany infection of the dorsum of the hand or palm. Hyperkeratotic tinea of the palms may be asymptomatic, and the patient may be unaware of the infection, attributing the dry, thick, scaly surface to hard physical labor. The diagnosis is easily missed.

LABORATORY

- The diagnosis is established by performing a microscopic examination of skin scrapings with a potassium hydroxide wet mount.
- Fungal cultures are required if the diagnosis cannot be confirmed by wet-mount examination.

COURSE AND PROGNOSIS

- Annular lesions on the back of the hand respond to treatment and tend not to recur.
- Hyperkeratotic scaling palms respond to treatment, but this condition may recur. The thickened palms may dry severely and develop cracks and fissures.

DISCUSSION

- Tinea of the hands may look like eczema or psoriasis, especially if the border is not distinct.
- If there is any doubt, skin scrapings should be obtained and a potassium hydroxide wet mount prepared.

TREATMENT

- Topical antifungal agents (butenafine [Mentax], econazole [Spectazole], terbinafine [Lamisil]) may be effective, but oral medication is more reliable.
- Infection on the back of the hand responds faster than infection on the palms.
- Adults are treated with griseofulvin ultramicrosize, 330 to 500 mg/day for 3 to 6 weeks.
- Alternative therapy includes itraconazole, 200 or 400 mg daily for 1 to 2 weeks; terbinafine, 250 mg/day for 2 or 4 weeks; or fluconazole, 150 mg/wk for 2 or 4 weeks. Treatment of nail infections require a longer course of treatment (see p. 190).
- Patients with palm infections should be reevaluated 6 months after treatment. There is a significant recurrence rate.

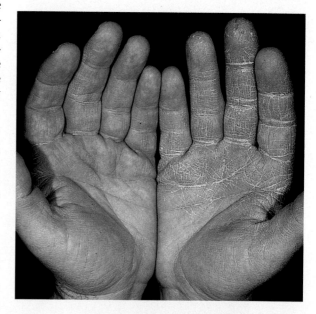

Tinea of the palm has the same appearance as the dry, diffuse, keratotic form of tinea on the soles. It may be asymptomatic, and the patient may be unaware of the infection, attributing the dry, thick, scaly surface to hard physical labor.

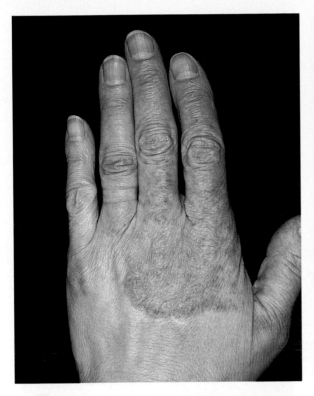

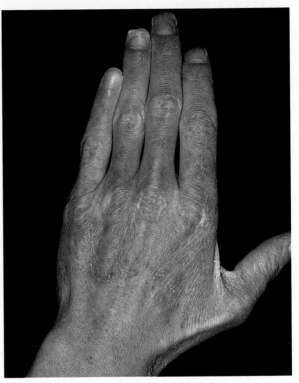

Tinea of the dorsal aspect of the hand (tinea manuum) has all of the features of tinea corporis. The nails are also frequently infected.

A diagnosis of eczema was made and the infection initially treated with topical steroids. It spread over a wide area before the infectious nature of the eruption was discovered.

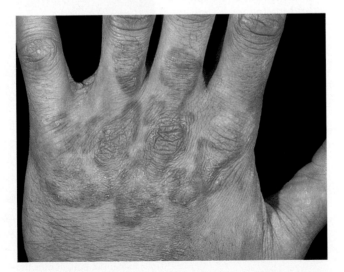

Tinea incognito. Fungal infections treated with topical steroids often lose some of their characteristic features. Multiple rings have appeared.

■ TINEA INCOGNITO

DESCRIPTION

- Cortisone creams applied to cutaneous fungal infections decrease inflammation, alter the usual clinical presentation, and produce unusual, atypical eruptions. This altered clinical picture is called *tinea incognito*.
- Lesion progression
  - Treatment is with topical steroids.
    - Topical steroids decrease inflammation and give the false impression that the rash is improving.
    - The fungus flourishes secondary to cortisone-induced immunologic changes.
  - Treatment is stopped.
    - The rash returns when treatment is stopped.
    - The rash has changed. Scaling at the margins may be absent. Diffuse erythema, diffuse scaling, scattered pustules or papules, and brown hyperpigmentation may all result.
    - A well-defined border may not be present, and a once-localized process may have expanded greatly.
  - The cycle continues.
    - Memory of the good initial response prompts reuse of the steroid cream, and the repetitive cycle continues.
    - The intensity of itching varies.
- Sites include the groin, face, and dorsal aspect of the hand. Tinea infections of the hands are often misdiagnosed as eczema and treated with topical steroids.

LABORATORY

- Potassium hydroxide wet-mount examination reveals numerous hyphae, especially a few days after use of the steroid cream is discontinued, when scaling reappears.
- Culture is usually unnecessary because the potassium hydroxide preparation is almost always positive.

DIFFERENTIAL DIAGNOSIS

- Eczema, boils
- Folliculitis, rosacea
- Pityriasis rosea
- Psoriasis

TREATMENT

- Superficial lesions respond to antifungal creams (clotrimazole, miconazole, econazole [Spectazole], butenafine [Mentax], terbinafine [Lamisil]) applied twice a day for a minimum of 2 weeks. Treatment is continued for at least 1 week after resolution of the infection.
- Extensive lesions or those with red papules require oral therapy, including griseofulvin ultramicrosize, 333 mg/day or 250 mg twice a day for adults and 5 to 7 mg/kg/day for 2 to 6 weeks for children; itraconazole (Sporanox), 200 mg/day for 2 weeks; terbinafine (Lamisil), 250 mg/day for 2 weeks; or fluconazole (Diflucan) 150 mg once a week for 3 to 4 weeks.
- Secondary bacterial infection is treated with oral antibiotics.
- Cool, wet compresses with water suppress inflammation and control itching.

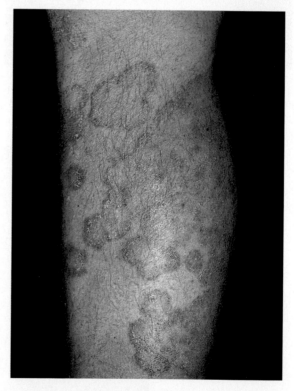

Tinea incognito. Fungal infections treated with topical steroids can lose some of their characteristic features. Here, a once-localized process has expanded greatly.

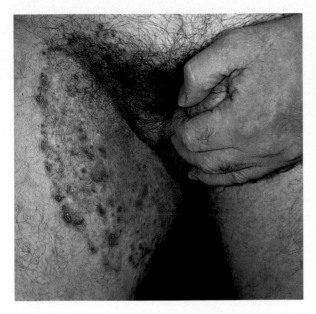

Tinea incognito. Topical steroid creams modify the typical clinical presentation of tinea. Red papules sometimes appear at the edges and center of the lesion. This modified form may not be immediately recognized as tinea.

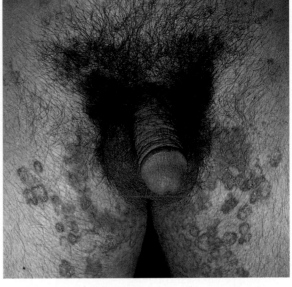

Tinea incognito. The eruption may be much more extensive, and the advancing, scaly border may not be present.

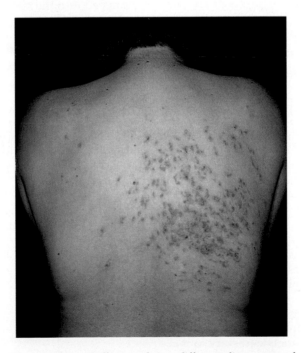

Tinea incognito. Diffuse erythema, diffuse scaling, scattered pustules or papules, and brown hyperpigmentation may all result. All of the characteristic features of tinea have been lost.

■ TINEA OF THE SCALP (TINEA CAPITIS)

DESCRIPTION

- Tinea of the scalp is caused by the invasion of the stratum corneum and the hair shaft with fungal hyphae.

HISTORY

- *Trichophyton tonsurans* is responsible for over 90% of cases of tinea of the scalp in the United States.
  - It occurs more often in prepubertal children and adults.
  - The source of infection is contact with a pet or an infected person.
  - Spores are shed in the air and remain viable for long periods on combs, brushes, blankets, and telephones.
  - Tinea of the scalp does not resolve spontaneously at puberty, resulting in a large population of infected carriers.
  - It is seen in the crowded inner cities, especially in African-Americans or Latinos.
- *Microsporum canis* infection is suspected in children who have a new cat; adults are not infected.

SKIN FINDINGS

- *T. tonsurans* has four patterns of clinical infection. An asymptomatic adult carrier state exists.

Inflammatory Tinea Capitis (Kerion)

- One or many inflamed, boggy, tender areas of alopecia with pustules appear. Scarring alopecia may occur.
- Fever, occipital adenopathy, and leukocytosis may occur.
- Potassium hydroxide wet-mount examination and fungal culture are often negative.
- Treatment may have to be initiated based on clinical appearance.

Seborrheic Dermatitis Type

- The seborrheic dermatitis type is common, is difficult to diagnose, and resembles dandruff.
- Diffuse or patchy, fine, white, adherent scales appear on the scalp.
- Adenopathy is often present.
- The results of a potassium hydroxide examination are often negative; culture is necessary to make the diagnosis.

Noninflammatory (Black-Dot) Pattern

- Large areas of alopecia are present without inflammation.
- There is a mild to moderate amount of scalp scaling.
- Occipital adenopathy may be present.
- Arthrospores weaken the hair and cause it to break off at the scalp surface, resulting in a black-dot appearance.

Pustular type

- Pustules or scabbed areas without scaling or significant hair loss occur.
- Cultures and potassium hydroxide wet-mount examination may be negative.

LABORATORY

- A systematic approach for investigation is presented in Box 9-1.
- The brush-culture method, a painless technique for children, involves gently rubbing a previously sterilized toothbrush in a circular motion over areas where scaling is present or over the margins of patches of alopecia. The brush fibers are then pressed into the culture media, and the brush is discarded.

DIFFERENTIAL DIAGNOSIS

- Seborrheic dermatitis
- Psoriasis
- Eczema
- Tinea amiantacea, a form of seborrheic dermatitis that occurs in children (A localized 2- to 8-cm patch of large, brown, polygonal scales adheres to the scalp and mats the hair. The matted scale grows out, attached to the hair. There is little or no inflammation.)

TREATMENT

- Management requires oral and topical approaches.

Box 9-1   Systematic Approach to the Investigation of Tinea Capitis

Determine Clinical Presentation

Most forms of tinea capitis begin with one or several round patches of scaling or alopecia.

Inflammatory lesions, even if untreated, tend to resolve spontaneously in a few months; the noninflammatory infections are more chronic.

Patchy alopecia + fine dry scale + no inflammation
  Short stubs of broken hair ("gray patch ringworm")
    Microsporum audouinii
  Hairs broken off at surface ("black-dot ringworm")
    T. tonsurans (most common), *Trichophyton violaceum*
  Patchy alopecia + swelling + purulent discharge
    M. canis, Trichophyton mentagrophytes (granular), *Trichophyton verrucosum*

Kerion is a severe inflammatory reaction with boggy induration. Any fungus, but especially *M. canis, T. mentagrophytes* (granular), *T. verrucosum.*

Wood's Light Examination

Blue-green fluorescence of hair—only *M. canis* and *M. audouinii* have this feature. Scales and skin do not fluoresce.

Potassium Hydroxide Wet Mount of Plucked Hairs

The pattern of hair invasion is characteristic for each species of fungus. Hairs that can be removed with little resistance are best for evaluation.

Large-spored endothrix pattern-chains of large spores (densely packed) within the hair, "like a sack full of marbles."
  T. tonsurans, T. violaceum
Large-spored ectothrix pattern-chains of large spores inside and on the surface of the hair shaft and visible with the low-power objective
  T. verrucosum, T. mentagrophytes
Small-spored ectothrix—small spores randomly arranged in masses inside and on the surface of the hair shaft, not visible with the low-power objective. Looks like a stick dipped in maple syrup and rolled in sand.
  M. canis, M. audouinii

Identification of Source after Species is Verified by Culture

Anthropophilic (parasitic on humans)—infection from other humans
  M. audouinii, T. tonsurans, T. violaceum
Zoophilic (parasitic on animals)—infection from animals or other infected humans
  M. canis—dog, cat, monkey
  T. mentagrophytes (granular)—dog, rabbit, guinea pig, monkey
  T. verrucosum—cattle

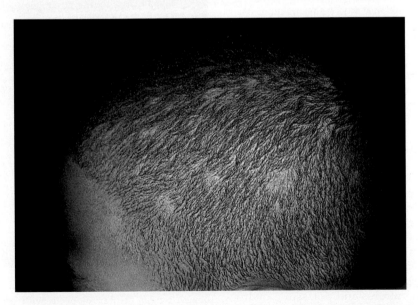

Most forms of tinea capitis begin with one or several round patches of scale or alopecia.

Oral Therapy

- Griseofulvin is usually the drug of first choice, but many children cannot tolerate the high doses, and some children do not respond. Terbinafine, itraconazole, and fluconazole are alternatives.
- Terbinafine, 3 to 6 mg/kg/day, is effective. The dosage ranges from 62.5 to 250 mg for 4 to 8 weeks. There is no liquid formulation. Terbinafine may be the most cost-effective treatment.

Body Weight	Daily Dosage
<20 kg	62.5 mg (one fourth of a tablet)
20-40 kg	125 mg (one half of a tablet)
>40 kg	250 mg (one tablet)

- Itraconazole, 25 to 100 mg/day (2.5 to 5 mg/kg/day), is taken with food for 4 to 8 weeks. The contents of a capsule is sprinkled into food (e.g., applesauce) for children who cannot swallow capsules.
  - Patients are seen 2 weeks from the start of treatment. If significant inflammation is present, the dosage is increased to the next weight category in the chart.
  - The oral solution contains cyclodextrin and is probably not suitable for children.

Body Weight	Dosage
22-40 lb (10-18 kg)	100 mg every other day
40-60 lb (18-27 kg)	100 mg/day
60-90 lb (27-41 kg)	100 mg/day or alternation of 100 and 200 mg/day
90-110 lb (41-50 kg)	Alternation of 100 and 200 mg/day
>110 lb	200 mg/day

- Fluconazole is available in a pediatric liquid formulation. A dosage of 6 to 8 mg/kg/day for 4 to 8 weeks is effective. A single 150-mg dose once a week for 4 weeks may also be effective for older children.
- Griseofulvin microsize, 20 to 25 mg/kg/day of the liquid formulation, or griseofulvin ultramicrosize, 15 to 20 mg/kg/day in a capsule, is administered once as a single dose or divided into two doses daily and taken for a minimum of 6 to 8 weeks. Some children require larger dosages.
  - Griseofulvin is absorbed more efficiently with a fatty meal; children can be given the medicine with ice cream or whole milk.
  - The patient should be treated 2 weeks beyond the time that cultures and potassium hydroxide preparations become negative. This generally requires 6 to 12 weeks.
- Suppressing the inflammation of a kerion may be accomplished with topical, oral, or intralesional steroids. Prednisone, 1 to 2 mg/kg/day, may hasten resolution and reduces or prevents scarring.

Topical Treatment

- Shampoo with selenium sulfide 1% (Selsun Blue, Head & Shoulders Intensive Treatment) or ketoconazole (Nizoral) is used every other day for the first 2 weeks and then twice weekly throughout the rest of the course of oral therapy. This reduces the risk of shedding of spores.
- The shampoo is applied, left on for 5 minutes, and rinsed.
- Other family members should also use the shampoo two to three times a week.

Prevention of Recurrence

- Scrupulous cleaning of all possibly contaminated objects helps prevent reinfection.
- All family members should be examined carefully for tinea capitis and tinea corporis.

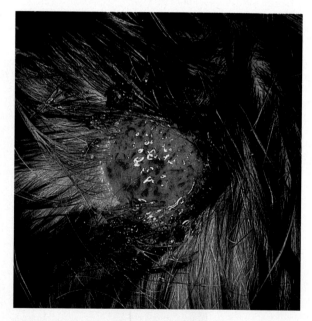

Inflammatory tinea capitis (kerion). There is an inflamed, boggy, tender area of alopecia with pustules. Occipital adenopathy was present.

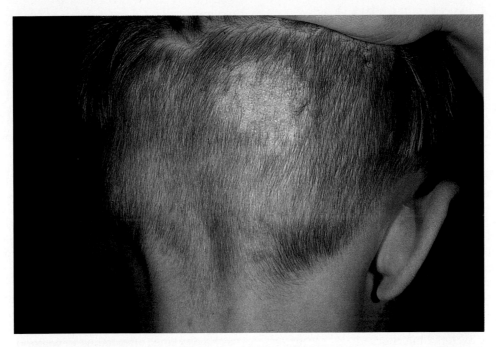

Noninflammatory lesions tend to be chronic and last for months. Hairs break off at or below the scalp surface, resulting in a "black-dot" appearance of the scalp surface.

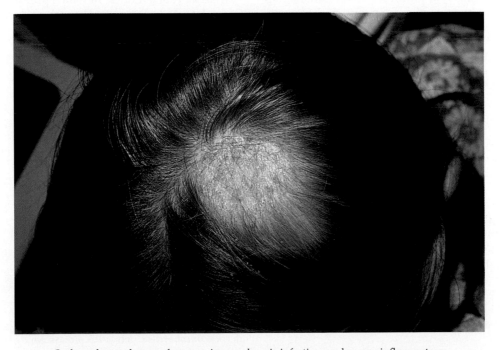

Scale and pustules may be seen. A once chronic infection can become inflammatory.

■ TINEA OF THE BEARD

DESCRIPTION

- Fungal infection of the skin and hair in the beard area is called *tinea barbae*.

HISTORY

- Tinea is a slowly evolving disease in contrast to bacterial infections.
- Infection of the skin causes some itching.
- Infection of the follicle causes pain and swelling.

SKIN FINDINGS

- There are two patterns of infection.
  - In the ringworm pattern, superficial infection resembles the annular lesions of tinea corporis with a sharply defined scaling border; the hair follicle is also usually infected.
  - In the follicular pattern, deep follicular infection resembles bacterial folliculitis.

NONSKIN FINDINGS

- Regional lymphadenopathy occurs when there is secondary bacterial infection.

LABORATORY

- Skin scrapings and plucked hair are obtained for potassium hydroxide examination. Hair is sometimes easily removed from follicles infected with fungi. It is more difficult to extract it from follicles infected with bacteria.
- Fungal cultures are required if the diagnosis is suspected but cannot be confirmed with the potassium hydroxide wet-mount preparation.

COURSE AND PROGNOSIS

- Unlike bacterial folliculitis, follicular fungal infection is slow to evolve and is usually restricted to one area of the beard.
- Bacterial folliculitis spreads rapidly over wide areas after shaving.
- Tinea begins insidiously with a small group of follicular pustules.
- The process becomes confluent in time with the development of a boggy, erythematous, tumorlike abscess covered with a dense, superficial crust similar to the fungal kerions seen in tinea capitis.
- Scarring may occur in advanced cases.

DIFFERENTIAL DIAGNOSIS

- Bacterial folliculitis and furunculosis
- Pseudofolliculitis produced by shaving
- Rosacea
- Acne

TREATMENT

- Topical antifungal agents are not reliably effective because they do not penetrate deep enough into the hair follicle.
- Men are treated with griseofulvin ultramicrosize, either 500 mg or 330 mg once or twice a day for 4 weeks. Alternative therapy includes itraconazole (Sporanox), 200 mg/day for 2 to 4 weeks; terbinafine (Lamisil), 250 mg/day for 2 to 4 weeks; or fluconazole (Diflucan), 150 mg once a week for 3 to 4 weeks.

CAVEAT

- Fungal infection of the beard area is often misdiagnosed as bacterial folliculitis. It is not unusual to see patients who have finally been diagnosed as having tinea after failing to respond to several courses of antibiotics.
- A positive culture for *Staphylococcus* organisms does not rule out tinea, in which purulent lesions may be infected secondarily with bacteria.

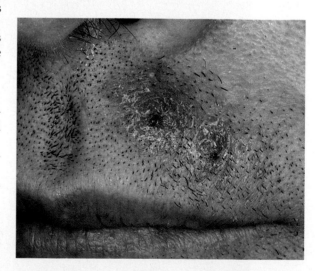

Tinea begins insidiously with a small group of follicular pustules. The process becomes confluent and resembles bacterial infection or seborrheic dermatitis. Potassium hydroxide examination proves the diagnosis.

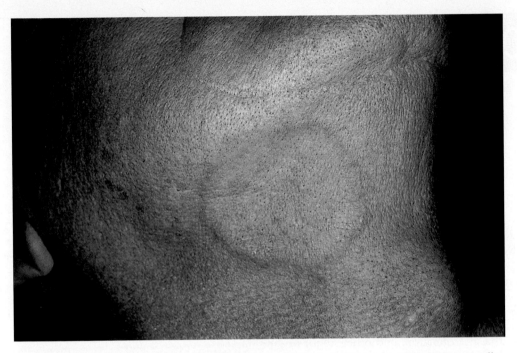

Superficial infection. This pattern resembles the annular lesions of tinea corporis. The hair is usually infected.

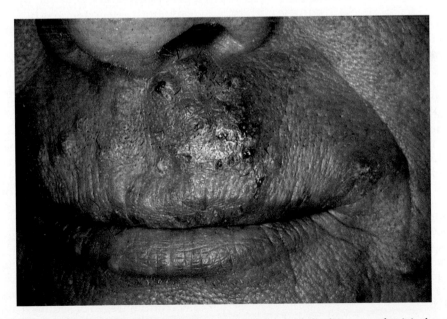

Deep follicular infection. This pattern clinically resembles bacterial folliculitis except that it is slower to evolve and is usually restricted to one area of the beard.

10

Exanthems and Drug Reactions

■ TOXIC SHOCK SYNDROME (TSS)

DESCRIPTION

- Toxic shock syndrome (TSS) is a rare, potentially fatal, multisystem illness associated with *Staphylococcus aureus* infection and the production of toxins (see Box 10-1).
- TSS is characterized by high fever, rash, mucosal erythema, hypotension, and other major organ damage.
- Cases may be menstrual related (MTSS) or non-menstrual related (NMTSS); nonmenstrual cases are frequently observed in children.
- Streptococcal toxic shock syndrome (STSS), caused by group A beta-hemolytic streptococcus, is a similar serious multisystem illness caused by bacterial exotoxins.

HISTORY

- From 50% to 70% of TSS cases occur in women of reproductive age. The onset is within 4 days of menses; there is a higher risk with high-absorbency tampons.
- From 20% to 30% of TSS cases are not menstrual related. High-risk settings include infected burn wounds and bacterial tracheitis (after an infection with influenza B virus). Other settings include surgical and nonsurgical wound infections, abortion, childbirth, and use of nasal packing and contraceptive sponges.
- In STSS, the infectious focus is often the skin or soft tissue; many patients have bacteremia.

SKIN FINDINGS

- In TSS, the early signs are diffuse scarlatiniform erythroderma, edema of the hands and feet (50%),

petechiae (27%), conjunctival injection (85%), oropharyngeal hyperemia (90%), and genital hyperemia (100%). Desquamation of the palms, soles, fingertips, and toes occurs 1 to 2 weeks after the onset.
- One of the signs of STSS is erythroderma with or without bullae.

NONSKIN FINDINGS

- In TSS, vomiting may precede illness. The creatine phosphokinase level may be elevated. Disorientation can occur, as can hypotension, adult respiratory distress syndrome, pulmonary edema, and myocarditis. (See also the section on laboratory.)
- In NMTSS, there is a delayed symptom onset after injury; more frequently, there is involvement of the central nervous system; less frequently, musculoskeletal manifestations occur.

LABORATORY

- In TSS, coagulase-positive staphylococci are cultured from infected sites, not usually blood. Assays for toxin and antibody can be performed.
- Hematologic findings include thrombocytopenia ($<100,000$ platelets/mm^3), left shift, and lymphopenia (<650 cells/mm^3).
- Calcium levels decrease to less than 7.8 mg/dl, albumin levels decrease to less than 3.1 gm/dl, and cholesterol levels decrease to less than 120 mg/dl.
- Bilirubin, serum aspartate transaminase, and serum alanine transaminase levels increase.
- Blood urea nitrogen or serum creatinine levels increase to two times normal; oliguria, pyuria, and proteinuria can also occur.

Box 10-1	Toxic Shock Syndrome Case Definition

Major Criteria (All Four Must Be Met)

Fever: Temperature >38.9° C (102° F)

Rash: Diffuse or palmar erythroderma progressing to subsequent peripheral desquamation (hands and feet)

Mucous membrane: Nonpurulent conjunctival hyperemia, or oropharyngeal hyperemia, or vaginal hyperemia or discharge

Hypotension: Systolic blood pressure (BP) less than 90 mm Hg for an adult (over 16 years of age) or less than 5th percentile for age for a child; or orthostatic hypotension as shown by a drop in diastolic BP greater than 15 mm Hg from recumbent to sitting; or history of orthostatic dizziness

Multisystem Involvement (Three or More Must Be Present)

Gastrointestinal: History of vomiting or diarrhea at onset of illness

Muscular: Creatinine phosphokinase (CPK) more than 2 times the upper limit of normal for laboratory values 4 to 20 days after onset

Central nervous system: Disorientation or alteration in consciousness without focal signs at a time when patient is not in shock or hyperpyrexic

Renal: BUN or serum creatinine clearance levels more than 2 times the upper limit of normal; and abnormal findings on urinalysis (>5 WBCs per HPF; >1 RBC per HPF; protein >1+); or oliguria defined as urine output <1 ml/kg/hr for 24 hr

Hepatic: Total serum bilirubin level greater than 1.5 times the upper limit of normal or SGPT levels more than 2 times the upper limit of normal

Hematologic: Thrombocytopenia (platelet: less than 100,000/mm^3)

Cardiopulmonary: Adult respiratory distress syndrome; or pulmonary edema; or new onset second- or third-degree heart block; or ECG criteria for myocarditis decreased voltage and ST-T wave changes; or heart failure shown by new onset of gallop rhythm, or by increase in size of cardiac silhouette from one chest roentgenogram to another during the course of the illness, or diagnosed by cardiologist

Metabolic: Serum calcium level less than 7.0 mg/dl with serum phosphate level less than 2.5 mg/dl, and total serum protein level less than 5.0 mg/dl

Evidence for Absence of Other Causes

When obtained: Negative blood, throat, urine, or CSF cultures

When obtained: Absence of serologic evidence of leptospirosis, rickettsial disease, or rubeola

Evidence for absence of Kawasaki syndrome; no unilateral lymphadenopathy or fever lasting more than 10 days

From Chesney PJ et al: *JAMA* 246:741, 1981.
CSF, Cerebrospinal fluid; *ECG,* electrocardiogram; *HPF,* high-power field; *RBC,* red blood cells; *SGPT,* serum glutamate pyruvate transaminase; *WBC,* white blood cell.

DIFFERENTIAL DIAGNOSIS

- Drug eruptions
- Kawasaki syndrome
- Scarlet fever
- Staphylococcal scalded skin syndrome
- Toxic epidermal necrolysis
- Viral exanthem

DISCUSSION

- TSS is mediated by five enterotoxins (A to E) and toxic shock syndrome toxin-1 (TSS toxin-1).
- STSS is mediated by toxins A, B, and C.
- The mortality rate is 3.7%. For men, it is 12.2%, and for women, it is 2.6%.

TREATMENT

- In TSS, beta-lactamase-resistant, antimicrobial antibiotics (oxacillin, nafcillin, cefoxitin, vancomycin, clindamycin) are administered intravenously. There is a conversion to oral therapy after resolution of acute illness (usually 3 to 5 days).
- Therapy should last at least 2 weeks. Intravenous fluids and pressers are given as necessary for blood pressure support.
- In STSS, early diagnosis, treatment with antibiotics, and operative débridement are required.

■ CUTANEOUS DRUG REACTIONS

DESCRIPTION

- A common complication of drug therapy, cutaneous drug reactions can occur in many forms and can mimic many dermatoses.

HISTORY

- Cutaneous drug reactions are seen in 2% to 3% of hospitalized patients, most of whom are on multiple medications.
- Fever may occur, and hours later a diffuse maculopapular rash, hives, generalized pruritus, or a combination thereof develop.
- There is no correlation between the development of an adverse reaction and the patient's age, diagnosis, or survival.
- Drugs may be taken for weeks or years without ill effect, but once sensitization occurs, a reaction may occur within minutes to 24 to 48 hours.
- Chemically related drugs may cross-react in a patient sensitized to one agent.
- Two groups of mechanisms are mostly involved: immunologic (with all four types of hypersensitivity reactions described) and nonimmunologic (more common).

Maculopapular Eruptions

- The most frequent of all cutaneous drug reactions, maculopapular eruptions are often indistinguishable from viral exanthems.
- The onset occurs 7 to 10 days after starting the drug but may not occur until after the drug is stopped. The rash lasts 1 to 2 weeks and fades, in some cases even if the drug is continued.
- Maculopapular eruption, red macules, and papules become confluent in a symmetric, generalized distribution that often spares the face. Itching is common. The mucous membranes, palms, and soles may be involved.
- Symptoms are treated with antihistamines and cooling lotions (e.g., Sarna lotion).

Urticarial Drug Reactions

- Aspirin, penicillin, and blood products are the most frequent causes of urticarial drug eruptions, but almost any drug can cause hives.
- Anaphylactic immunoglobulin E–dependent reactions occur within minutes (immediate reactions) to hours (accelerated reactions) of drug administration.

- In circulating immune complex disease (serum sickness), urticaria occurs 4 to 21 days after drug ingestion; hives typically fade in less than 24 hours, only to recur in another area. Once the drug is stopped, this problem resolves over several weeks.
- Nonimmunologic histamine reactions can occur in minutes; the allergenic drug or agent (e.g., morphine, codeine, polymyxin B, lobster, strawberries) may exert a direct action on the mast cell.
- Symptoms are treated with antihistamines and cooling lotions (e.g., Sarna lotion); topical steroids do not help.
- Hospitalization, observation, intubation, and epinephrine all may be called for in severe reactions.

Internal-External Reactions

- The patient first develops a contact dermatitis with a topical agent and subsequently develops either a focal flare or a generalized eruption when exposed orally to the same or chemically related medication.
- Continued use of the medication can intensify the reaction and lead to generalization of the eruption.
- Eczematous internal-external reaction usually presents as areas of redness, particularly in the axillae or groin.
- Topical or oral steroids control these eruptions.

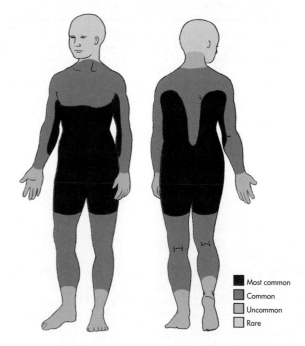

■ Most common
■ Common
□ Uncommon
□ Rare

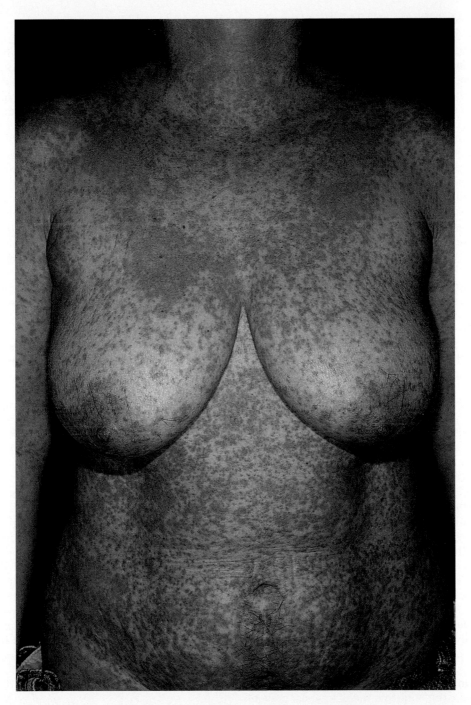

Maculopapular eruption. Maculopapular eruptions are often indistinguishable from viral exanthems. They are the classic ampicillin rashes, but several other drugs also cause this pattern.

Erythema Multiforme and Toxic Epidermal Necrolysis Reactions

- The lesions of erythema multiforme look like targets. Bullae develop in severe forms of the disease.
- These reactions may be limited to the skin or mucous membranes but can be generalized.
- Severe forms are often caused by medications. Less severe forms are caused by mycoplasmal pneumonia, herpes simplex infections, and medication.
- Toxic epidermal necrolysis can be severe and fatal. The cause of death is loss of large areas of skin, resulting in fluid loss and sepsis.
- Severe reactions are best managed in burn or intensive care units.
- The use of oral steroids is controversial.

Exfoliative Erythroderma

- There are generalized redness and desquamation.
- The reaction is potentially life threatening.

Fixed Drug Eruptions

- Single or multiple, round, sharply demarcated, dusky red plaques appear soon after drug exposure and reappear in exactly the same site each time the drug is taken.
- The lesions are generally preceded or accompanied by itching and burning, which may be the only manifestations of reactivation in an old patch.
- The area often blisters and then erodes; desquamation or crusting (after bullous lesions) follows, and brown pigmentation forms with healing.
- Lesions can occur on any part of the skin or mucous membrane, but the glans penis is the most common site. Tetracycline and co-trimoxazole frequently cause lesions on the glans penis.
- The length of time from reexposure to a drug and the onset of symptoms is 30 minutes to 8 hours.
- After each exacerbation, some patients experience a refractory period (weeks to several months) during which the offending drug does not activate the lesions.
- A careful history is important because patients often do not relate their complaints to the use of a drug.
- "Provoking" the appearance of the lesion with the suspected drug confirms the diagnosis, prevents recurrences, and allays the anxiety of the patient regarding a venereal origin of disease.

Drug-Induced Hyperpigmentation

- Drug-induced hyperpigmentation is caused by many different drugs, including antiarrhythmics (amiodarone), antimalarials, antibiotics (minocycline), antivirals (zidovudine), antiseizure agents (hydantoin), chemotherapy agents, heavy metals, hormones, and antipsychotics (chlorpromazine). The discoloration often fades with time (months to years).
- Amiodarone causes a dusky red coloration that with time becomes blue-gray or ashen. This is usually in photodistributed areas.
- Minocycline (Minocin) causes a blue-gray or slate-gray discoloration, often in acne lesions but also on gingiva and perhaps on teeth.
- Zidovudine causes brown longitudinal pigmentation on the nails and a similar brown color on the lips and oral mucosa.
- Antimalarial agents typically cause a brown discoloration on the shins or elsewhere.
- Hydantoin may cause melasma-like brown pigmentation on the face.
- Bleomycin causes a dramatic reaction, causing a flagellate, streaking hyperpigmentation on the trunk and extremities.
- Melasma, associated with oral contraceptive use, is a typical brown pigmentation on the cheeks and central face. The use of a broad-spectrum ultraviolet B and A sun screen is advisable in many of these cases.

Lichenoid Drug Reactions

- The clinical and histologic patterns mimic those of lichen planus.
- The latent period between the beginning of administration of a drug and the eruption is 3 weeks to 3 years.
- There are multiple flat-topped, itchy violaceous papules; oral lesions may be present.
- Lesions heal with brown pigmentation.
- Gold and antimalarial agents are most often associated with drug-induced lichen planus.
- The lesions are chronic and persist for weeks or months after the offending drug is stopped.

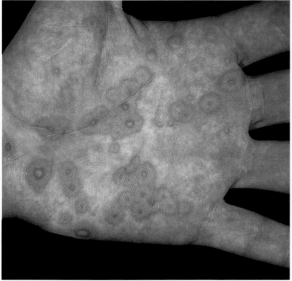

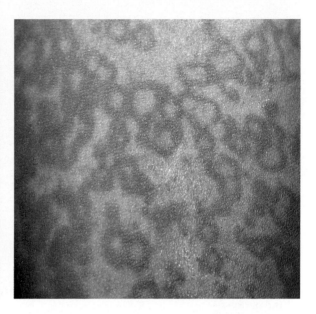

Erythema multiforme. The classic ringlike eruption on the palms.

Urticarial eruption. Drugs are a common cause of hives.

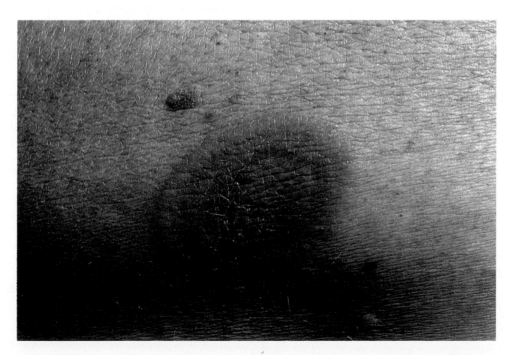

Fixed drug eruption. Single or multiple, round, sharply demarcated, dusky red plaques appear soon after drug exposure and reappear in exactly the same site each time the drug is taken.

Photosensitivity Drug Eruptions

- Both systemic and topical medications can induce photosensitivity.
- There are two main types: phototoxicity and photoallergy.
  - Phototoxic reactions are related to drug concentration and can occur in anyone. They can occur on first administration and subside when the drug is stopped. The eruption is confined to sun-exposed areas. There is erythema within 24 hours of light exposure.
  - Photoallergic reactions are less common and are not concentration related. There is a delay of 48 hours after exposure before the eruption appears. The eruption can spread to non-sun-exposed regions.

Onycholysis

- Onycholysis is separation of the nail plate from the nailbed.
- It may occur from drug photosensitivity and has occurred after the administration of tetracyclines, psoralens, and fluoroquinolones.

Small-Vessel Necrotizing Vasculitis (Palpable Purpura)

- Small-vessel necrotizing vasculitis may be precipitated by drugs.
- Lesions are most often concentrated on the lower legs.
- The kidneys, joints, and brain may be involved.

Chemotherapy-Induced Acral Erythema

- Tingling on the palms and soles is followed in a few days by painful, symmetric, well-defined swelling and erythema.
- The hands are more severely affected than the feet.
- Areas of pallor develop, blister, desquamate, and reepithelialize.
- Chemotherapy-induced acral erythema occurs most commonly after the administration of cytosine arabinoside, fluorouracil, and doxorubicin.
- The reaction is dose dependent, and a direct toxic effect of the drug is likely.

- The time of onset is 24 hours to 10 months, and the severity varies.
- Cytosine arabinoside has a predilection to progress to blisters.
- Treatment is supportive and includes elevation and cold compresses.
- Systemic steroids have been used with variable success.
- Cooling the hands and feet during treatment to decrease blood flow may attenuate the reaction.
- Modification of the dosage schedule may also help.

Gold Rashes

- There are many different forms of gold rashes. The most common is a nonspecific, eczematous, papular, itchy eruption.
- Some 25% of gold rashes resemble lichen planus, but the distribution is atypical.
- A pityriasis rosea–like eruption occurs also.
- The rate of resolution correlates with the extent of the rash and not with the specific morphologic form. The median duration to resolution is 10 weeks. There is no increased risk of developing the rash when gold therapy is resumed.
- Group V topical steroids provide symptomatic relief for gold dermatitis.
- Systemic steroids may be required for severe reactions.

Acute Generalized Exanthematous Pustulosis

- Acute generalized exanthematous pustulosis (AGEP) is a newly described clinical entity. There are multiple tiny, superficial pustules over most of the body.
- The most common drugs are the antibacterial agents (mostly penicillin).
- There is a short interval between drug ingestion and the eruption (mean, 5 days), and resolution occurs in less than 15 days.
- Fever, leukocytosis, and an ill-appearing patient are common.
- Desquamation occurs with no scarring.
- Simple lubrication of the skin along with removal of offending drug is all that is needed.

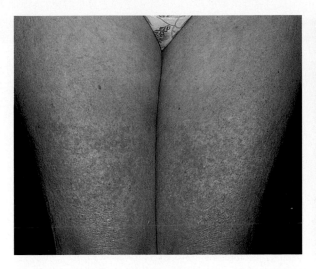

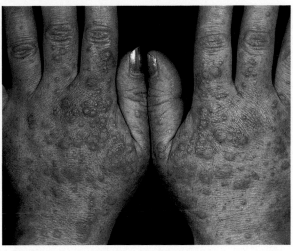

Photosensitivity drug eruption. Erythema and papules occurred on exposed areas in this patient who had been taking a thiazide antihypertensive medication.

Photosensitivity drug eruption. Red papules in a symmetric photodistribution in a patient taking amiodarone.

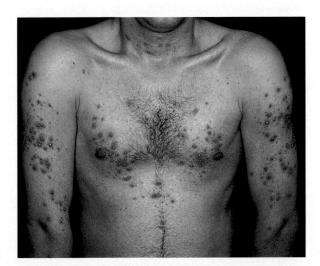

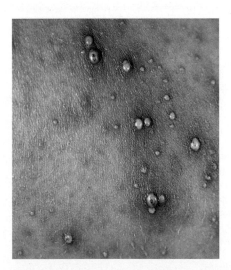

Acute generalized exanthematous pustulosis. Antibiotics, especially beta-lactams and macrolides, are the main culprits.

Acute generalized exanthematous pustulosis. Numerous pustules appeared 5 days after penicillin was started. The medication was stopped, and the pustules cleared spontaneously in 2 weeks.

Box 10-2   Drug Reactions and the Drugs That Cause Them

Maculopapular (Exanthematous) Eruptions

Ampicillin
Barbiturates
Diflunisal (Dolobid)
Gentamicin
Gold salts
Isoniazid
Meclofenamate (Meclomen)
Phenothiazines
Phenylbutazone
Phenytoin
  (5% of children—dose dependent)
Quinidine
Sulfonamides
Thiazides
Thiouracil
Trimethoprim-sulfamethoxazole
  (in patients with acquired immunodeficiency
  syndrome)

Anaphylactic Reactions

Aspirin   Sera (animal derived)
Penicillin   Tolmetin (Tolectin)
Radiographic dye

Serum Sickness

Aspirin   Sulfonamides
Penicillin   Thiouracils
Streptomycin

Acneiform (Pustular) Eruptions

Bromides   Iodides
Hormones   Isoniazid
  Adrenocorticotropic   Lithium
    hormone   Phenobarbital
  Androgens   (aggravates acne)
  Corticosteroids   Phenytoin
  Oral contraceptives

Alopecia

Allopurinol   Indomethacin
Anticoagulants   Levodopa
Antithyroid drugs   Oral contraceptives
Chemotherapeutic agents   Propranolol
  Alkylating agents   Quinacrine
  Antimetabolites   Retinoids
  Cytotoxic agents   Thallium
Colchicine   Vitamin A
Hypocholesteremic drugs

Erythema Nodosum

Iodides
Oral contraceptives
Sulfonamides

Exfoliative Erythroderma

Allopurinol   Hydantoins
Arsenicals   Isoniazid
Barbiturates   Lithium
Captopril   Mercurial diuretics
Cefoxitin   Paraaminosalicylic acid
Chloroquine   Phenylbutazone
Cimetidine   Sulfonamides
Gold salts   Sulfonylureas

Fixed Drug Eruptions

Aspirin   Phenylbutazone
Barbiturates   Sulfonamides
Methaqualone   Tetracyclines
Phenazones   Trimethoprim-
                              sulfamethoxazole
Phenolphthalein   Many others reported

Lichen Planus–Like Eruptions

Antimalarials   Methyldopa
Arsenicals   Penicillamine
Beta-blockers   Quinidine
Captopril   Sulfonylureas
Furosemide   Thiazides
Gold salts

Erythema Multiforme–Like Eruptions

Allopurinol   Penicillin
Barbiturates   Phenolphthalein
Carbamazepine   Phenothiazines
Hydantoins   Rifampin
Minoxidil   Sulfonamides
Nitrofurantoin   Sulfonylureas
Nonsteroidal anti-   Sulindac
  inflammatory agents

Lupus-Like Eruptions

Common   *Probable*
Hydralazine   Acebutolol
Procainamide   Carbamazepine
Uncommon   Ethosuximide
Chlorpromazine   Lithium carbonate
Hydrochlorothiazide   Penicillamine
Isoniazid   Phenytoin
Methyldopa   Propylthiouracil
Quinidine   Sulfasalazine

Photosensitivity

Amiodarone
Carbamazepine
Chlorpropamide
Furosemide
Griseofulvin
Lomefloxacin
Methotrexate
  (sunburn reactivation)
Nalidixic acid
Naproxen
Phenothiazines
Piroxicam (Feldene)
Psoralens
Quinine
Sulfonamides
Tetracyclines
  Demeclocycline
  Doxycycline
    (less frequently with tetracycline and minocycline)
Thiazides
Tolbutamide

Skin Pigmentation

Adrenocorticotropic hormone
  (brown as in Addison's disease)
Amiodarone (slate-gray)
Anticancer drugs
  Bleomycin (30%—brown, patchy, linear)
  Busulphan (diffuse as in Addison's disease)
  Cyclophosphamide (nails)
  Doxorubicin (nails)
Antimalarials (blue-gray or yellow)
Arsenic (diffuse, brown, macular)
Chlorpromazine (slate-gray in sux-exposed areas)
Clofazimine (red)
Heavy metals (silver, gold, bismuth, mercury)
Methysergide maleate (red)
Minocycline (patchy or diffuse blue-black)
Oral contraceptives (chloasma-brown)
Psoralens
Rifampin—very high dose (red man syndrome)

Pityriasis Rosea–Like Eruptions

Arsenicals	Gold compounds
Barbiturates	Methoxypromazine
Bismuth compounds	Metronidazole
Captopril	Pyribenzamine
Clonidine	

Toxic Epidermal Necrolysis

Large areas of skin become bright red, then slough at
  the dermoepidermal border. This is a life-threatening
  reaction
Allopurinol
Phenylbutazone
Phenytoin
Sulfonamides
Sulindac

Small-Vessel Cutaneous Vasculitis

Allopurinol
Diphenylhydantoin
Hydralazine
Penicillin
Piroxicam (Feldene) (Henoch-Schönlein purpura)
Propylthiouracil
Quinidine
Sulfonamides
Thiazides

Vesicles and Blisters

Barbiturates (pressure areas—comatose patients)
Bromides
Captopril (pemphigus-like)
Cephalosporins (pemphigus-like)
Clonidine (cicatricial pemphigoid–like)
Furosemide (phototoxic)
Iodides
Nalidixic acid (phototoxic)
Naproxen (like porphyria cutanea tarda)
Penicillamine (pemphigus foliaceus–like)
Phenazones
Piroxicam (Feldene)
Sulfonamides

Ocular Pemphigoid

Demecarium bromide	Idoxuridine
Echothiophate iodide	Pilocarpine
Epinephrine	Timolol

Chemotherapy-Induced Acral Erythema

Cyclophosphamide
Cytosine arabinoside
Doxorubicin
Fluorouracil
Hydroxyurea
Mercaptopurine
Methotrexate
Mitotane

■ ROSEOLA INFANTUM

DESCRIPTION

- Roseola infantum is caused by human herpesvirus 6.
- The childhood exanthem is characterized by high fever, followed by the sudden appearance of a macular rash.

HISTORY

- The age range is 6 months to 4 years.
- The incubation period is 12 days (range, 5 to 15 days).
- The condition lasts 6 days.
- Prodromal symptoms include a sudden onset of high fever of 103° to 106° F.
- Most children appear to be inappropriately well.
- There is slight anorexia or one or two episodes of vomiting, runny nose, cough, and hepatomegaly.
- Seizures (but more frequently general cerebral irritability) may occur before the eruptive phase.
- Most cases are asymptomatic or present with fever of unknown origin and occur without a rash.

SKIN FINDINGS

- The rash begins as the fever subsides.
- The lesions appear on the trunk and neck.
- Pink, almond-shaped macules remain discrete or become confluent and then fade in a few hours to 2 days without scaling.

NONSKIN FINDINGS

- Mild to moderate lymphadenopathy, usually in the occipital regions, begins at the onset of the febrile period and persists until after the eruption has subsided.

COURSE AND PROGNOSIS

- The high fever is worrisome, but the onset of the characteristic rash is reassuring.
- Roseola is a major cause of visits to the emergency department, febrile seizures, and hospitalizations.

LABORATORY

- Leukocytosis develops at the onset of fever.
- Leukopenia with a granulocytopenia and relative lymphocytosis appears as the temperature increases and persists until the eruption fades.
- Human herpesvirus 6 antibody is present in 90% to 100% of the population over age 2. Seroconversion occurs during the convalescent phase.

DIFFERENTIAL DIAGNOSIS

- Rubella
- Measles
- Drug eruptions

TREATMENT

- The temperature should be controlled.
- The child and parents should receive reassurance.

CAVEAT

- Human herpesvirus 6 infection should be suspected in infants with febrile convulsions, even those without the exanthem.

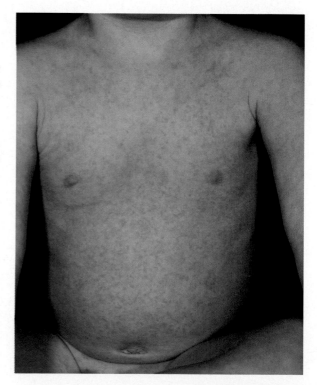

Numerous pale pink, almond-shaped macules.

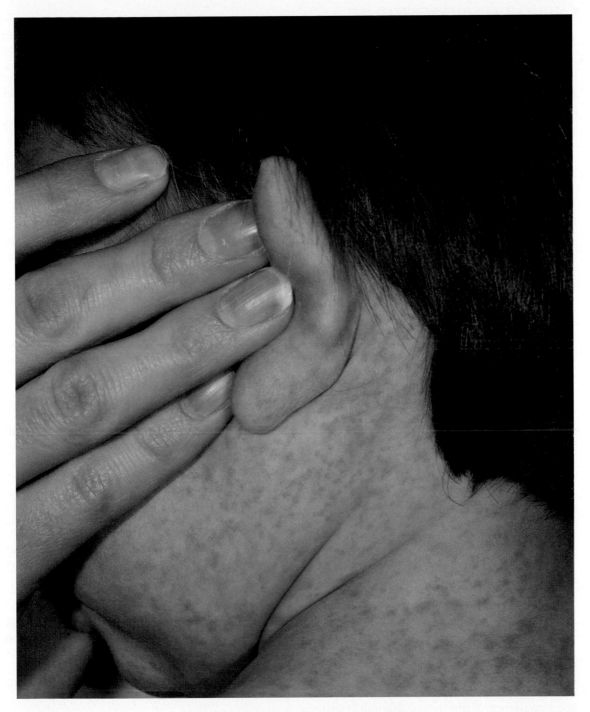

Pale pink macules may first appear on the neck.

■ ERYTHEMA INFECTIOSUM (FIFTH DISEASE)

DESCRIPTION

- Erythema infectiosum is caused by parvovirus B19.
- It is common, is mildly contagious, and appears sporadically or in epidemics.
- Peak attack rates occur in children between 5 and 14 years of age; more than 50% of adults have serologic evidence of past infection. Asymptomatic infection is common.
- Parvovirus B19 infection can cause severe complications in pregnant women.

HISTORY

- The incubation period is 13 to 18 days.
- Prodromal symptoms are usually mild or absent. Pruritus, low-grade fever, malaise, and sore throat precede the eruption in approximately 10% of cases. Lymphadenopathy is absent. Older individuals may complain of joint pain.

SKIN FINDINGS

- There is facial erythema ("slapped-cheek" appearance). Red papules on the cheeks rapidly coalesce in hours, forming red, slightly edematous, warm, erysipelas-like plaques that are symmetric on both cheeks and spare the nasolabial fold and the circumoral region. The slapped-cheek appearance fades in 4 days.
- Erythema in a fishnetlike pattern begins on the extremities approximately 2 days after the onset of facial erythema and extends to the trunk and buttocks, fading in 6 to 14 days.
- In the recurrent phase, the eruption may fade and then reappear in previously affected sites on the face and body during the next 2 to 3 weeks.
- The rash fades without scaling or pigmentation.

NONSKIN FINDINGS

- Arthritis and pruritus occur.

Adults

- Women may develop itching and arthritis. The itching varies from mild to intense and is localized or generalized.
- A nonspecific macular eruption occurs without the appearance of the typical fishnetlike pattern before the arthritis.

- Women develop moderately severe, symmetric polyarthritis that evolves to a form often indistinguishable from rheumatoid arthritis. It lasts 2 weeks to 4 years. Men are not affected.
- It usually starts in the small joints of the hand. In most patients, there is involvement of the knees and other joints as well as migratory arthritis.
- No patients with parvovirus B19 infection develop chronic arthritis.
- Influenza-like symptoms and arthropathies begin with immunoglobulin G antibody production 18 to 24 days after exposure and are probably immune-complex mediated.

Children

- Both boys and girls may develop joint symptoms. Most children briefly experience acute arthritis; a few have arthralgias.
- The large joints are affected more often than the small joints. The knee is the most common joint affected (82%).
- Laboratory findings are normal.
- The duration of joint symptoms is usually less than 4 months, but some have persistent arthritis for 2 to 13 months, which fulfills the criteria for the diagnosis of juvenile rheumatoid arthritis.

Pregnant Women

- In pregnant women, infection can, but usually does not, lead to fetal infection.
- Fetal infection sometimes causes severe anemia, congestive heart failure, generalized edema (fetal hydrops), and death.
- The overall risk of fetal loss after maternal exposure may be less than 3% in the first 20 weeks of gestation.
- Parvovirus B19–associated congenital abnormalities have not been reported among live newborns of infected mothers.

LABORATORY

- Immunoglobulin M antibodies are the most sensitive indicator of acute parvovirus B19 infection in immunologically normal persons and can persist for up to 6 months.
- There may be a slight lymphocytosis or eosinophilia.

- A pregnant woman's immune status should be evaluated. If she is already immune (immunoglobulin G positive), there is no risk. Fetal surveillance by repeated ultrasonographic examination and immune status reevaluation is recommended for pregnant women at risk of infection.

DIFFERENTIAL DIAGNOSIS

- Diagnosis is difficult when the classic features are not present.
- This infection should be considered in the differential diagnosis of early rheumatoid arthritis.

TREATMENT

- Patients should be assured that this unusual eruption will fade and does not require treatment.
- Most health departments do not recommend exclusion from school for children with fifth disease.
- If a fetus is affected, intrauterine evaluation and treatment are available at tertiary care centers.

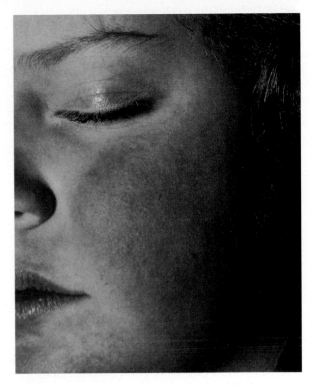

Facial erythema "slapped cheek." The red plaque covers the cheek and spares the nasolabial fold and the circumoral region.

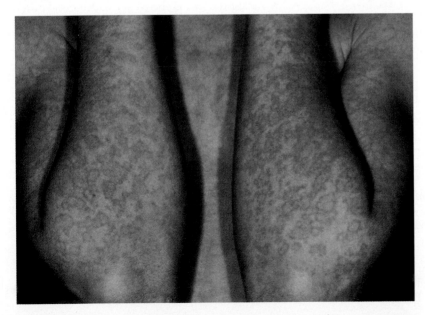

Netlike pattern of erythema.

■ KAWASAKI DISEASE (MUCOCUTANEOUS LYMPH NODE SYNDROME)

DESCRIPTION

- Children have a high fever for 1 to 2 weeks, rashes, and edema of the extremities that is painful and interferes with walking. They are extremely irritable.
- Kawasaki disease was first described in Japan in 1967.
- There is an acute multisystem vasculitis of unknown etiology.
- The major causes of short- and long-term morbidity are the cardiovascular manifestations.
- Vasculitis involving the arterioles, capillaries, and venules appear in the earliest phase of the disease.
- An infectious agent is strongly suggested.
- This condition occurs in both endemic and epidemic forms worldwide.
- Ages range from 7 weeks to 12 years (mean, 2.6 years); adult cases are rarely reported.
- Recurrences are rare.

CLINICAL PRESENTATION

Fever

- Fever without chills or sweats is a constant feature; it lasts 5 to 30 days (mean, 8.5 days).
- The fever begins abruptly and spikes from 101° to 104° F and does not respond to antibiotics or antipyretics.

Conjunctival Injection

- Bilateral congestion of the bulbar and sometimes the palpebral conjunctivae is an almost constant feature.
- Uveitis occurs in 70% of cases.
- There is no discharge or ulceration.

Changes in the Oral Mucous Membrane

- The lips and oral pharynx become red 1 to 3 days after the onset of the fever.
- The lips become dry, fissured, cracked, and crusted.
- Hypertrophic tongue papillae result in the "strawberry tongue" typically seen in scarlet fever.
- Cough occurs in 25% of patients.

Extremity Changes

- Within 3 days of the onset of fever, the palms and soles become red, and the hands and feet become edematous (nonpitting). The tenderness can be severe enough to limit walking and use of the hands. The edema lasts for approximately 1 week.
- Peeling of the hands and feet occurs 10 to 14 days after the onset of fever. The skin peels off in sheets, beginning about the nails and fingertips and progressing down to the palms and soles.
  - Beau's lines appear in the nails weeks later.

Rash

- A rash appears soon after the onset of fever.
- Several symptoms have been described. An urticarial eruption and a diffuse, deep red, maculopapular eruption are the most common.
- Dermatitis in the diaper area is common and occurs in the first week. Red macules and papules become confluent. Desquamation occurs within 5 to 7 days.
- In children with inflammation of the diaper area, the skin peels at the margins of the rash and on the labia and scrotum.
- Perineal desquamation occurs 2 to 6 days before desquamation of the fingertips and toes.

Cervical Lymphadenopathy

- Firm, nontender, nonsuppurative lymphadenopathy is often limited to a single node and occurs in 50% of patients.

Cardiac Involvement

- Kawasaki disease is the major cause of acquired heart disease in children in the United States. Clinical cardiac involvement occurs in 16.3% of patients.
- In the acute phase, myocarditis with tachycardia and gallop rhythms is seen in more than 50% of patients.
- In the subacute phase, aneurysm formation in medium-sized arteries, particularly the coronary arteries, is found in about a fourth of patients; these lesions may persist, scar with stenosis, or resolve angiographically. Aneurysms and thrombi form between 12 and 25 days after the onset and may result in congestive heart failure, pericardial effusions, arrhythmias, and death from myocardial ischemia or aneurysmal rupture.
- The abnormalities peak in the third week and often resolve thereafter.
- The prevalence of cardiac sequelae is high in male patients, infants younger than 1 year of age, and children older than 5 years of age.

- Boys younger than age 1 year who have prolonged fever, elevated platelet counts, and high erythrocyte sedimentation rates are at greatest risk for coronary involvement.

LABORATORY

- No diagnostic test exists.
- The acute phase is characterized leukocytosis (20,000 to 30,000 cells/mm^3) with a left shift (80%), thrombocytosis, and anemia.
- The erythrocyte sedimentation rate (90%), C-reactive protein levels, and serum alpha1-antitrypsin levels are elevated with the onset of fever and persist for up to 10 weeks.

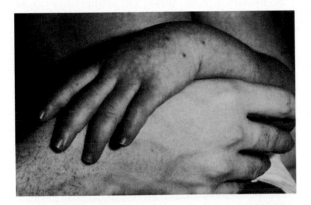

The hands become red and swollen. (*Courtesy Nancy B. Esterly, M.D.*)

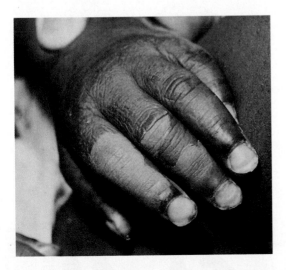

The hands peel approximately 2 weeks after the onset of fever. (*Courtesy Nancy B. Esterly, M.D.*)

- The platelet count begins to rise on the tenth day of the illness, peaks at 600,000 to 1.6 million cells/mm^3, and returns to normal by the thirtieth day.

TREATMENT

- Intravenous gamma-globulin (IVGG), 200 or 400 mg/kg/day for 2 to 5 consecutive days, and aspirin are the treatments of choice.
- Prednisolone, 2 mg/kg/day for 1 week followed by tapering over 2 weeks, may be indicated in some patients during the acute phase.
- Coronary artery aneurysms or ectasia develop in approximately 15% to 25% of children. Treatment with IVGG, in the acute phase reduces this risk threefold to fivefold.
- A total of 1 to 3 days of pulsed doses of methylprednisolone or the readministration of IVGG has been recommended for patients with IVGG-resistant disease.

COURSE AND PROGNOSIS

- The worst prognosis occurs in children with so-called giant aneurysms (i.e., those with a maximum diameter >8 mm).
- Almost 10% of children do not improve clinically with treatment.

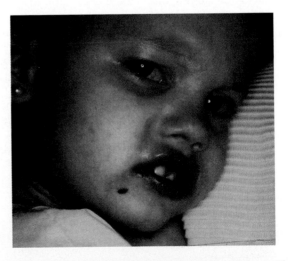

Nonpurulent conjunctival injection and "cherry red" lips with fissuring and crusting are early signs of the disease. (*Courtesy Anne W. Lucky, M.D.*)

11

Infestations and Bites

■ SCABIES

DESCRIPTION

- Scabies is an intensely pruritic contagious disease.
- It is caused by the mite *Sarcoptes scabiei* var *hominis*.

HISTORY

- Itching is worse at night.
- In untreated scabies, there is unremitting itching.
- Ultimately, others in the household become infected.
- In treated scabies, the itch subsides over a month or more.
- Nodular lesions take longest to heal.
- Crusted scabies (thousands to millions of mites) may be the source of epidemic scabies.
- Persistent itching after treatment is due to reinfestation or inadequate treatment.

SKIN FINDINGS

- A burrow is the classic lesion; it is linear, curved, or S-shaped; 1 to 2 mm wide; up to 15 mm long; pink-white; and slightly elevated.
- Typical locations are the wrists, web space of the hands, sides of hands and feet, genital area, warm intertriginous regions, and abdomen.
- In infants, the scalp, palms, and soles are affected; pustules may be seen.

- Secondary lesions (most common) have an eczematous reaction pattern with many excoriations.
- In the secondary infection, there is a honey-colored crust of impetigo.
- Nodules occur on the buttocks, genitals, or axillae; they last for weeks even after adequate therapy.
- A unique clinical variant is crusted (Norwegian) scabies. Patients, usually those with senile dementia, Down syndrome, and immunosuppression, experience asymptomatic crusting and eczematous dermatitis, especially on the hands and feet. Numerous mites are present.

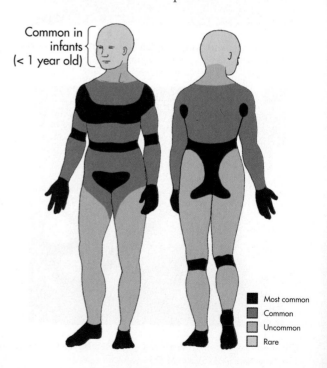

Common in infants (< 1 year old)

Most common
Common
Uncommon
Rare

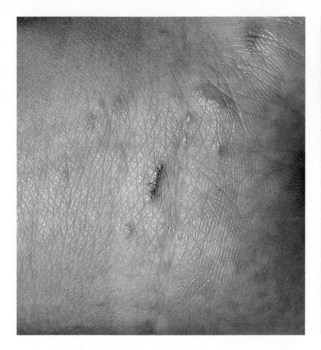

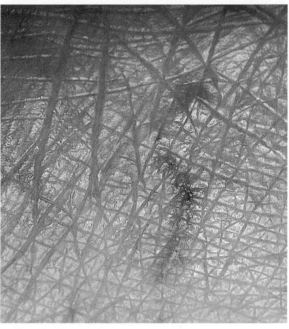

Burrow. Burrows are most likely to be found in the finger webs, wrists, sides of the hands and feet, penis, buttocks, scrotum, and the palms and soles of infants.

Burrow. The linear, curved, or S-shaped burrows are approximately as wide as #2 suture material and are 2 to 15 mm long. A drop of ink can accentuate them.

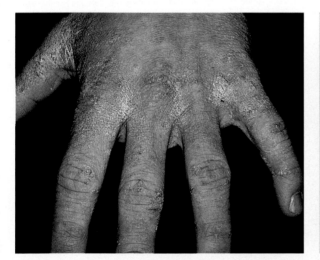

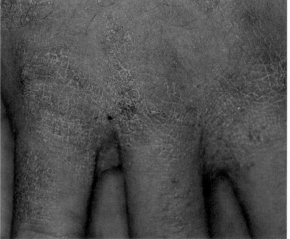

Vesicles and papules. Vesicles are isolated, pinpoint, and filled with serous rather than purulent fluid. The fact that they remain discrete is a key point in differentiating scabies from other vesicular diseases such as poison ivy.

Secondary lesions result from infection or are caused by scratching. Scaling, erythema, and all stages of eczematous inflammation occur as a response to excoriation or to irritation caused by overzealous attempts at self-medication.

LABORATORY

- Mites, eggs, or feces should be identified.
- Mineral oil is applied to a burrow, vesicle, or papule to preserve the mite feces. The burrow is scraped with a #15 blade and applied to a slide. A coverslip is set in place.
- The mites can also be seen in a potassium hydroxide or saline wet-mount preparation.

DIFFERENTIAL DIAGNOSIS

- Insect bites
- Eczema
- Impetigo

TREATMENT

- Permethrin (Elimite, Acticin) is applied to the entire skin surface below the neck, including under the fingernails and toenails, and in the umbilicus. The head and neck may need treatment in children. This regimen is repeated in 1 week. Pretreatment with a hot bath or shower is not needed. This is the best treatment for children younger than 2 years of age.

- All clothes and bed clothes must be washed the morning after the application.
- Lindane (Kwell) lotion is safe when used as directed. It is applied with the same technique and frequency as permethrin but may be less effective.
- There is no need for fumigation or extermination of the house.
- A single dose of oral ivermectin (Stromectol, 6-mg scored tablet) (200 µg/kg) is effective and may soon become a standard therapy. Repeating the dose 2 weeks later may provide a higher cure rate.
- Group V topical steroids may be used to control inflammation after treatment with a scabicide.
- Itching is controlled with lotions (e.g., Sarna lotion) and antihistamines.
- Persistent nodular lesions are treated with intralesional steroids.
- Oral or topical antibiotics (mupirocin [Bactroban]) are used for secondary infection.

CAVEAT

- Scabies should be considered for any generalized itchy eruption unresponsive to prednisone.

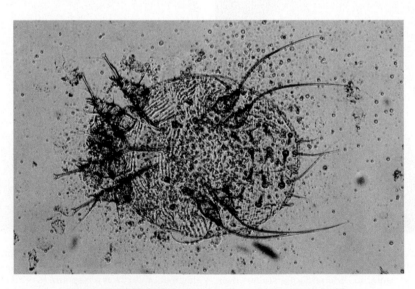

Sarcoptes scabiei in a potassium hydroxide wet mount (×40).

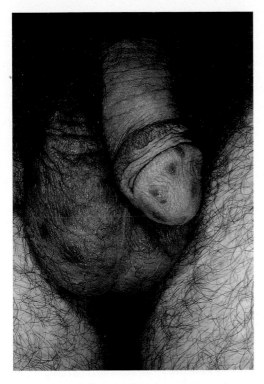

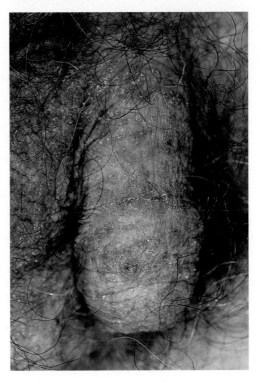

Secondary lesions. Nodules occur in covered areas such as the buttocks, groin, scrotum, penis, and axillae. Nodules on the penis and scrotum are highly characteristic of scabies.

Secondary lesions dominate the clinical picture in this case. Pustules, scaling, and erythema, accompany this heavy infestation of mites.

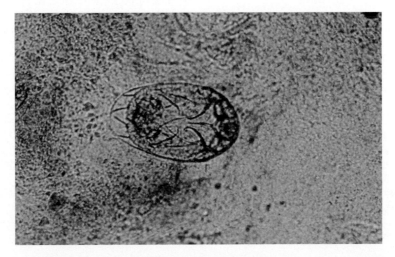

Sarcoptes scabiei. Egg containing mites. A potassium hydroxide wet mount (×40).

■ LICE (PEDICULOSIS)

DESCRIPTION

- An infestation by *Pediculus humanus* var *capitis* is head lice.
- An infestation by *Phthirus pubis* is pubic lice (see p. 144).
- An infestation by *Pediculosis corporis* is also called *body lice.*
- Pruritic bumps appear on the nape of the neck.
- Nits (eggs) attach to the hair shaft.

HEAD LICE

- Lice appear in the scalp hair, typically in children.
- Lice infestation is highly contagious.
- Direct contact is the primary source of transmission.
- Lice are obligate human parasites; they cannot survive on other animals.
- The head louse does not carry any human disease.
- Lice suck blood every 3 to 6 hours.
- Lice live for 1 month, and females lay 7 to 10 eggs a day.
- Eggs (nits) are cemented to the shaft 1 cm from the scalp surface.
- Nits hatch in 8 to 10 days.
- Additional information can be found at the website for the National Pediculosis Association (www.headlice.org).

HISTORY

- Lice infestation is typically diagnosed by the school nurse.
- Girls are affected more than boys.
- Fomite transmission is common (hats, brushes, earphones).
- Infestation is rare in African-Americans.
- No symptoms appear, or there is only itching at the nape of the neck.
- Posterior cervical adenopathy is occasionally noted.

SKIN FINDINGS

- The nits are firmly cemented to the hair.
- Pruritic papules appear on the neck.
- Honey-colored crusting and secondary adenopathy occur if the papules become infected.
- Infestation may occur rarely in the eyelashes.

DIFFERENTIAL DIAGNOSIS

- Seborrheic dermatitis (Dandruff scales are not firmly attached but can easily slip up and down the hair shaft.)

TREATMENT

- Strains resistant to synergized pyrethrins (e.g., permethrin 1% [Nix], permethrin 5% [Elimite]) have emerged.
- All agents attack the louse's nervous system; young nits are not affected.
- The use of all agents should be repeated in 1 week.
- Fomite control is essential.

Standard Therapies

- Permethrin rinse 1% (Nix creme rinse), an over-the-counter (OTC) preparation, is often the drug of first choice.
- Synergized pyrethrin shampoos (RID, A-200, R & C) can be purchased OTC.
- Pyrethrin liquids (TISIT, Pyrinyl, Barc) are available OTC.
- Permethrin 5% (Elimite) is administered for treatment failures. It is left on the hair overnight under a shower cap.
- Lindane (Kwell) shampoo is left in for 5 minutes and then washed out; treatment is repeated in 1 week. It is used if OTC treatment fails. Lindane-resistant lice have emerged.
- Malathion lotion 0.5% (Ovide) is rapidly pediculicidal and ovidicidal. It is useful for the treatment of head lice resistant to pyrethrins and permethrin. The lotion is applied for 8 to 12 hours; it should be applied 7 to 9 days later if necessary.

Alternative Therapies ("Home Remedies")

- Petrolatum (Vaseline), mayonnaise (not the nonfat kind), or pomades applied to scalp overnight under a shower cap smother lice. These are difficult to remove, however. (Shampooing with Dawn dishwashing liquid should be tried.) Copious amounts must be used to smother all lice. This treatment does not kill nits, so it should be repeated each week for 4 weeks.
- HairClear 1-2-3 hair gel is an oil that kills lice in 20 minutes.
- As a last resort, the head is shaved.

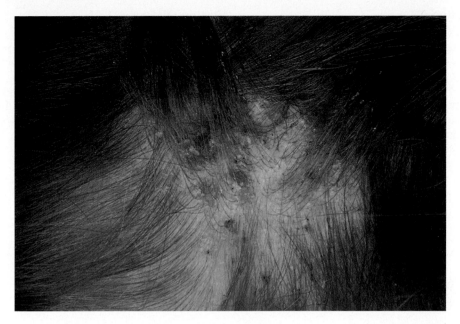

Pediculosis capitis.

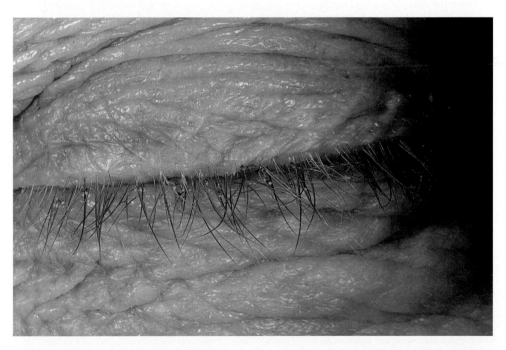

Eyelash infestation. Infestation of the eyelashes is seen almost exclusively in children. It may induce blepharitis with lid pruritus, scaling, crusting, and purulent discharge. Eyelash infestation may be a sign of childhood sexual abuse.

Oral Medication

- Ivermectin (Stromectol, 6-mg scored tablet), 200 μg/kg, is prescribed in a single oral dose and is repeated in 10 days. It attacks invertebrate nerve and muscle cells and causes paralysis and death. It has selective activity against parasites but no systemic effects on mammals.
- Trimethoprim-sulfamethoxazole (Bactrim, Septra) kills synergistic bacteria in lice. A prolonged course may be necessary. There are no studies documenting its efficacy.
- Antibiotics are administered for secondary infection.

Nit Removal

- It is important to remove nits.
- LiceMeister comb (1-888-542-3634 or www.lice-meister.org) can be used to more effectively comb lice from the hair.
- Clear lice egg–remover gel is applied to the hair and combed with a plastic comb (included).
- Hair saturated with a solution of 50% vinegar and 50% water, applied and removed in 15 minutes, may help "unglue" nits.

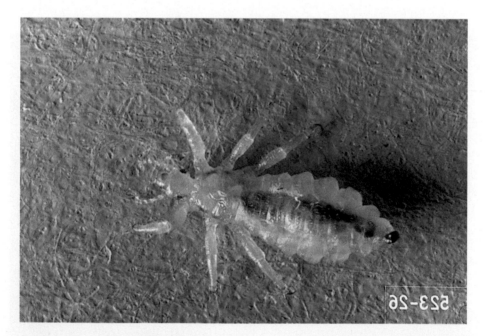

Three kinds of lice infest humans. All three have similar anatomic characteristics. Each is a small (less than 2 mm), flat, wingless insect with three pairs of legs located on the anterior part of the body directly behind the head. The legs terminate in sharp claws that are adapted for feeding and permit the louse to grasp and hold firmly on to hair or clothing. The body louse is the largest and is similar in shape to the head louse.

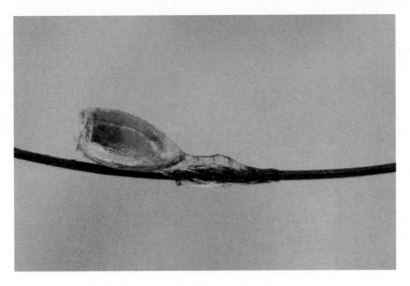

The louse egg (nit) is cemented to a hair shaft.

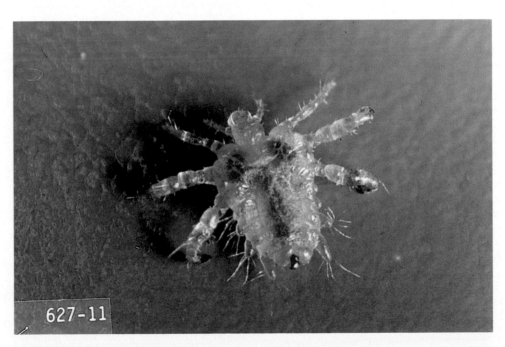

Pthirus pubis (pubic or crab louse). The crab louse is the smallest louse, with a short, oval body and prominent claws resembling those of sea crabs.

■ MYIASIS

DESCRIPTION

- Myiasis is an infestation of the body tissues of animals or humans by the larval stage of nonbiting flies.

HISTORY

- There are two main types of skin invaders: *Dermatobia hominis* (human botfly infestation) and *Tunga penetrans* (tungiasis).
- The human botfly infestation is seen in travelers returning from Central and South America, whereas tungiasis is seen in those returning from Africa.
- Fly larvae are deposited on the skin and penetrate to the subcutaneous tissue, where they mature into maggots.
- The larva is alive in an erythematous papule that resembles an insect bite.
- Within the papule is a central punctum consisting of the larva's breathing tube.
- The time to maturation is species specific.
- Pain is created by the inflammation.
- Many patients report a moving sensation within the skin.
- At maturation, the larva exits the body and drops to the ground and matures into an adult fly.

SKIN FINDINGS

- The red papule is 2 to 4 mm in diameter.
- A furuncle forms as the larva matures. This inflamed, cystlike structure is known as a *warble*.
- Close inspection shows the maggot moving up and down, with its head and respiratory apparatus (spiracles) appearing at the surface about once a minute.
- Serous or seropurulent material can be discharged from the opening.
- In tungiasis, an inflammatory papule is usually located in the web space of the toes. This is followed by an intensely painful furuncle.

LABORATORY

- After extraction, the botfly larva appears as a juicy larva with spiracles (breathing apparatus) at one end.

TREATMENT

- Larvae require oxygen. The human botfly larva can be forced to the surface by the application of petroleum jelly (Vaseline) or bacon fat over the opening. The larva is smothered and enters the greasy trap while coming up for air. Larvae can be removed with forceps, often within 3 hours after application.
- Another technique is to inject lidocaine below the larva. The pressure forces it out of the orifice.
- On occasion the opening needs to be enlarged with a #11 blade. There is just one maggot in each lesion.
- In tungiasis, the maggot needs to be excised, so the application of petroleum jelly or bacon fat does not help.
- A topical formulation containing ivermectin 1% in propylene glycol (pharmacist compounded) directly applied to the area with a syringe and covered with a dry dressing for 2 hours is reported to be highly effective.

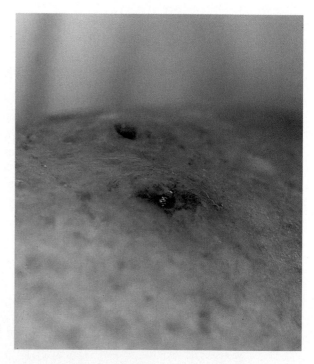

The lesion resembles a furuncle or inflamed cyst. The head of the larva rises to the surface for air about once a minute through a small central pore. Movement of the larval spiracle (respiratory apparatus) may be observed.

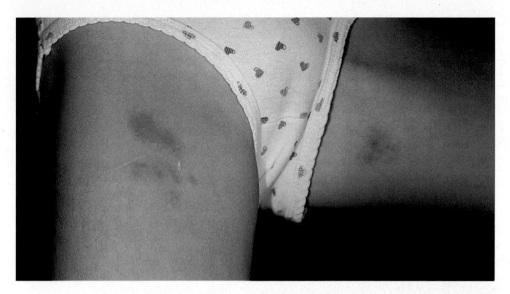

Myiasis. Lesions are found on the face, scalp, chest, arms, or legs. A red papule 2 to 4 mm in diameter develops. An intense inflammatory reaction occurs in the tissue surrounding the larvae.

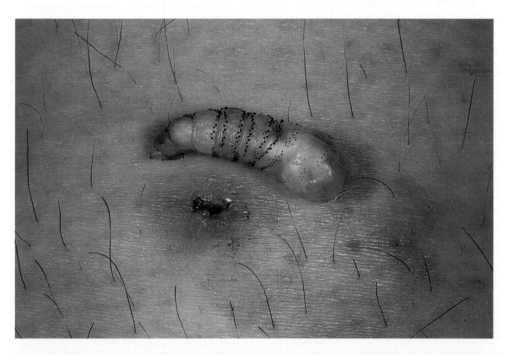

It is usually not necessary to enlarge the hole, but in this case, a #11 surgical blade was used to enlarge the hole so that this very large maggot could be extracted with forceps. Xylocaine was injected into the cavity to aid in the extraction.

■ BEE AND WASP STINGS

DESCRIPTION

- Honey bees are the most common source of insect stings.
- A honey bee stinger separates from the bee's abdomen when stinging and remains embedded in vertebrate tissue. Stingers of other bees and wasps do not detach. The detached stinger is a useful diagnostic feature for distinguishing honey bee stings from the stings of other bees and wasps. Accurate identification of the Hymenoptera is critical to an allergy evaluation.

HISTORY

- The initial sharp or painful sting lasts a few minutes and is followed by moderate burning. Symptoms resolve in a few days.
- Most reactions in children are mild.
- Children with deeper dermal reactions still have a benign course and are unlikely to have recurrent reactions.
- Severe reactions are more common in adults.
- Localized or systemic allergic reaction may develop.
- Patients sensitized by prior stings may develop large, local reactions, with edematous swelling forming hours after the sting and resolving in a few days. Edema is more prominent with head and neck stings.
- A toxic systemic reaction may develop hours after the sting. Vomiting, diarrhea, headache, fever, muscle spasm, and loss of consciousness can occur.
- Allergic anaphylactic reactions involve itching, hives, shortness of breath, wheezing, nausea, and abdominal cramps. They occur within minutes to an hour after the sting.
- Most fatal bee and wasp stings occur in a hypersensitive person older than 40 years of age and who has received a single sting on the head or neck. Deaths are caused by respiratory dysfunction or anaphylaxis.
- Delayed-onset allergic symptoms (up to a week after the sting) range from anaphylaxis to serum sickness.

SKIN FINDINGS

- A raised white wheal with a central red spot appears minutes after the sting and lasts for about 20 minutes.
- A local reaction and hives appear with thick, hard swelling (angioedema) as large as 10 to 50 cm or more.

Multiple Stings

- Large numbers of stings can cause death in nonallergic people.
- The median lethal dose of bee venom is estimated to be 500 to 1500 stings.
- Humans have survived more than 1000 stings.

DIFFERENTIAL DIAGNOSIS

- Hives
- Angioedema
- Bites from other insects

TREATMENT

- The stinger must be removed as fast as possible. The degree of envenomation does not differ if the stinger is scraped or pinched off. Delays of a few seconds in removing the stinger leads to greater venom delivery.
- Localized nonallergic reactions are treated with ice.
- Localized allergic reactions are treated with cool, wet compresses and oral antihistamines.
- Severe generalized reactions are treated with aqueous epinephrine 1:1000 (0.3 to 0.5 ml subcutaneously). This is repeated once or twice at 20-minute intervals if needed.
- If the patient is hypotensive, an intravenous 1:10,000 dilution of epinephrine is administered.
- Preloaded epinephrine syringes kits (e.g., EpiPen Auto-Injector, Anakit) are available.
- An antihistamine (e.g., Benadryl), 25 to 50 mg, is administered orally or intramuscularly.
- Venom immunotherapy is highly effective for those with systemic reactions.

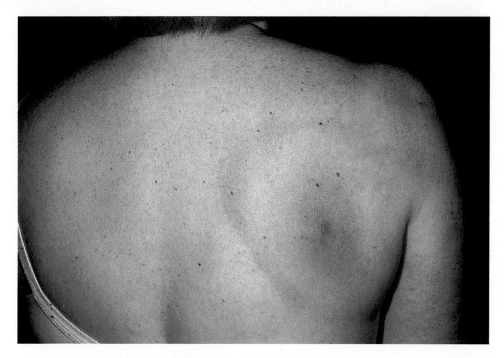

A large local allergic reaction larger than 10 cm in diameter.

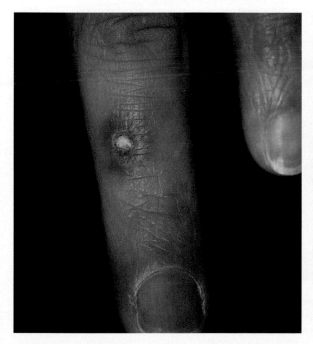

Severe local reaction with necrosis and ulceration at the site of a bee sting.

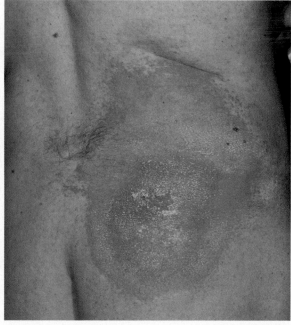

Huge urticarial plaque in a patient with a known history of bee sting allergy.

■ BLACK WIDOW SPIDER BITE

DESCRIPTION

- The adult female spider *(Latrodectus mactans)* is about 4 cm in length and has a shiny, fat abdomen that looks like a big black grape, with the longest legs extending out in front.
- The black widow spider has a red hourglass marking on the ventral surface of her globular abdomen.
- This spider is not aggressive but spins a web and waits for her prey.
- The web makes a crackling sound when it is torn apart.
- *Latrodectus mactans* is found from the South to southern New England, but related widow spiders are found in other areas of the United States and around the world.
- Systemic disease is due to the envenomations of a neurotoxin.
- The protein component of venom (alpha-latrotoxin) causes acetylcholine depletion at motor nerve endings and catecholamine release at adrenergic nerve endings.

HISTORY

- Humans encounter the spider in her web, which is located in protected areas such as under a log, in the crevice of a barn, or in a lumber pile.
- The initial bite reaction may be asymptomatic or mildly painful.
- Abdominal pain (100%), hypertension (92%), muscle complaints (75%), a target lesion (75%), and irritability or agitation (66%) are the most common symptoms.
- Migratory muscle cramps and spasm, headache, nausea, vomiting, hypertension, weakness, tremors, paresthesias, and ultimately paralysis may occur.
- Cramping abdominal pain is common and is the classic presenting complaint; it mimics an acute abdomen and occurs minutes to hours after the bite.
- All symptoms are collectively known as *latrodectism.*
- Symptoms may increase in severity for up to 24 hours and then slowly subside over 2 to 7 days.

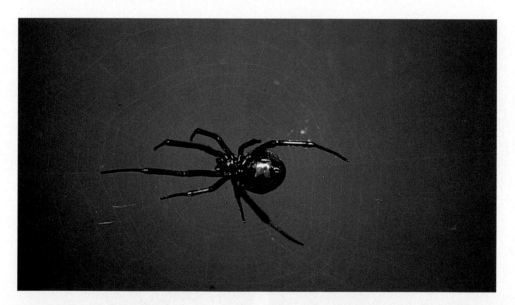

Adult females have a total length of 4 cm and are the only spiders capable of envenomation. The female has a smooth, black body; a globose abdomen that resembles an old-fashioned shoe button; long, slender legs; and a red hourglass marking on the underside of the abdomen. Black widow spiders place their webs close to the ground in protected places near logs and in dark, sheltered areas such as crevices in old barns, lumber piles, and privies. They usually do not bite when away from the web because they are clumsy and need the web for support.

- Residual weakness, tingling, nervousness, and muscle spasms may persist for weeks to months.
- In the young and elderly, convulsion, paralysis, and shock may occur. Death is rare.

SKIN FINDINGS

- Mild erythema or swelling occurs at the bite site.
- Red fang mark may be seen.
- The nodes draining the bite site may become painful and enlarged.

DIFFERENTIAL DIAGNOSIS

- Brown recluse spider bite
- Acute abdomen

TREATMENT

- Ice is applied to restrict the spread of venom.
- Antivenin *(Latrodectus mactans)* for acute symptoms is given intramuscularly or intravenously. It may also be useful days after a bite for patients with persistent symptoms (e.g., weakness, muscle cramping, orthostatic tachycardia, increased blood pressure). The severity of symptoms abates within 3 hours after treatment. Occasionally, re-treatment is indicated.
- Calcium gluconate, given intravenously for acute abdomen, acts as a muscle relaxant.
- Pain is relieved with intravenous opioids and benzodiazepines.
- Muscle relaxants (diazepam [Valium], methocarbamol [Robaxin]) may help.

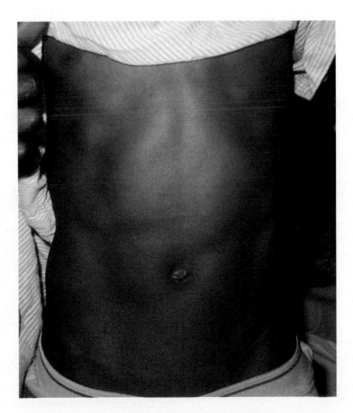

Latrodectism after a black widow spider bite.

■ BROWN RECLUSE SPIDER BITE

DESCRIPTION

- The bite of the brown recluse spider (*Loxosceles reclusa*) may cause necrotic arachnidism.
- The spider is identified by a dark brown, violin-shaped marking on its cephalothorax (fiddleback spider). Its color is yellow-tan to brown.
- The body length is 10 to 15 mm, and the leg span is about 25 mm.
- The brown recluse spider is a shy, nocturnal, nonaggressive arachnid.
- It lives in dark areas such as woodpiles, under rocks, or in dark corners of attics, garages, or basements.
- Most are located in the south central United States.

HISTORY

- Humans come in contact with the spider accidentally.
- Many bites are painless and go unnoticed.
- Localized pain, burning, and stinging occur at the bite site.
- Systemic symptoms, including fever, chills, nausea, vomiting, weakness, and joint and muscle pain, are uncommon; they occur 12 to 24 hours after the bite.
- A bite is associated with rashes that look like hives or measles.
- Death rarely occurs; most patients respond well to treatment.

SKIN FINDINGS

- The bite site may show localized reaction with minimal redness and swelling. Sphingomyelinase D is the toxin responsible for the necrosis.
- Some 10% of cases develop significant necrosis. A cyanotic color, followed by expanding necrosis of the skin, develops at the bite site. The most severe reaction occurs in fatty areas such as the thighs, abdomen, and buttocks. The necrosis can be deep and ultimately leaves an ulcer that takes weeks to months to heal.

DIFFERENTIAL DIAGNOSIS

- Ecthyma gangrenosum
- Necrotizing vasculitis
- Necrotizing fasciitis
- Pyoderma gangrenosum

TREATMENT

- The majority of bites heal with supportive care alone.
- For localized reactions, the patient should rest, ice and cold compresses should be applied, mild analgesics should be administered, and the bite site should be elevated. Heat and strenuous exercise should be avoided.
- Immediate surgical excision of bite sites is not routinely performed and may lead to more complications.
- Necrotic skin needs local wound and ulcer care.
- Antibiotics and tetanus toxoid are given when indicated.
- Dapsone, 50 to 100 mg/day orally, may be helpful in preventing severe necrosis.
- Prednisone, 1 mg/kg/day, may be prescribed if the necrotic area is larger than 2 cm. Treatment lasts for 2 to 3 weeks.
- An antivenin is being developed.
- Hyperbaric oxygen treatment within 48 hours has been reported to be effective for necrotic lesions.

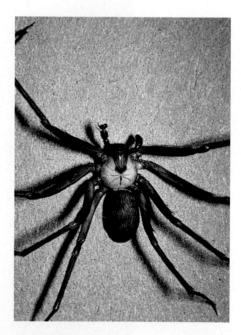

The brown recluse spider, *Loxosceles reclusa* ("fiddle-back spider"), is small, approximately 1.5 cm in overall length. Its color ranges from yellow-tan to dark brown.

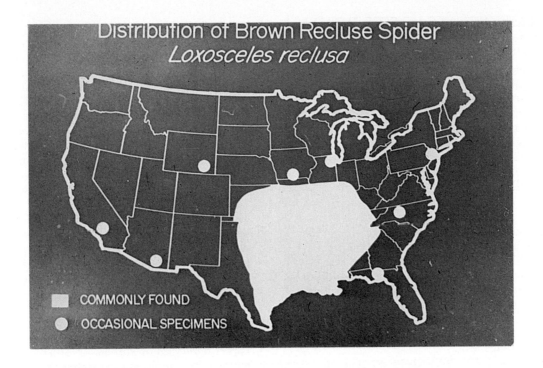

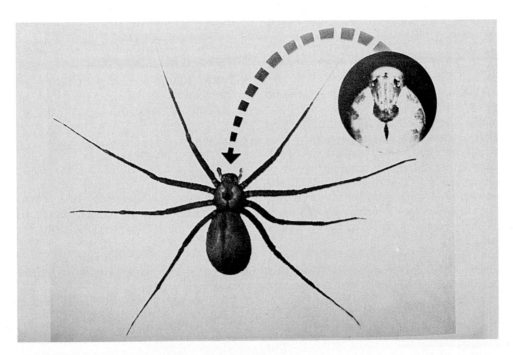

A characteristic, dark, violin- or fiddle-shaped marking is located on the spider's back. The broad base of the violin is near the head and the violin stem points toward the abdomen.

■ LYME DISEASE WITH ERYTHEMA MIGRANS

DESCRIPTION

- Lyme disease with erythema migrans is a three-stage tick-borne disease.
- It is due to the spirochete *Borrelia burgdorferi*.
- There is a marked potential for overdiagnosis of Lyme disease. A different disorder was diagnosed in 80% of cases initially diagnosed as Lyme disease.

HISTORY

- Like syphilis, Lyme disease with erythema migrans affects many systems; it occurs in stages and mimics other diseases.
- It begins 3 to 21 days after a tick bite.
- The three stages overlap or occur alone.
  - In stage 1, an expanding skin lesion (erythema migrans) and influenza-like symptoms (malaise, fatigue, fever up to 105° F, headache, stiff neck, myalgias, arthralgias) occur.
  - In stage 2, there are cardiac and neurologic diseases.
  - In stage 3, arthritis and chronic neurologic syndromes appear.
- Symptoms may intensify 24 hours after treatment.

SKIN FINDINGS

- The initial tick bite inflicts a local reaction: pain, erythema, and a papule.
- Secondary adenopathy may occur after a bite on the scalp.
- Skin lesions, erythema migrans being the most characteristic, are not present in all cases.
- Erythema migrans involves a spontaneously healing erythematous lesion occurring at the site of *Borrelia* inoculation. It begins as a small papule with a slowly enlarging ring; central erythema gradually fades, leaving a normal to light blue surface. The ring remains flat, blanches with pressure, and does not desquamate, vesiculate, or have scale at the periphery, like tinea.
- The erythema migrans border may be slightly raised. It enlarges to form a broad, round to oval area of erythema measuring 5 to 10 cm. The border advances for days or weeks.
- Some 20% to 50% of patients have multiple concentric rings at sites of subsequent hematogenous dissemination.
- The lesions of erythema migrans usually fade within 3 to 4 weeks.

LABORATORY

- Diagnosis without erythema migrans is difficult.
- Routine laboratory studies are not helpful.
- Serologic testing is the only practical laboratory method of diagnosing Lyme disease, but insensitivity and interlaboratory variability are frequent problems.
- The results of serologic testing for anti-*Borrelia* antibodies by enzyme-linked immunosorbent assay (ELISA) are positive at the initial presentation in 25% of infected patients and are positive in 75% of infected patients 4 to 6 weeks later, even with antibiotic therapy.
- The more specific Western immunoblot test is used to corroborate equivocal or positive results obtained with the ELISA assay.
- High titers of immunoglobulin G or M indicates disease, but lower titers can be misleading.
- A culture of *B. burgdorferi* is possible. A punch biopsy is placed in a modified Barbour-Stoenner-Kelly medium and sent via overnight mail to a reference laboratory.
- Direct detection of *Borrelia* organisms by polymerase chain reaction can establish the diagnosis early in the acute phase. The diagnosis can be made with punch biopsy and analysis of blood and urine specimens.

DIFFERENTIAL DIAGNOSIS

- Tinea
- Insect bites
- Granuloma annulare
- Urticaria
- Cellulitis
- Fixed drug eruption

TREATMENT

- Preventing tick bites is first line of defense.
- The patient should wear protective garments, tuck the pants into the socks, and wear closed-toed shoes.
- *N,N*-diethyl-meta-toluamide (DEET) can be used on the skin or permethrin (Permanone) on the clothing.
- Ticks should be detected and removed as soon as possible.
- A special instrument for tick removal (TICKED OFF) is available.
- Adults with early Lyme disease should receive 21 days of treatment with doxycycline (100 mg twice

a day), amoxicillin (500 mg three times a day), or cefuroxime axetil (Ceftin) (500 mg twice a day).

- Erythromycin, penicillin V, and azithromycin are less effective.
- Amoxicillin (25 to 50 mg/kg/day divided into three doses) or cefuroxime axetil (250 mg twice a day) is used for children. Doxycycline is an alternative. A short course of doxycycline is safe for children.
- The duration of treatment is guided by the clinical response and the disease stage.
- Disease that has progressed to stage 2 or 3 requires more intensive treatment.
- The prophylactic antibiotic treatment of tick bites is common but controversial. In most circumstances, treating a person for tick bite alone is not recommended.
- The management of asymptomatic patients with elevated Lyme titers has not yet been defined.
- Immunization should be considered for high-risk patients but the long-term safety and the duration of the vaccine's effectiveness are unknown.

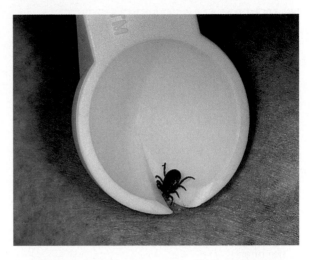

TICKED OFF. A simple plastic tool called TICKED OFF removes ticks, including the mouth parts. These inexpensive tools are generally available.

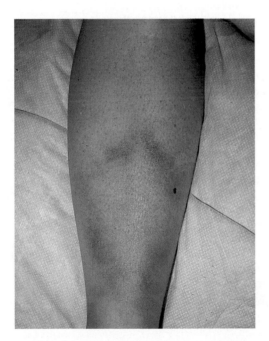

The lesion begins as a small papule at the bite site. The papule forms into a slowly enlarging ring, whereas the central erythema gradually fades and leaves a surface that is usually normal. Even in untreated patients, erythema migrans lesions usually fade within 3 to 4 weeks.

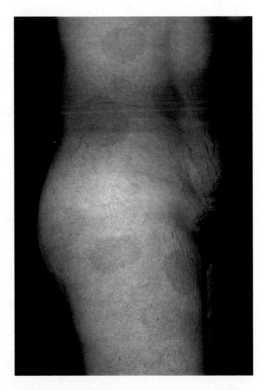

The most common configuration of the lesion is circular, but as migration proceeds over skinfolds, distortions of the configuration occur. Multiple lesions may occur.

■ ROCKY MOUNTAIN SPOTTED AND SPOTLESS FEVER

DESCRIPTION

- Rocky mountain spotted or spotless fever is a potentially lethal disease characterized by an acute onset of fever, a severe headache, myalgia, vomiting, and a petechial rash.
- It is transmitted by ticks and caused by *Rickettsia rickettsii*.
- Organisms disseminate via the bloodstream and multiply in vascular endothelial cells.
- This condition occurs most commonly in Oklahoma and the south Atlantic states.

HISTORY

- The incubation period is, on average, 7 days after the bite.
- An abrupt onset of fever (94%), a severe headache (88%), myalgia (85%), and vomiting (60%) occur.

SKIN FINDINGS

- The rash is discrete and macular, blanches with pressure, and becomes petechial in 2 to 4 days. It is difficult to see in African-Americans.
- The rash begins on about the third day, erupting first on the wrists and ankles. In hours, it involves the palms and soles (73%), and then it becomes generalized.
- The rash does not appear in about 15% of cases. Rashless disease is much more common in adults.

NONSKIN FINDINGS

- Splenomegaly is present in half of cases.

DISCUSSION

- The pulmonary system (cough or rales), the gastrointestinal system (nausea, vomiting, abdominal pain, diarrhea), and the central nervous system (stupor, meningismus) are also affected.
- Visceral and central nervous system dissemination can lead to shock and death.
- Many of those who die have a fulminant course and are dead in 1 week.

COURSE AND PROGNOSIS

- The fever subsides in 2 to 3 weeks, and the rash fades with residual hyperpigmentation.
- The mortality rate in treated patients is 4%; in untreated patients, it is about 20%.

LABORATORY

- The diagnosis must rely on clinical (fever, headache, rash, myalgia) and epidemiologic (tick exposure) criteria, since laboratory confirmation cannot occur before 7 to 14 days after the onset of illness.
- Indirect fluorescent antibody tests on acute and convalescent sera are fairly accurate and can be used later to confirm the diagnosis.
- The leukocyte count is normal or low; there are thrombocytopenia, an elevated serum hepatic aminotransferase level, and hyponatremia.
- The blood urea nitrogen level may be elevated, indicating prerenal azotemia or interstitial nephritis.

DIFFERENTIAL DIAGNOSIS

- Measles
- Mononucleosis and other viral exanthems
- Drug eruptions
- Meningococcemia
- Toxic shock syndrome
- Typhoid fever
- Vasculitis
- Kawasaki's syndrome

TREATMENT

- Doxycycline, 100 mg twice a day, and tetracycline, 25 to 50 mg/kg/day in four divided doses, can be administered. Doxycycline is the most favorable agent for children younger than 9 years of age. Treatments lasts for a minimum of 5 to 7 days. It is continued for at least 48 hours after the resolution of fever. Up to five courses of doxycycline may be administered with minimal risk of dental staining.
- Chloramphenicol, 50 mg/kg/day, is an alternative.

CAVEAT

- A therapeutic trial of doxycycline or tetracycline should be considered for any adult who has been in an endemic geographic area during the summer months and who has fever, myalgia, and headache.

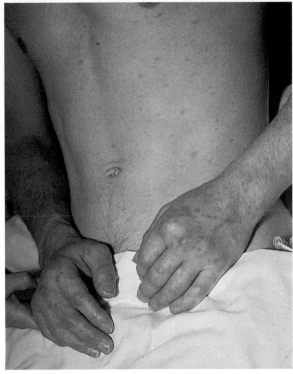 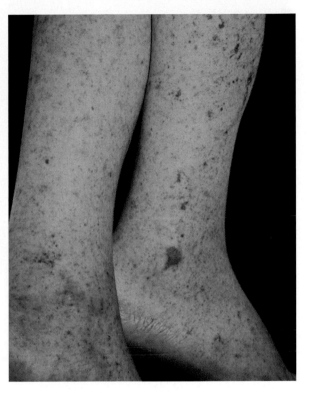

The rash is reported in 83% of cases and typically begins on the fourth day, erupting first on the wrists and ankles. In hours, it involves the palms and soles (73%) and then becomes generalized. The rash is discrete and macular and blanches with pressure at first; it becomes petechial in 2 to 4 days.

A generalized petechial eruption that involves the entire cutaneous surface, including the palms and soles.

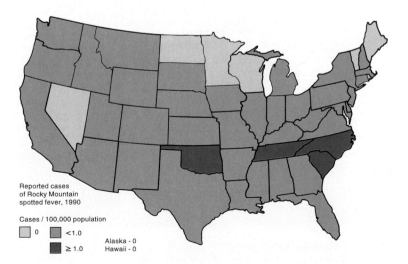

Reported cases
of Rocky Mountain
spotted fever, 1990

Cases / 100,000 population

☐ 0   ▨ <1.0

■ ≥ 1.0   Alaska - 0
Hawaii - 0

Reported cases and incidence rates of Rocky Mountain spotted fever.

■ FLEA BITES

DESCRIPTION

- A pruritic eruption is typically found on the legs.

HISTORY

- Clusters of pruritic papules develop on the legs; they are often grouped around the ankles.
- Pants and socks offer some protection.
- This is a self-limited, itchy eruption. Depending on the patient's sensitivity, it may subside in days to weeks.
- The flea eggs can lie dormant for over a year and can reactivate because of the vibrations from footsteps.

SKIN FINDINGS

- Initially, tiny red dots or bite puncta may be seen, often grouped around the ankles.
- Red, raised urticarial lesions known as *papular urticaria* develop in hypersensitive patients, especially children.
- Pruritus is intense in hypersensitive patients. Scratching causes infected, crusted lesions.
- The persistent scratching can lead to round, white scars after healing.

DESCRIPTION

- The flea itself is a small red-brown, hard-bodied, wingless insect.
- It is flattened laterally so that it can squeeze between the hairs of its host.

TREATMENT

- The bites are treated symptomatically.
- Topical antipruritics such as Sarna lotion can help. Sometimes, oral antihistamines are useful.
- Infected lesions require antibiotics.
- Group I to III topical steroids are useful for treating papular urticaria.
- Fleas must be eradicated. The infested animal, its bedding, and rugs must be treated.

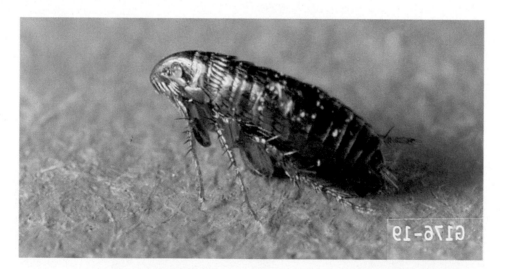

Fleas are tiny, red-brown, hard-bodied, wingless insects that are capable of jumping approximately 2 feet. They have distinctive, laterally flattened abdomens that allow them to slip between the hairs of their hosts. They live in rugs and on the bodies of animals and may jump onto humans.

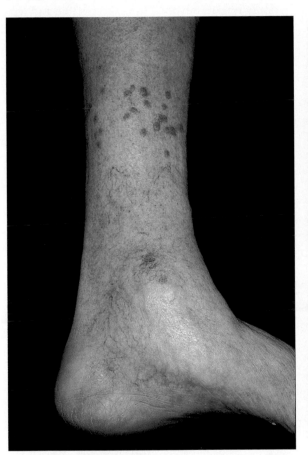

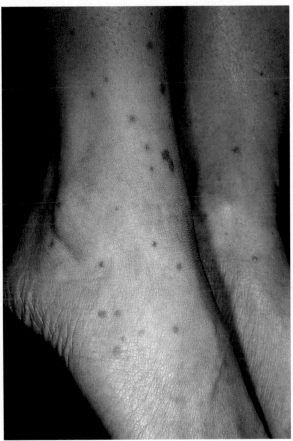

Flea bites occur in a cluster or group.

Most lesions are grouped around the ankles or lower legs, areas within easy leaping distance of the floor.

◼ CUTANEOUS LARVA MIGRANS (CREEPING ERUPTIONS)

DESCRIPTION

- Cutaneous larva migrans is a migratory, inflammatory condition most often seen on the feet; it is caused by the aimless wandering of the hookworm larvae within the skin.

HISTORY

- The lesions typically begin about 3 weeks after a vacation in the Caribbean, Africa, South America, Southeast Asia, or even the Southeastern United States.
- The patient notes itchy, inflammatory lesions that migrate in a snakelike fashion.
- The larvae are indiscriminate, and the parasite can penetrate the skin when humans walk on moist, feces-contaminated sand.
- If untreated, the larvae die in 2 to 8 weeks, but persistence up to a year has been reported.
- The larvae is eventually sloughed away as the epidermis matures.
- Typically, the resolution of migration and itching occurs within 2 to 3 days after therapy has begun.
- It may take a week or so for the more intense allergic inflammatory response to resolve.

SKIN FINDINGS

- A local inflammatory response to the larval secretions occurs within 3 weeks.
- The larvae cause the classic lesion, which is a wavy, twisted, red to purple, snakelike, 3-mm-wide tract.
- Itching is moderate to intense, and sometimes, secondary infection and eczematous inflammation can occur.

LABORATORY

- Up to 30% blood eosinophil count has been reported.
- A transitory, patchy infiltration of the lung along with eosinophilia in blood and sputum (Löffler's syndrome) is reported.

TREATMENT

- Freezing of the leading edge of the lesion with liquid nitrogen is often ineffective.
- Ivermectin, 200 μg/kg (average dose, 12 mg) administered as a single oral dose, is effective. Lesions heal within 5 days. A second round of treatment with the same dose is given for relapses.
- Albendazole, either 400 mg/day orally or 200 mg orally twice a day for 7 days, is effective and well tolerated. Its action is rapid, pruritus disappears in 3 to 5 days, and cutaneous lesions disappear after 6 to 7 days of treatment.
- Thiabendazole 15% in a liquid or a cream compound is applied topically three times a day for 5 days. It is applied to affected areas and 2 cm beyond the leading edge because the parasite is often located beyond the clinical lesion. The preparation is often difficult to obtain.
- Antibiotics are used for secondary infection.
- Topical or systemic steroids may be needed to treat severe pruritus.

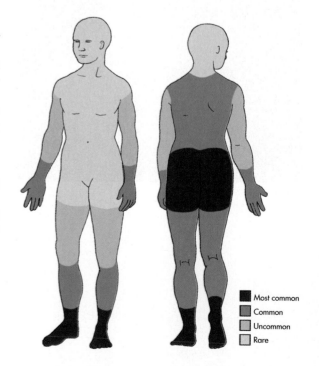

■ Most common
■ Common
▨ Uncommon
□ Rare

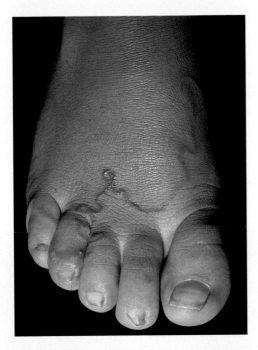

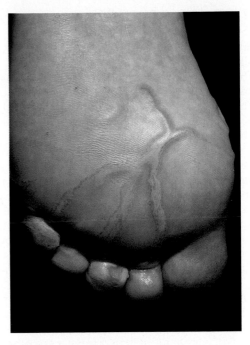

The trapped larva struggles a few millimeters to a few centimeters each day laterally through the epidermis in a random fashion, creating a tract reminiscent of the trail of a sea snail wandering aimlessly over the sand at low tide.

The 1-cm larva stays concealed directly ahead of the advancing tip of the wavy, twisted, red-to-purple, 3-mm tract. Any skin surface can be affected.

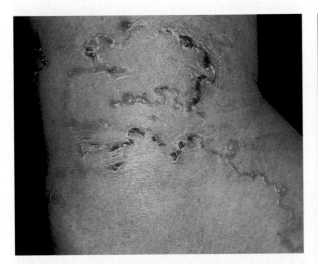

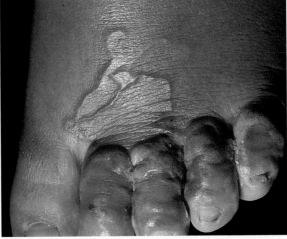

Many larvae may be present in the same area, creating several closely approximated wavy lines.

During larval migration, a local inflammatory response is provoked by the release of larval secretions. Itching is moderate to intense, and secondary infection or eczematous inflammation occurs.

■ FIRE ANT STINGS

DESCRIPTION

- Imported fire ants are small, are yellow to red or black, and have large heads.
- They have prominent incurved jaws and stingers on their tails.
- They were imported from South America and are now established in Southeastern United States.
- They form large colonies with giant mounds.
- The bite causes a painful pustular eruption.
- Sting reactions range from local pustules and large, late-phase responses to life-threatening anaphylaxis.
- Even brief exposures to endemic areas result in significant sting rates and the concurrent rapid development of fire ant–specific immunoglobulin E in 16% of stung subjects.
- Fire ant stings are common on the legs of children.

HISTORY

- Initially, burning and a sharp pain occur at the sting site. Ants can inflict multiple stings. They either run across the skin and leave a line of stings or rotate around the point of mandible attachment and leave a ring of stings.
- Children, who are unaware of the danger, are common victims.
- An infestation of buildings with fire ants may be associated with indoor attacks.
- Occasionally, a systemic allergic reaction occurs. Death from anaphylactic shock from 1 to fewer than 150 stings has been documented.
- Victims have survived 5000 to 10,000 stings.

SKIN FINDINGS

- The classic lesion is two tiny red dots (the bite) surrounded by a ring of pustules (the sting).
- A 10-mm wheal forms and is accompanied by edema and itching. Sterile vesicles form in 4 hours, evolve into pustules in 24 hours, and resolve in 3 to 10 days. Lesions may scar.
- Occasionally, there is a large, local, late-phase reaction (a red, edematous, indurated, and pruritic plaque). It resolves in 24 to 72 hours.

LABORATORY

- Skin testing is the most common diagnostic method for diagnosing allergy.
- Imported fire ant venom–specific immunoglobulin E antibodies can be measured in patients suspected of allergic reactions.

DIFFERENTIAL DIAGNOSIS

- Other insect bites
- Folliculitis
- Pustular psoriasis

TREATMENT

- Cool, wet compresses are applied.
- Topical antipruritics (Sarna lotion) are used.
- Oral antihistamines are administered.
- A short course of prednisone is used for severe local reactions.
- Immunotherapy should be considered for severe cases.

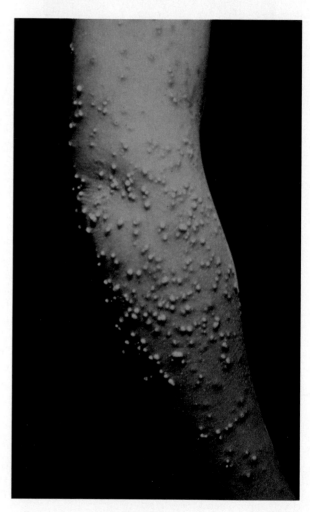

Fire ant stings. Numerous pustules occurred after a child was attacked by a large colony of ants.

■ SWIMMER'S ITCH

DESCRIPTION

- Swimmer's itch is an annoying inflammatory response to penetration of the skin by larval form of nonhuman schistosome parasites while swimming or wading in lakes. Unlike schistosomiasis, swimmer's itch is limited and follows a benign course.
- The diagnosis is often missed when this condition occurs sporadically, because of its unspecific characteristics.

HISTORY

- Indiscriminate larvae released from the snail seek out a warm-blooded host such as a bird or a rodent but accidentally penetrate human skin.
- The larvae are restricted primarily to fresh water; this condition occurs worldwide, but the Great Lakes area has the highest incidence in the United States.
- Cercariae die after penetration, resulting in a skin reaction.
- The intensity of the eruption depends on the degree of sensitization.
- Initial symptoms are minor after the first exposure.
- Papules occur only after sensitization (approximately 5 to 13 days after the penetration).
- A typical eruption occurs with subsequent exposures.
- The eruption begins as bathing water evaporates and cercariae begin penetrating.

- Pruritus and rash reach maximal intensity in 2 to 3 days.
- This condition subsides in 2 to 3 weeks.

SKIN FINDINGS

- Itching begins in approximately 1 hour.
- It is followed hours later by discrete, highly pruritic papules.
- Occasionally, pustules are surrounded by erythema.
- A highly sensitive individual develops secondary urticaria, vesicles, or even eczematous plaques.
- Secondary infection occurs after excoriation.

DIFFERENTIAL DIAGNOSIS

- Seabather's eruption (occurs under the bathing suit) after swimming in salt water

TREATMENT

- Symptoms should be relieved while the eruption fades.
- Itching is controlled with antihistamines, cool compresses, and "shake" lotions (calamine).
- Intense inflammation is suppressed with group II through V topical steroids.
- Antibiotics are administered for secondary infection.
- Immediate towel drying might be effective, since most larvae penetrate the skin as water is evaporating.

■ ANIMAL AND HUMAN BITES
HISTORY
- The type of animal, as well as the animal's behavior, should be determined.
- Time elapsed since injury is important.
- The patient's health status (e.g., immunosuppression by disease or medication, diabetes) should be determined.
- Cats have long, sharp teeth that often penetrate down to tendon and bone.
- Rabies transmission should be considered in the unprovoked attack of a wild or unvaccinated domestic animal.
- Seemingly trivial bites can result in severe complications.

PHYSICAL EXAMINATION
- The bite site is checked for depth and crush injury.
- Tendon and nerve function is tested.
- Vessel integrity is determined.
- Body cavities and joints are evaluated for penetration.

SKIN FINDINGS
- Pain and swelling suggest infection.

LABORATORY
- Infected wounds (aerobic and anaerobic) are cultured. *Pasteurella* species are the most common isolates from dog and cat bites.
- Cultures taken at the time of injury are of little value.
- Crush injuries, suspected fractures, and foreign body penetrations are examined radiographically.

TREATMENT
- A culture is obtained before irrigation.
- Tetanus immune globulin and tetanus toxoid are given to patients who have two or fewer primary immunizations. Tetanus toxoid alone is given to those who have completed a primary immunization series but who have not received a booster for more than 5 years.
- Any animal that behaves wildly or erratically after biting a person should be killed and its brains examined for rabies. A healthy animal should be confined and observed for 10 days; if signs of illness appear, the animal should be killed and its brains studied.
- Rabies prophylaxis is indicated if the laboratory evaluation found that the animal was rabid or if the animal was not captured. Patients not previously vaccinated are given both human rabies vaccine (a series of five doses administered in the deltoid area) and rabies immune globulin (20 IU/kg, with as much as possible infiltrated in and around the wound and the remainder given intramuscularly at a site distant from that used for vaccine administration).
- Rabies prophylaxis is given after exposure to bats in a confined setting, particularly for children, even when no bites are visible.
- Vaccination is prophylactic; once signs of rabies occur, the chance of survival is diminished.
- Wounds are irrigated with normal saline or povidone-iodine 1% solution at high pressure. Cleaning a bite with soap is as effective as cleaning with quaternary ammonium compounds in lowering the risk of transmission of rabies.
- Devitalized tissue is débrided.
- The decision whether to close the wound is made based on the increased risk of infection vs. the cosmetic benefits.
- Puncture wounds may be left open if they are not disfiguring; are infected by a human; involve the arms, hands, or legs; or occurred more than 6 to 12 hours before presentation in the case of bites to the arms and legs and 12 to 24 hours before presentation in the case of bites to the face.
- Facial lacerations from dog or cat bites are usually closed.

- Antibiotics are not routinely given.
- Antibiotics are used for severe wounds; crush injuries; deep puncture wounds; wounds near a bone; wounds that may have penetrated a joint; wounds that require surgical repair; wounds involving the hands, head, and neck; and most cat bites. Asplenic, immunocompromised, and diabetic patients are also treated with antibiotics.
- Empirical therapy for dog and cat bites should be directed against *Pasteurella* organisms, streptococci, staphylococci, and anaerobes.

- Empirical therapy should include a combination of a beta-lactam antibiotic and a beta-lactamase inhibitor (e.g., amoxicillin/clavulanate [Augmentin]), a second-generation cephalosporin with anaerobic activity (cefprozil [Cefzil]), or combination therapy with either penicillin and a first-generation cephalosporin (e.g., Cefadroxil [Duricef]) or clindamycin and a fluoroquinolone; when given alone, azithromycin, trovafloxacin, and the new ketolide antibiotics may also be useful.

12

Vesicular and Bullous Diseases

■ DERMATITIS HERPETIFORMIS

DESCRIPTION

- Dermatitis herpetiformis is a rare, chronic, intensely pruritic vesicular dermatosis associated with a gluten-sensitive enteropathy.

HISTORY

- The male/female ratio is 2:1.
- Dermatitis herpetiformis is rare in African-Americans and Asians.
- There are associations with HLA-DRw3, HLA-B8, HLA-DQw2.
- The prevalence is 11 to 39 per 100,000.
- Mean age of onset is the second to the fifth decade. It is rare in children.

SKIN FINDINGS

- Severe itching and burning occur.
- Clustered vesicles or excoriations are symmetrically distributed on the elbows, knees, sacrum, and base of the scalp but may be generalized.
- Intact vesicles are often destroyed by scratching and are thus often difficult to identify.
- Though more commonly vesicles, the lesions may be erythematous papules or urticarial papules.
- Oral lesions are very uncommon.

NONSKIN FINDINGS

- Gastrointestinal involvement is usually asymptomatic. A change seen on an upper gastrointestinal scan with small bowel follow-through is blunting of intestinal villi; although it is not routinely indicated, small bowel biopsy shows villous atrophy.
- Malabsorption of fat, D-xylose, or iron occurs in less than 20% of patients.

- The severity of skin disease does not correlate with the degree of intestinal involvement.
- There is an increased risk of small bowel lymphoma and nonintestinal lymphoma. The risk is reduced with a gluten-free diet.
- Hypothyroidism or thyroid disorders may be associated.

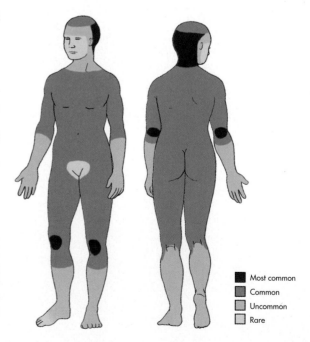

Most common
Common
Uncommon
Rare

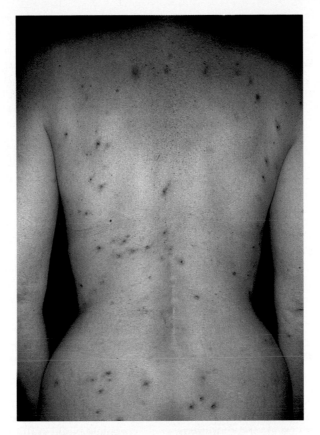

The vesicles are symmetrically distributed and appear on the elbows, knees, scalp and nuchal area, shoulders, and buttocks. The distribution may be more generalized.

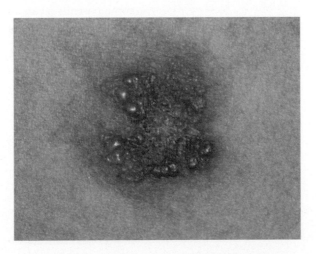

Herpetiform refers to the typical grouping of vesicles.

LABORATORY

- Skin biopsy shows subepidermal clefting and papillary dermal tips stuffed with neutrophils and few eosinophils. An inflammatory infiltrate of neutrophils and occasionally, eosinophils is typical in the upper dermis.
- An immunofluorescence skin biopsy is the gold standard for diagnosis. Taken from adjacent normal (perilesional) skin, the biopsy specimen shows granular or fibrillar immunoglobulin A (IgA) deposits in dermal papillae in 90% of cases.
- IgA antiendomysial antibodies (IgA-EmA) are found in 70% of patients not on a gluten-free diet. Serum IgA-EmA titers correlate with the severity of jejunal villous atrophy.

DIFFERENTIAL DIAGNOSIS

- Insect bites
- Papular urticaria
- Scabies
- Neurotic excoriations
- Primary pruritus
- Linear IgA disease
- Vesicular bullous pemphigoid

COURSE AND PROGNOSIS

- Dermatitis herpetiformis is typically chronic, with spontaneous remission in about a third of cases.
- Systemic iodides may aggravate the condition.
- Disease is recurrent but usually well controlled with oral sulfones such as dapsone or a strict gluten-free diet.

TREATMENT

Dietary

- A gluten-free diet can control the disease alone or allow decreased requirement for oral medication. Strict adherence to a gluten-free diet is required for many months for effective control.
- Gluten is present in all grains except rice and corn. Gluten-free foods can be ordered from: ENER-G Foods, Inc., 6901 Fox Ave SO, P.O. Box 24723, Seattle, WA 98124-0723, 1-800-331-5222.
- Motivation and dietary instruction are required for successful adherence to gluten-free diet. The Gluten Intolerance Group of North America offers a newsletter and other services: P.O. Box 23053, Seattle, WA 98102-0353, 1-206-325-6980.

Medication

- Treatment does not alter disease duration but allows for disease control and remission.
- Dapsone, 100 to 150 mg/day orally, typically relieves itching and burning within 48 to 72 hours. The daily maintenance dose varies from 25 to 200 mg/day. Glucose-6-phosphate dehydrogenase levels should be determined before treatment because there is an increased risk of severe hemolysis in deficient patients.
- Monitoring of dapsone for hemolysis, anemia, and methemoglobinemia is recommended. A complete blood count should be done weekly for 1 month, then monthly for 6 months, and semiannually thereafter.
- Sulfapyridine (1.0 to 1.5 gm/day) is effective in some patients as an alternative to dapsone. Tetracycline (500 mg one to four times a day) or minocycline (100 mg twice a day) and nicotinamide (500 mg two or three times a day) have been reported to be effective.

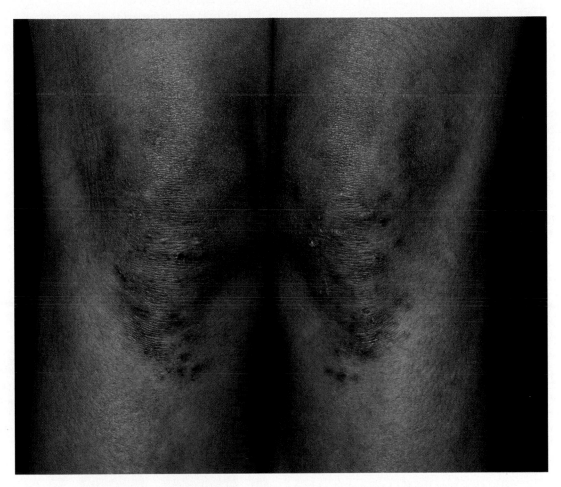

Symmetric distribution of vesicles in dermatitis herpetiformis.

■ PEMPHIGUS VULGARIS

DESCRIPTION

- Pemphigus vulgaris is a rare, potentially lethal, autoimmune, intraepidermal blistering disease involving the skin and mucous membranes.
- Keratinocyte desmosomal molecules are the target of autoantibodies associated with this disease.

HISTORY

- The mean age of onset is 60 years. Many patients are Jewish.
- Oral erosions usually precede the onset of skin blisters by weeks or months.
- Itching is minimal.

SKIN FINDINGS

Blisters

- The size of blisters varies from 1 cm to several centimeters.
- They appear gradually and may be localized for a considerable length of time but become generalized if untreated.
- They rupture easily because the vesicle roof, which consists of a thin portion of the upper epidermis, is very fragile.
- The application of pressure to small, intact bullae causes the fluid to dissect laterally into the mid-epidermal areas altered by bound immunoglobulin G (IgG) (positive Nikolsky's sign).
- Exposed erosions last for weeks before healing with brown hyperpigmentation but without scarring.

Oral Mucosa

- Oral erosions occur in most patients and typically precede the skin blisters by weeks or months.
- Blisters, erosions, and lines of erythema may appear in the esophageal mucosa.

LABORATORY

- A small, early vesicle or the skin adjacent to a blister or erosion, which is biopsied with a 3- or 4-mm punch, shows an intraepidermal bulla, acantholysis (separation of epidermal cells), and a mild to moderate infiltrate of eosinophils.
- Two biopsy specimens, one from the edge of a fresh lesion and the second from an adjacent normal area, are deposited in special transport media available from specialized laboratories. IgG and often complement C3 are found in the intercellular substance areas of the epidermis.

- Serum IgG antibodies are present in approximately 75% of patients with active disease. The level of antibody reflects the activity of disease. Periodic serum tests performed to detect changes in titers are helpful in evaluating the clinical course.

COURSE AND PROGNOSIS

- Death formerly occurred in all cases, usually from cutaneous infection, but now occurs in only 10% of cases, usually from complications of steroid therapy.

DIFFERENTIAL DIAGNOSIS

- Pemphigus foliaceus
- Paraneoplastic pemphigus (neoplasia-associated pemphigus)
- Bullous pemphigoid

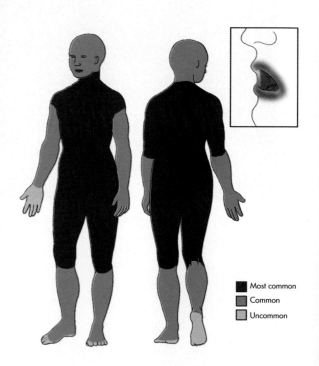

	Most common
	Common
	Uncommon

TREATMENT

- Treatment is very complicated and best accomplished with the help of experts.
- Prednisone with an immunosuppressive adjuvant agent such as azathioprine or cyclophosphamide is standard treatment.
- Adjuvant drugs have a "steroid-sparing" effect.
- Therapeutic choices are affected by the patient's age and the degree of involvement.
- Starting dosages of prednisone typically vary between 40 and 120 mg/day. Prednisone is tapered to establish a minimum dose that controls most disease activity.

- Cyclophosphamide (1.5 to 2.5 mg/kg/day) or azathioprine (1.5 to 2.5 mg/kg/day) is initiated with or after starting corticosteroids.
- Plasmapheresis, pulse intravenous corticosteroids, gold, dapsone, and intralesional steroids may be more effective in some patients than the other regimens.
- Direct immunofluorescence should be performed before therapy is discontinued. A negative finding is a good indication of remission.

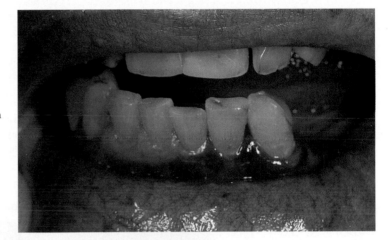

Oral erosions usually precede the onset of skin blisters by weeks or months.

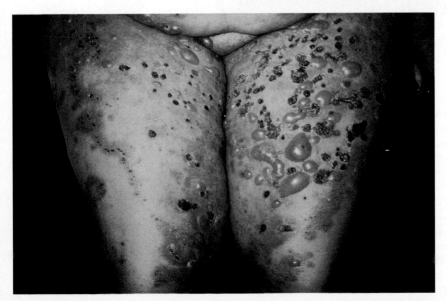

Flaccid blisters rupture easily because the roof, which consists only of a thin portion of the upper epidermis, is very fragile. Healing is with brown pigmentation but without scarring.

■ PEMPHIGUS FOLIACEUS

DESCRIPTION

- Pemphigus foliaceus is an autoimmune, intraepidermal blistering disease characterized by crusted lesions.

HISTORY

- The age of onset varies more widely than in pemphigus vulgaris.
- Pemphigus foliaceus occurs in middle-aged and older patients. There is no racial prevalence.
- Pain and burning are reported more often than itching.
- Sun or heat may worsen the signs and symptoms.

SKIN FINDINGS

- Lesions appear in a "seborrheic distribution" on the face or first appear on the scalp, chest, or upper back.
- Intact blisters are not usually seen. The vesicle roof is so thin that it ruptures. Serum leaks out and desiccates, forming localized or broad areas of crust.
- Intact, thin-walled blisters are sometimes seen near the edge of the erosions.
- The upper portion of the epidermis can be dislodged with lateral finger pressure (positive Nikolsky's sign).

LABORATORY

- A small, early vesicle or skin adjacent to a blister or erosion is biopsied with a 3- or 4-mm punch and on light microscopy, shows an intraepidermal bulla, acantholysis (separation of epidermal cells) in the upper epidermis, and a mild to moderate infiltrate of eosinophils.
- For direct immunofluorescence, two biopsies, one from the edge of a fresh lesion and another from an adjacent normal area, are taken.
- Specimens are deposited in special transport media available from specialized laboratories. Immunoglobulin G and often complement C3 are found in the intercellular substance areas of the epidermis.
- In indirect immunofluorescence, serum immunoglobulin G antibodies are present in approximately 75% of patients with active disease. The level of antibody reflects the activity of disease. Antibodies of pemphigus vulgaris can be distinguished from those of pemphigus foliaceus via testing on two tissue substrates.

COURSE AND PROGNOSIS

- Pemphigus foliaceus may be localized for years or may progress rapidly and become generalized, evolving into an exfoliative erythroderma.
- It may last for years and be fatal if not treated.

DISCUSSION

- Oral lesions are rarely present.
- Lesions are well demarcated and do not extend into large, eroded areas like those of pemphigus vulgaris.
- Fogo selvagem (Portuguese for "wild fire") is an endemic form of pemphigus foliaceus found in certain rural areas of Brazil and Colombia.
- Pemphigus erythematosus (Senear-Usher syndrome), may be a combination of localized (face and other seborrheic areas) pemphigus foliaceus and systemic lupus erythematosus. In many of these patients, the results of antinuclear antibody tests are positive, but few patients have any other signs or symptoms of lupus.
- Pemphigus foliaceus has been reported in approximately 5% of patients taking D-penicillamine or captopril.

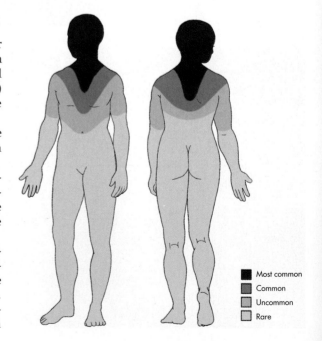

Most common
Common
Uncommon
Rare

- Most cases are mild. Many patients experience spontaneous recovery once the drug is stopped. Other drugs have been reported to induce pemphigus.
- The pemphigus-like eruption is not always limited, and the mortality rate approaches 10%.

TREATMENT

- Early localized disease may be managed with group I to III topical steroids. Active widespread disease is treated like pemphigus vulgaris (see p. 269).

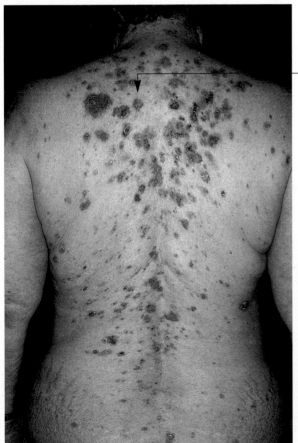

The disease begins gradually on the face in a "butterfly" distribution or first appears on the scalp, chest, or upper back as localized or broad, continuous areas of erythema, scaling, crusting, or, occasionally, bullae.

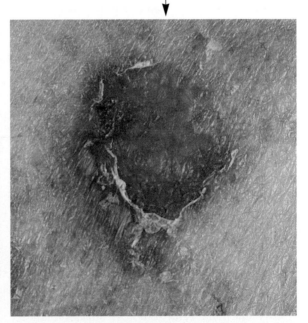

The vesicle roof is so thin that it ruptures. Serum leaks out and desiccates, forming the localized or broad areas of crust. Intact, thin-walled blisters are sometimes seen near the edge of the erosions.

■ BULLOUS PEMPHIGOID
DESCRIPTION

- Bullous pemphigoid is an uncommon subepidermal blistering disease typically presenting on the flexor surfaces of elderly patients.

HISTORY

- A disease of the elderly, bullous pemphigoid usually occurs after age 60; childhood cases have been reported, but they are rare.
- There is no racial or gender prevalence. Drugs are often implicated. There is little evidence of an association with malignancy.
- Itching is usually moderate to severe.

SKIN FINDINGS

- Bullous pemphigoid begins with a localized area of erythema or with pruritic urticarial plaques.
- A diagnosis of hives is frequently made in this preblistering stage.
- Plaques turn dark red in 1 to 3 weeks as vesicles and bullae rapidly appear on their surfaces.
- The bullae are tense with good structural integrity. They rupture within a week, leaving an eroded base that does not spread and heals rapidly.
- Flexor surface involvement is typical, but the eruption may be localized or generalized.
- Oral blisters, if present, are mild and transient.

LABORATORY

- Peripheral blood eosinophilia occurs in 50% of patients.
- Lesions arise from inflamed (infiltrate-rich) or noninflamed (infiltrate-poor) skin; the most information is provided through a biopsy on an early bulla on inflamed skin. Subepidermal bullae occur with eosinophils in the dermis and bullae cavities.
- Another 3- or 4-mm punch biopsy is taken and submitted in special transport media. The highest diagnostic yield for direct immunofluorescence (DIF) comes from biopsies of inflamed skin next to a blister. The results of DIF are positive in a high percentage of patients, even after treatment is initiated. DIF shows immunoglobulin G (IgG), complement C3, or both in a linear band at the basement membrane zone. DIF studies relate to treatment responses. As the disease subsides, complement C3 deposits disappear. The normal skin of the forearm can be used for such studies.

- Circulating IgG antibodies are present in approximately 70% of cases; the level of IgG does not correlate with disease activity as it does in pemphigus.

COURSE AND PROGNOSIS

- In treated patients, the duration of the disease varies from 9 weeks to 17 years. The remission rate is 30% at 2 years and 50% at 3 years. Late relapse can be observed after disease-free intervals of more than 5 years. The mortality rate at 1 year is 19%.
- Untreated bullous pemphigoid remains localized and undergoes spontaneous remission or may become generalized. Recurrences may be less severe than the initial episode.

DISCUSSION

- Bullae are tense with good structural integrity, in contrast to the large, flaccid, easily ruptured bullae of pemphigus. Pemphigoid is more common than pemphigus.
- Firm pressure on the blister does not result in extension into normal skin as occurs in pemphigus; therefore Nikolsky's sign is negative.

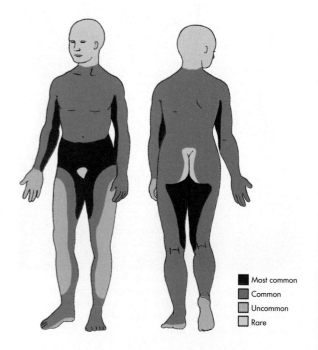

■ Most common
■ Common
■ Uncommon
□ Rare

Differential Diagnosis

- Dermatitis herpetiformis
- Pemphigus
- Bullous systemic lupus erythematosus
- Bullous drug eruptions

Treatment

- Drugs are often suspected; stopping medication or changing to a different medication may help.
- Ultraviolet light and scratching may induce bullae and should be avoided.
- Itching is controlled with hydroxyzine (10 to 50 mg every 4 hours as needed).
- Topical steroids are used to control limited disease. Group I or II steroids are applied twice a day until lesions are healed and for 2 weeks thereafter.
- Excellent responses may occur when localized or generalized bullous pemphigoid is treated with tetracycline or erythromycin, 1.0 to 2.5 gm/day, or minocycline, 200 mg/day. Niacinamide, 1.5 to 2.5 gm/day, may enhance the efficacy of the antibiotics. These drugs may suppress the inflammatory response at the basement membrane zone.
- Some 40% of cases respond to dapsone, 100 mg/day.
- Disease that does not respond to antibiotics and dapsone is treated with prednisone, 1.0 to 1.5 mg/kg per day in two daily doses. Most cases are controlled in 28 days, and the dosage can be gradually tapered (0.5 mg/kg/day at 3 months and 0.2 mg/kg/day at 6 months). The time required for resolution with prednisone depends on the number of blisters on the first day. The addition of dapsone may help produce a remission.
- Adjuvant immunosuppressive therapy with cyclophosphamide or azathioprine may be considered if dapsone and prednisone fail (see section on the treatment for pemphigus).

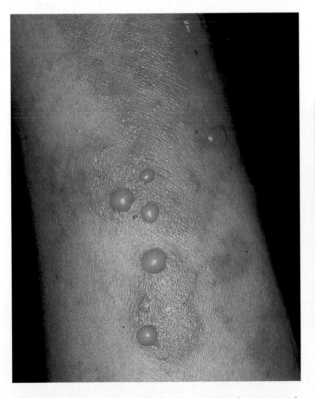

Pemphigoid begins with a localized area of erythema or with pruritic urticarial plaques that gradually become more edematous and extensive.

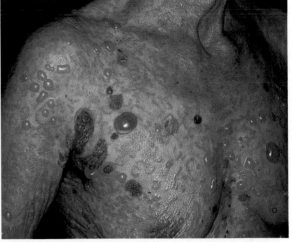

The eruption is often generalized, but the most common sites are the lower part of the abdomen, the groin, and the flexor surfaces of the arms and legs. The palms and soles are affected. The plaques turn dark red or cyanotic in 1 to 3 weeks, resembling erythema multiforme, as vesicles and bullae rapidly appear on their surface.

13

Connective Tissue Diseases

■ LUPUS ERYTHEMATOSUS

Description

- Lupus erythematosus is a multifaceted disease with a wide spectrum of manifestations ranging from solitary chronic skin lesions in chronic discoid lupus erythematosus (DLE) to widespread polymorphous lesions in subacute cutaneous lupus erythematosus (SCLE) to multiple organ involvement in systemic lupus erythematosus (SLE). A dysregulation of T cells causes the activation of B cells, producing a variety of autoantibodies directed to cellular antigens such as DNA, RNA, and RNA-protein complexes.

Treatment

- There are many treatment options.
- Skin disease often occurs with systemic disease in patients with SLE. Such patients respond to the systemic immunosuppressive therapy required to treat this form of lupus.
- Cyclic use of group I to II topical steroids are administered twice a day for 2 weeks; moisturizers are used for 1 week.
- Steroids (e.g., triamcinolone [Kenalog], 10 mg/ml) are injected into DLE lesions.
- Corticosteroid-impregnated tape (Cordran tape) is used for DLE lesions.
- Hydroxychloroquine, 200 to 400 mg/day, may be combined with quinacrine.
- Other medications that may be prescribed include dapsone, 100 to 200 mg/day; thalidomide, 50 to 300 mg/day; prednisone, 0.5 to 1.5 mg/kg/day; retinoids (acitretin, 10 to 50 mg/day, or isotretinoin, 1 mg/kg/day); gold (oral or parenteral); azathioprine; methotrexate; and cyclophosphamide.
- Sun-protective clothing is available from Sun Precautions, 2815 Wetmore Avenue, Everett, WA 98201, 1-800-882-7860, www.sunprecautions.com.
- Sun exposure (especially between 11 AM and 3 PM) should be minimized.
- Broad-spectrum, ultraviolet A–blocking sunscreens, especially those containing avobenzone (Parsol 1789) and titanium dioxide, should be used.

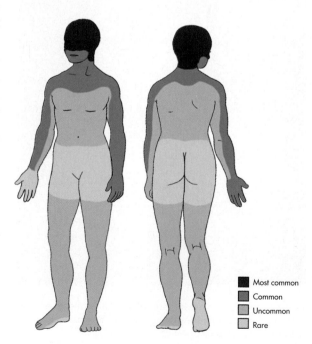

- ■ Most common
- ■ Common
- ■ Uncommon
- ■ Rare

■ CHRONIC CUTANEOUS LUPUS (DISCOID LUPUS ERYTHEMATOSUS)

DESCRIPTION

- DLE is the most common form of cutaneous lupus erythematosus.

HISTORY

- Discoid lupus erythematosus (DLE) is more common in female patients.
- It is perhaps more common in African-Americans.
- The peak incidence is in the fourth decade.
- Trauma and ultraviolet B may initiate and exacerbate lesions.
- There is a lower incidence of systemic disease; 1% to 5% of cases progress to systemic lupus erythematosus.
- Scarring alopecia permanent.

SKIN FINDINGS

- Lesions may occur on any body surface, but the scalp, face, and ears are the most common areas.
- DLE begins asymptomatically; there are well-defined, elevated, red to violaceous, 1- to 2-cm, flat-topped plaques with firmly adherent scaling.
- Follicular plugs are prominent; peeling the scale reveals an undersurface that looks like a carpet penetrated by several carpet tacks.
- Epidermal atrophy gives the surface either a smooth white or a wrinkled appearance.
- Lesions endure for months; they either resolve spontaneously or progress with further atrophy, ultimately forming smooth, white or hyperpigmented, depressed scars with telangiectasia and scarring alopecia.
- Scalp disease begins with erythema, scaling, and follicular plugging.
- Hair follicles are destroyed, resulting in irreversible, scarring alopecia. Hair loss is haphazard in distribution.

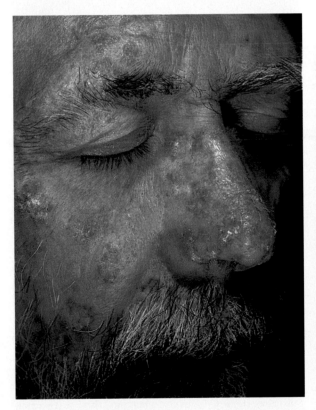

The face is the most commonly affected area. Epidermal atrophy occurs early and gives the surface either a smooth and white or a wrinkled appearance.

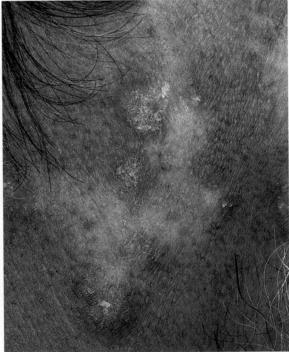

Follicular plugs may be prominent. These lesions progress, ultimately forming smooth and white or hyperpigmented depressed scars with telangiectasia and scarring alopecia.

■ SUBACUTE CUTANEOUS LUPUS ERYTHEMATOSUS

DESCRIPTION

- Subacute cutaneous lupus erythematosus (SCLE) is a clinical spectrum of cutaneous lupus erythematosus between the chronic destructive discoid lupus and the erythema of acute cutaneous lupus erythematosus.

HISTORY

- SCLE is most common in white, young to middle-aged women.
- Sudden eruption occurs after sun exposure.
- Lesions appear on the upper trunk, arms, and dorsal hands.
- Internal involvement is less severe than in systemic lupus erythematosus.
- The individual lesions may last for months.
- This condition tends to be chronic and recurrent.
- Ro antibody–positive women may have babies with neonatal lupus and congenital heart block.

SKIN FINDINGS

- There are two patterns: papulosquamous and annular-polycyclic.
- Lesions occur most often on the sun-exposed trunk; they are rarely seen below the waist.
- A subtle gray hypopigmentation and telangiectasia are seen in the center of annular lesions; this becomes more obvious as lesions resolve. Hypopigmentation fades in several months, but the telangiectasia persists.
- Follicular plugging, adherent hyperkeratosis, scarring, and dermal atrophy are not prominent features.
- Other signs include photosensitivity, periungual telangiectasia, discoid lupus erythematosus, and vasculitis.

LABORATORY

- The antinuclear antibody titer is elevated in 50% to 72% of cases.
- Anti-Ro (anti–SS-A) antibody titer is elevated in 50% to 100% of cases.
- Anti-La (anti–SS-B) coexist with anti-Ro (anti–SS-A) and are usually not present as a unique antibody.
- Leukopenia is present in 25% to 50% of patients with SCLE.

DIFFERENTIAL DIAGNOSIS

- Drug eruptions (thiazides)
- Dermatomyositis
- Secondary syphilis
- Psoriasis
- Seborrheic dermatitis
- Tinea corporis

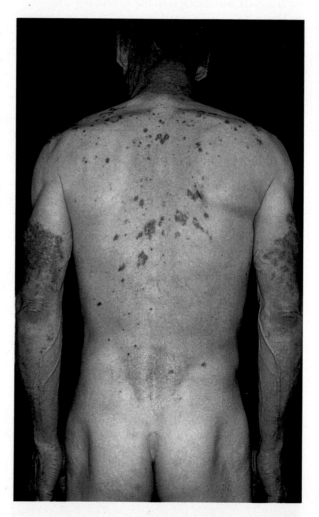

Subacute cutaneous lupus erythematosus. There are two morphologic varieties: a papulosquamous pattern and an annular-polycyclic pattern. Both occur most often on the trunk; one predominates.

■ ACUTE CUTANEOUS LUPUS ERYTHEMATOSUS

DESCRIPTION

- Acute cutaneous lupus erythematosus is a serious multisystem disease.

HISTORY

- Women are affected more often than men (8:1).
- It occurs most frequently in the 30- to 40-year age range.
- Sunlight exacerbates acute cutaneous lupus erythematosus and may induce it.
- Drugs (hydralazine, procainamide, anticonvulsants) may case a lupuslike syndrome.
- Acute cutaneous lupus erythematosus is a multisystem disease; there may be fever, arthritis, and renal, cardiac, pulmonary, and central nervous system involvement.

SKIN FINDINGS

- Superficial to indurated, nonpruritic, erythematous to violaceous plaques appear on the sun-exposed chest, shoulders, extensor arms, and backs of the hands.
- There may be fine scaling on the surface.

- In 10% to 50% of patients, a butterfly rash appears over the malar and nasal bridge.
- Atrophy does not occur.
- Nailfold capillary microscopy reveals tortuous, "meandering" capillary loops.
- The patient may have excess vellus hair at the frontal margin (lupus hair) or diffuse hair thinning.
- Alopecia (scarring and nonscarring) occurs in 20% of cases.

DIFFERENTIAL DIAGNOSIS

- Contact dermatitis
- Rosacea
- Erysipelas
- Seborrheic dermatitis
- Tinea
- Polymorphous light eruption

LABORATORY

- Biopsy of lesional skin is obtained for routine study and for immunofluorescence.
- Underlying systemic lupus erythematosus (SLE) is screened for by using an antinuclear antibody titer, a complete blood count, a serum chemistry profile, and urinalysis.

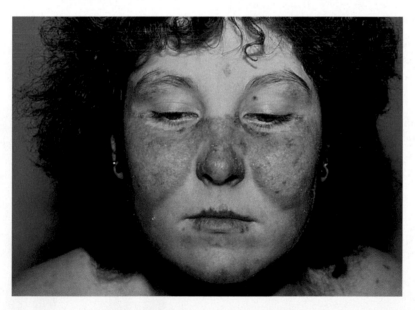

The rash of acute cutaneous lupus erythematosus consists of superficial to indurated, nonpruritic, erythematous to violaceous plaques; these occur primarily on sun-exposed areas. The classic butterfly rash over the malar and nasal area occurs in 10% to 50% of patients with acute lupus erythematosus, but it is not the most common cutaneous presentation.

14

Hypersensitivity Syndromes and Vasculitis

■ ERYTHEMA MULTIFORME

DESCRIPTION

- Erythema multiforme is a relatively common, acute, often recurrent inflammatory disease.
- It is commonly associated with a preceding herpes simplex infection, *Mycoplasma pneumoniae* infection, and acute upper respiratory tract disease.
- Many other factors, including numerous infectious agents, contact allergens, drugs, connective tissue diseases, physical agents, x-ray therapy, pregnancy, and internal malignancies, have been implicated in the etiology.
- In approximately 50% of cases, no cause can be found.

HISTORY

- The disease may be preceded by malaise, fever, or itching and burning at the site where the eruption will occur.
- The entire episode lasts for approximately 1 month.
- Only a few of the many individuals who experience recurrent herpes simplex virus infection also develop recurrent herpes-associated erythema multiforme. Some adults and children develop erythema multiforme after each episode of herpes simplex.

SKIN FINDINGS

- The cutaneous eruptions are most distinctive, and classification is based on their form.

Target Lesions and Papules

- Target lesions and papules are the most characteristic findings.
- Dusky red, round maculopapules appear suddenly in a symmetric pattern on the backs of the hands and feet and the extensor aspect of the forearms and legs.

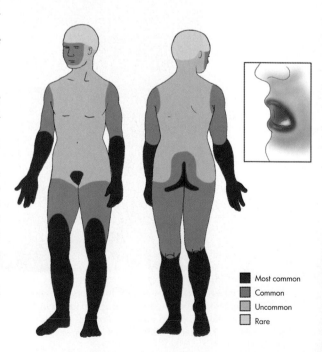

Most common
Common
Uncommon
Rare

- The diagnosis may not be suspected until the nonspecific early lesions evolve into target lesions during a 24- to 48-hour period.
- The classic "iris" or target lesion results from centrifugal spread of the red maculopapule to a circumference of 1 to 3 cm as the center becomes cyanotic, purpuric, or vesicular.
- Individual lesions heal in 1 or 2 weeks without scarring but with hypopigmentation or hyperpigmentation, whereas new lesions appear in crops.
- Bullae and erosions may be present in the oral cavity.

Urticarial Plaques

- Urticarial plaques may occur without the classic target lesions in the same distribution as target lesions.
- Unlike hives, all lesions are approximately the same size (1 to 2 cm) and remain unchanged for days.

TREATMENT

- Mild cases are not treated.
- Patients with many target lesions respond rapidly to a 1- to 3-week course of prednisone. Prednisone, 40 to 80 mg/day, is continued until control is achieved and is then tapered rapidly in 1 week.
- Treatment with prednisone can successfully abort a recurrence.
- Oral acyclovir, 200 mg two or three times a day or 400 mg twice a day, or valacyclovir (Valtrex), 500 mg/day, used continually prevents herpes-associated recurrent erythema multiforme in many cases.
- Herpes-associated erythema multiforme is not prevented if oral acyclovir is administered after a herpes simplex recurrence is evident, and acyclovir is of no value after erythema multiforme has occurred.
- The trunk may be involved in more severe cases.
- Early lesions itch, burn, or are asymptomatic.

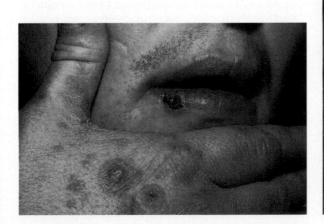

An episode may be precipitated by herpes simplex infection.

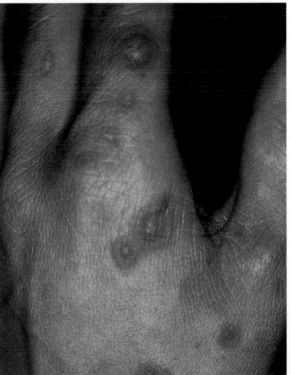

Classic iris lesions.

■ STEVENS-JOHNSON SYNDROME

DESCRIPTION

- Stevens-Johnson syndrome, also called *erythema multiforme major*, is a symmetric, severe vesicobullous eruption on at least two mucous membranes (oral, anogenital, and ocular mucous membranes; lips) with frequent atypical target lesions affecting in some cases up to 15% of the body surface area.
- This condition may be within the spectrum of toxic epidermal necrolysis, although it is often distinguished by a less extensive area of skin involvement.
- The mortality rate is less than 5%.

HISTORY

- The onset is sudden, although a 1-to 3-week prodrome of fever, malaise, myalgias or upper respiratory infection–like symptoms may precede the appearance of the eruptions.
- Stevens-Johnson syndrome occurs at all ages but is most commonly seen in children and young adults.
- The most common causes are herpes simplex virus, mycoplasmal infection, and drugs. (Approximately 50% of cases are deemed drug induced.)
- Frequently implicated drugs (similar to those associated with toxic epidermal necrolysis) are phenytoin, phenobarbital, carbamazepine, sulfonamides, and aminopenicillins.
- Other causes are upper respiratory infections, gastrointestinal disorders, and cranial radiation therapy.

SKIN FINDINGS

- Skin lesions are variable. Erythematous papules, small vesicles on dusky purpuric macules, or erythema multiforme target lesions can appear.
- Skin lesions may be painful or burning.
- On the oral mucosa, bullae erode and result in gray-yellow fibrinous exudate with a thick hemorrhagic crust.
- In the ocular form, there is conjunctivitis with or without purulence. Bullae, corneal ulceration, and uveitis may occur.
- On the genital and perianal mucosa, bullae result in erosions.
- The lesions appear mainly on the extremities but may be widely distributed and prominent on the trunk and face.

NONSKIN FINDINGS

- There is a high fever during the eruptive phase (10% to 30% of cases).
- Organ involvement can occur but is not common.
- Pneumonitis (23% of cases) and bronchitis (6%) are among the most common findings.
- Renal failure is unusual.

LABORATORY

- Skin biopsy should be performed. Frozen section may allow rapid diagnosis, showing full-thickness epidermal necrosis and a relatively normal underlying dermis.
- Direct immunofluorescence may be helpful in nontypical cases.

DIFFERENTIAL DIAGNOSIS

- Anticonvulsant hypersensitivity syndrome
- Paraneoplastic pemphigus
- Pemphigus vulgaris
- Toxic epidermal necrolysis
- Herpetic gingivostomatitis

TREATMENT

- Treatment of Stevens-Johnson syndrome is supportive and includes hydration and a soft diet.
- Frequent mouth rinses and frequent application of petroleum jelly (Vaseline) or Aquaphor to the lips are soothing. Viscous xylocaine or Benadryl elixir can be applied topically for comfort and to ease the discomfort of eating.
- An ophthalmologist should be consulted.
- Cutaneous blisters are treated with cool, wet compresses with Burow's solution. A bland emollient such as Aquaphor may promote comfort and healing.
- The complicating infection should be assessed and treated.
- The role of corticosteroids remains controversial. No double-blinded, controlled study exists; most authorities argue against their use. Small studies suggest that treatment with systemic corticosteroids may be associated with delayed recovery and significant side effects. Other studies conclude that corticosteroids are beneficial and may be lifesaving. Prednisone, 20 to 30 mg twice a day, is given for 1 week until new lesions no longer appear; it is then tapered rapidly.
- Recurrent cases related to herpes simplex can be treated early with oral acyclovir, famciclovir, or valacyclovir.

- Possible causes should be diligently sought so that recurrence can be avoided.

DISCUSSION

- Crops of lesions occur over 10 to 14 days; fewer appear typically over 3 to 4 weeks.
- For patients with limited disease, the prognosis is good with conservative treatment.

- The disease is self-limited and resolves in about a month if there are no complications. The mortality rate approaches 10% for patients with extensive disease.
- Recurrence is not common unless there is reexposure to an offending drug or the recurrence is caused by herpes simplex.

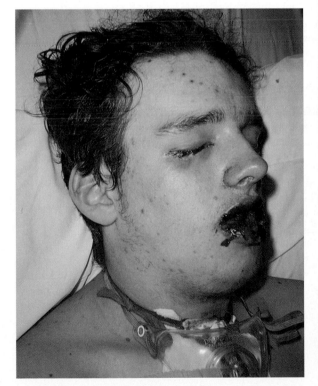

Severe bullous form. Bullae are present on the conjunctiva and in the mouth.

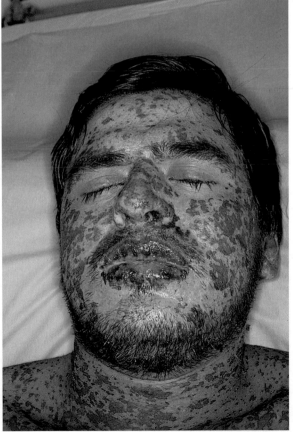

Skin lesions are flat, atypical targets or purpuric maculae that are widespread or distributed on the trunk. Lesions in this extensive case have become eroded and infected.

■ TOXIC EPIDERMAL NECROLYSIS

DESCRIPTION

- Toxic epidermal necrolysis is a rare, life-threatening exfoliative disease of the skin and mucous membranes; it affects 30% to 100% of the skin surface.
- Ocular involvement may lead to scarring.
- The mortality rate is 25% to 50%.

HISTORY

- Some 80% of cases may be drug induced. Drugs most frequently associated with toxic epidermal necrolysis are hydantoins, barbiturates, carbamazepine, sulfonamides, aminopenicillins, allopurinol, and nonsteroidal antiinflammatory drugs (piroxicam, phenylbutazone). Also associated are cephalosporins, fluoroquinolones, vancomycin, rifampin, ethambutol, fenbufen, tenoxicam, tiaprofenic acid, diclofenac, sulindac, ibuprofen, ketoprofen, naproxen, and thiabendazole.
- The time course is 1 to 3 weeks from first dose to disease onset.
- Other implicated causes are immunizations (diphtheria-pertussis-tetanus, measles, poliomyelitis, influenza), viral infections (cytomegalovirus infection, Epstein-Barr virus infection, herpes simplex, varicella zoster, hepatitis A, infectious mononucleosis), mycoplasmal infection, orf, psittacosis, streptococcal infection, syphilis, histoplasmosis, coccidioidomycosis, and tuberculosis.
- Graft-versus-host disease is also associated.
- Individuals infected with the human immunodeficiency virus and patients with other altered immune diseases such as systemic lupus erythematous are at greater risk for drug-induced toxic epidermal necrolysis.

SKIN FINDINGS

- Targetoid lesions or bullae form suddenly on either normal or erythematous skin. These lesions involve more than 30% of the body surface area. Skin erythema is often confluent.
- Widespread, full-thickness detachment (necrolysis) results in a glistening, raw, denuded, tender surface.
- Nikolsky's sign is positive (the skin denudes and sloughs with lateral pressure).
- Blisters and erosions often appear on the mouth, nose and conjunctivae. Genital and perianal skin may also be involved.

NONSKIN FINDINGS

- General findings include fever, malaise, arthralgias, and myalgias.
- Keratitis, conjunctivitis, photophobia, ectropion, symblepharon, corneal neovascularization, and lacrimal duct scarring can occur.
- Leukopenia, thrombocytopenia, and anemia may occur.
- Ulcerations may appear.
- Some 30% of the upper airway can be damaged. Pneumonia or pneumonitis can also occur.
- Urinary findings include urethritis, urinary retention, and prerenal azotemia.
- Hypovolemia may occur.
- Wound infections can lead to sepsis, electrolyte imbalance, and massive transepidermal fluid loss.

LABORATORY

- Vacuolization along the dermoepidermal junction, necrotic keratinocytes, and full-thickness epidermal necrosis can lead to subepidermal blister formation and separation. Dermal inflammation is minimal.
- The results of liver function tests may be elevated.
- Histologic testing is helpful for distinguishing toxic epidermal necrolysis from staphylococcal scalded skin syndrome, in which skin separation is more superficial and is in the granular layer of the epidermis.
- Direct immunofluorescence is performed on a skin biopsy specimen to distinguish paraneoplastic pemphigus from toxic epidermal necrolysis.

DIFFERENTIAL DIAGNOSIS

- Staphylococcal scalded skin syndrome
- Graft-versus-host disease
- Staphylococcal toxic shock syndrome
- Kawasaki syndrome
- Acute-onset paraneoplastic pemphigus
- Stevens-Johnson syndrome, in which two mucosal sites are also involved but less than 10% of the body surface is affected with small blisters or dusky purpuric macules

TREATMENT

- Recently introduced drugs are discontinued. Related illnesses are treated.
- Treatment is supportive; care provided by a burn center is optimal.
- Intravenous fluids are administered. Nutritional support is given. The patient is monitored closely for infection. Pain control is provided.
- An ophthalmologist should be consulted.
- Physical therapy is given for range of motion.
- Corticosteroid administration is generally not recommended. Strong arguments against their use include lack of any prospective, randomized, controlled trials assessing their use and outcome; an increased risk of infection; delayed healing; and masking of signs of infection.

DISCUSSION

- The extent and course of toxic epidermal necrolysis are unpredictable; the first 8 to 10 days are characterized by fever and mucous membrane and generalized skin sloughing.
- Recovery occurs over 1 to 2 weeks as the skin reepithelializes.
- Important prognostic factors include the extent of necrolysis, elevated urea and creatinine levels, thrombocytopenia, neutropenia, and sepsis.
- Elderly patients have greater mortality rates.
- This condition is considered by some to be a more extensive form of erythema multiforme major (Stevens-Johnson syndrome).
- The pathophysiology is unknown; the disease may be immune mediated.

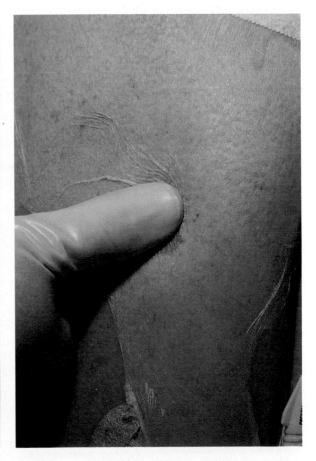

Shedding of full-thickness epidermis in toxic epidermal necrolysis.

Wrinkling with slight pressure in toxic epidermal necrolysis.

■ ERYTHEMA NODOSUM

DESCRIPTION

- Erythema nodosum is a nodular erythematous eruption usually limited to the extensor aspects of the extremities.
- Most cases are caused by nonmycobacterial infectious diseases or by noninfectious inflammatory diseases.

HISTORY

- The female/male ratio is 5:1, and the mean age at onset is 31 years.
- The incidence has decreased in the antibiotic era.
- Erythema nodosum is a hypersensitivity reaction to a variety of antigenic stimuli.
- It is associated with several diseases and drugs.
- Most common causes in the modern era are streptococcal infections, sarcoidosis, enteropathies (ulcerative colitis, regional ileitis), coccidioidomycosis, chlamydial infections, mycoplasmal infections, *Yersinia* infections, hepatitis B, and drugs.
- Tuberculosis is a rare cause of erythema nodosum today.
- Half of cases are idiopathic.
- The prodromal symptoms of fatigue, malaise, and arthralgia or the symptoms of an upper respiratory infection precede the eruption by 1 to 3 weeks.
- The eruptive phase begins with influenza-like symptoms, including low-grade fever and generalized aching.
- Individual lesions last approximately 2 weeks.
- New lesions sometimes appear for 3 to 6 weeks.
- Aching of the legs and swelling of the ankles may persist for weeks.
- This condition may recur for months or years.
- The course is benign in most patients.

SKIN FINDINGS

- Erythema nodosum begins as red, nodelike swellings over the shins.
- Both legs are usually affected.
- Lesions may appear on the extensor aspects of the forearms, thighs, and trunk.
- The border is poorly defined, the size varying from 2 to 6 cm.
- The oval lesions have a long axis corresponding to that of the limb.
- Within a week, the lesions become tense, hard, and painful.

- In the second week, they become fluctuant but never suppurate.
- The color changes in the second week from bright red to bluish or livid.
- The color gradually fades to a yellowish hue, resembling a bruise.
- The lesion disappears in 1 or 2 weeks as the overlying skin desquamates.

LABORATORY

- The initial evaluation includes a throat culture, antistreptolysin-O titer, chest film, purified protein derivative skin test, and erythrocyte sedimentation rate.
- Patients with gastrointestinal symptoms should have a stool culture for *Y. enterocolitica, Salmonella* species, and *Campylobacter* species.
- The rheumatoid factor is negative.
- Erythema nodosum is easily recognized clinically; biopsy is not required in most cases. An excisional rather than a punch biopsy is better for sampling the subcutaneous fat.

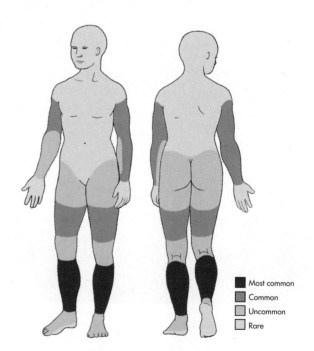

Most common

Common

Uncommon

Rare

DIFFERENTIAL DIAGNOSIS

- Cellulitis
- Infected insect bites
- Minor trauma
- Nodular vasculitis
- Henoch-Schönlein purpura
- Weber-Christian panniculitis (more on the thigh and trunk than on the leg)
- Superficial and deep thrombophlebitis
- Panniculitis secondary to pancreatic disease
- Erythema induratum (dull, red, tender nodules on the calves of women)

TREATMENT

- This self-limited disease requires only symptomatic relief.
- Nonsteroidal antiinflammatory drugs (indomethacin, naproxen) may be more effective than aspirin.
- Compressive bandages are applied and bed rest is ordered if the lesions are very inflamed.
- Potassium iodide, 300 mg three times a day for 3 to 4 weeks, is administered in severe cases.
- Oral corticosteroids are seldom necessary.
- Recurrence may follow discontinuation of treatment.
- Dapsone may be effective, but experience with this medication in this setting is limited.

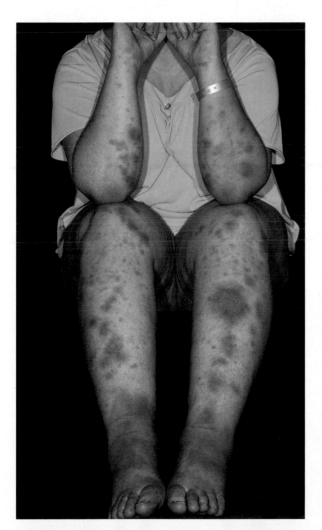

Red nodelike swelling in the characteristic distribution.

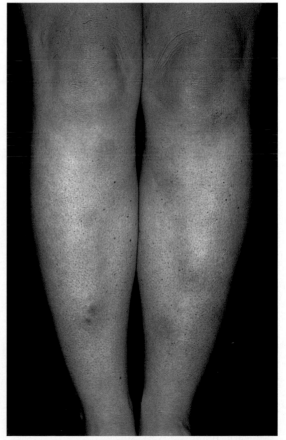

Lesions begin as red, nodelike swellings over the shins; as a rule, both legs are affected. The border is poorly defined, with size varying from 2 to 6 cm.

■ HYPERSENSITIVITY VASCULITIS (LEUKOCYTOCLASTIC VASCULITIS)

DESCRIPTION

- Vasculitis is an inflammation initiated by immune complex deposition in dermal postcapillary venules.
- Its triggers are diverse and include drugs and infectious agents.

HISTORY

- This condition is limited to the skin or may involve other organs (20% of cases).
- Prodromal symptoms include fever, malaise, myalgia, and joint pain.
- Smaller lesions itch and are painful.
- Nodules, ulcers, and bullae may be very painful.
- Lesions appear in crops, last 1 to 4 weeks, and heal with residual scarring and hyperpigmentation.
- This disease is usually self-limited.
- Some 10% of patients have recurrent disease for months to years.
- The duration of lesions does not correlate with the likelihood of systemic disease and is not a predictor of the prognosis.
- Most patients have a single episode that resolves spontaneously within several weeks or a few months.
- Other systems may be involved; these include the renal system (glomerulonephritis), central nervous system (hypoesthesia, paresthesia), gastrointestinal tract (abdominal pain, nausea, vomiting, diarrhea, melena), pulmonary system (cough, shortness of breath, hemoptysis), musculoskeletal (arthritis), and cardiac system (myocardial angiitis, arrhythmias, congestive heart failure).

ETIOLOGY

- The etiology is determined in two thirds of cases.
- Drugs cause 10% of the cases; penicillin, aminopenicillins, sulfonamides, allopurinol, thiazides, retinoids, quinolones, hydantoins, propylthiouracil, and many others are listed in single case reports. Drug-induced vasculitis develops within 7 to 21 days after treatment begins.
- Infections can also cause vasculitis; these can include streptococcal upper respiratory tract infections and hepatitis A, B, and C.
- Alternative causes are connective tissue disease, malignant neoplasms, and other systemic illnesses.

SKIN FINDINGS

- Lesions begin as asymptomatic, localized areas of cutaneous hemorrhage.
- The lesions may acquire substance and becomes palpable as blood leaks out of damaged vessels.
- They may coalesce, producing large areas of purpura.
- Nodules and urticarial lesions may appear.
- Hemorrhagic blisters and ulcers arise from purpuric areas (indicative more severe vessel involvement).
- Few to numerous discrete, purpuric lesions are most common on the lower extremities.
- The lesions may occur on any dependent area (e.g., the back or arms).
- Ankle and lower leg edema occurs with lower leg lesions.

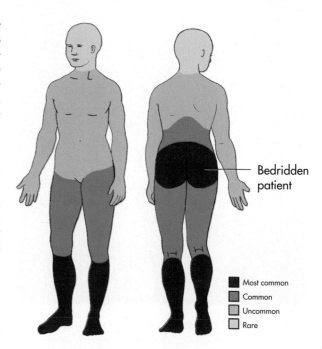

Bedridden patient

Most common
Common
Uncommon
Rare

LABORATORY

- The following tests should be considered: throat culture, antistreptolysin-O titer, erythrocyte sedimentation rate, platelet count, complete blood count, serum creatinine level, urinalysis, antinuclear antibody, antineutrophil cytoplasmic autoantibody titer, titer for antibodies to hepatitis B and C, cryoglobulins, total hemolytic complement (CH_{50}), and rheumatoid factor.
- The erythrocyte sedimentation rate is always elevated during active vasculitis.
- Punch biopsy taken from an early active lesion confirms the diagnosis.
- Immunofluorescent studies are indicated if the diagnosis is uncertain; biopsy can be used in all stages of vasculitis.

DIFFERENTIAL DIAGNOSIS

- Thrombocytopenic purpura
- Drug eruptions
- Disseminated intravascular coagulation
- Purpura fulminans
- Septic vasculitis
- Septic emboli
- Bacteremia

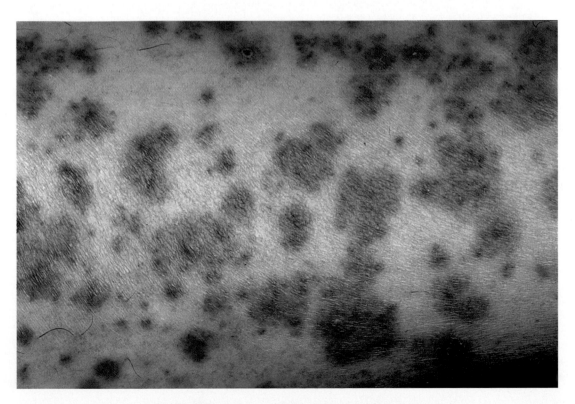

Lesions may coalesce, producing large areas of purpura.

TREATMENT

- Triggers should be identified and removed; these cases clear spontaneously.
- Antihistamines and nonsteroidal antiinflammatory drugs help the skin symptoms and arthralgias.
- For persistent, extensive or recurrent lesions, prednisone, 40 to 80 mg/day, is administered. The dose is slowly reduced over 3 to 6 weeks.
- Colchicine, 0.6 mg two or three times a day, may help if the disease becomes chronic.
- Dapsone, 100 to 200 mg/day, is usually used in disease confined to the skin.
- Immunosuppressive agents (cyclophosphamide, 2 mg/kg/day; methotrexate, 10 to 25 mg/wk; azathioprine, 50 to 200 mg/day) are used in cases with systemic involvement or rapid progression.

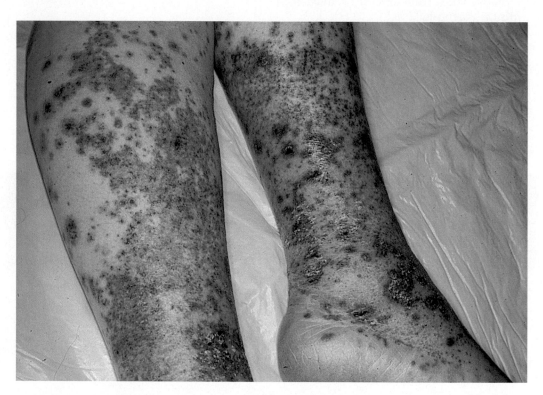

Hemorrhagic blisters and ulcers may arise from these purpuric areas and indicate more severe vessel inflammation and necrosis.

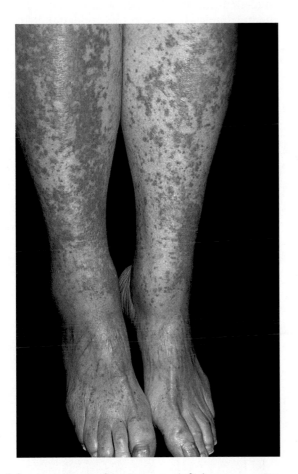

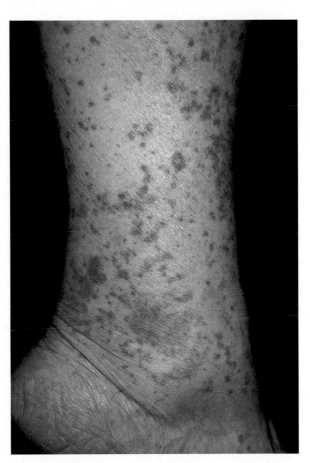

A few to numerous discrete, purpuric lesions are most commonly seen on the lower extremities but may occur on any dependent area, including the back if the patient is bedridden or the arms.

The characteristic lesions are referred to as *palpable purpura*.

■ HENOCH-SCHÖNLEIN PURPURA

DESCRIPTION

- Henoch-Schönlein purpura (HSP) occurs mainly in children. It is characterized by palpable purpura over the legs and buttocks, abdominal pain, gastrointestinal bleeding, arthralgia, and hematuria; histologically, it is characterized by leukocytoclastic vasculitis.
- It is the most common vasculitis syndrome of childhood.

HISTORY

- A streptococcal or viral upper respiratory infection may precede the disease by 1 to 3 weeks. The etiology of HSP remains unknown in many cases.
- The prodromal symptoms are anorexia and fever.
- The classic triad of purpuric rash, abdominal cramping, hematuria occurs.
- The spectrum varies from minimal petechial rash to severe gastrointestinal, renal, neurologic, pulmonary, and joint disease.
- Features are attributable to entrapment of circulating immunoglobulin A–containing immune complexes in the blood vessel walls, skin, kidneys, and gastrointestinal tract.
- Recurrences, typically in the first 3 months, occur in half of cases; recurrent disease is milder.
- The course is usually benign and self-limiting.
- Childhood Henoch-Schönlein nephritis requires long-term follow-up; the degree of renal involvement determines the long-term prognosis.

SKIN FINDINGS

- In nonthrombocytopenic palpable purpura, lesions appear on the lower extremities and buttocks and can appear on the arms, face, and ears; the trunk is usually spared.
- Acute scrotal swelling may be a presenting manifestation; lesions evolve from urticarial papules to purpura within 48 hours.
- Lesions are 2 to 10 mm in diameter and appear in crops among coalescent ecchymoses and pinpoint petechiae.
- Lesions fade in several days (more rapidly with bed rest), leaving brown macules.
- New lesions appear with ambulation.

LABORATORY

- Throat cultures are taken.
- Urinalysis demonstrates proteinuria and hematuria.
- Biopsy reveals acute vasculitis of arterioles and venules in the superficial dermis and bowel.
- Intestinal ultrasound demonstrates edematous hemorrhagic changes in the duodenal, jejunal, and ileal segments.
- Renal biopsy reveals mild focal glomerulitis to necrotizing or proliferative glomerulonephritis.
- Immunofluorescence shows immunoglobulin A in the walls of arterioles and in renal glomeruli.
- The serum immunoglobulin A level is frequently elevated.

DIFFERENTIAL DIAGNOSIS

- Leukocytoclastic vasculitis

TREATMENT

- The offending antigen (e.g., infections, malignancies, foods, drugs) must be identified and removed.
- Corticosteroids or dapsone may be useful in the early stages.
- Plasmapheresis may be effective.

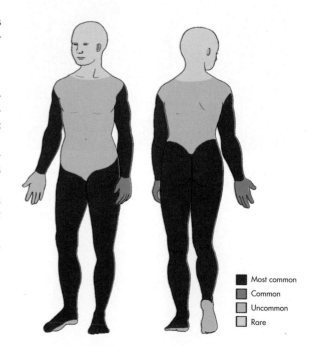

Most common
Common
Uncommon
Rare

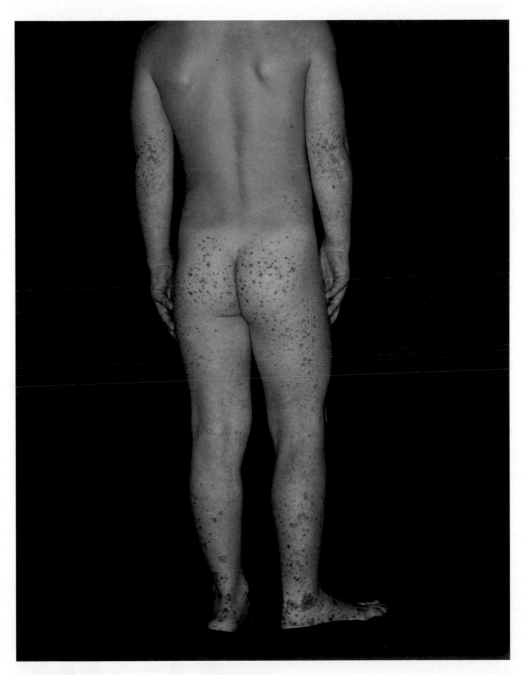

Henoch-Schönlein purpura.

■ SCHAMBERG'S DISEASE

DESCRIPTION

- Schamberg's disease is a lymphocytic capillaritis of unknown etiology.
- This is an uncommon eruption with petechiae and patches of brownish pigmentation (hemosiderin deposits).
- It occurs most often on the lower extremities.

HISTORY

- Male patients are affected more often than female patients.
- The lesions are insidious and slow to evolve.
- They are usually asymptomatic but may itch.
- The drug-induced variant develops and spreads more rapidly than the other types. Drugs implicated include acetaminophen, ampicillin, diuretics, and nonsteroidal and antiinflammatory agents.
- Lesions remain months or years; they are primarily a cosmetic problem.
- The drug-induced type may disappear more rapidly.

SKIN FINDINGS

- There are irregular, orange-brown patches of varying shapes and sizes.
- The characteristic feature is orange-brown, pinhead-sized "cayenne pepper" spots.
- Mild erythema and scaling cause slight itching.
- The spots appear more often on the lower legs but can appear on the upper body.
- New spots appear as older ones fade.

LABORATORY

- Biopsy reveals inflammation and hemorrhage without fibrinoid necrosis of vessels.

DIFFERENTIAL DIAGNOSIS

- Changes in chronic venous stasis
- Cutaneous T-cell lymphoma
- Nummular eczema
- Scurvy
- Senile purpura
- Trauma

TREATMENT

- The patient should be reassured that Schamberg's disease is not systemic but told that the pigmentation lasts for years.
- The spots can be covered with cosmetics (e.g., Dermablend).
- Mild itching and erythema respond quickly to group V topical steroids.
- This condition may improve with pentoxifylline (Trental), 300 mg per day for 8 weeks. A significant response may be observed within 2 to 3 weeks. Patients with recurrence after discontinuation of this treatment may respond to resumption of therapy.

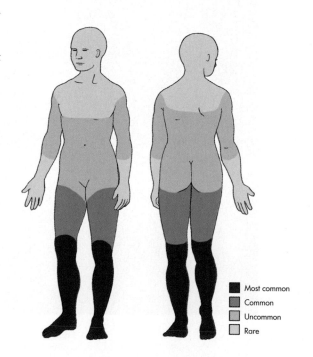

Most common
Common
Uncommon
Rare

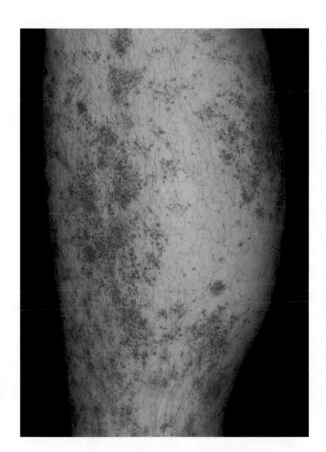

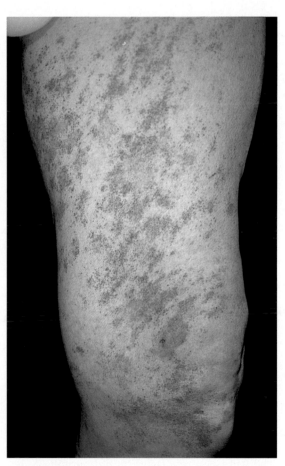

Asymptomatic, irregular patches of varying shapes and sizes occur most often on the lower extremities. The most characteristic feature is the orange-brown, pin-sized "cayenne pepper" spots.

The lesions begin as asymptomatic, localized areas of cutaneous hemorrhage that acquire substance and become palpable as blood leaks out of damaged vessels.

■ SWEET'S SYNDROME

DESCRIPTION

- Sweet's syndrome is an acute, idiopathic inflammatory eruption of multiple, discreet, erythematous, tender plaques with pseudovesiculation; it is often associated with fever, malaise, and leukocytosis.

HISTORY

- The mean age of onset is 56 years but can range from 22 to 82 years. Sweet's syndrome is uncommon in children.
- The male/female ratio is 3.7:1.
- The annual incidence in Scotland is 2.7 cases per million.
- This syndrome is regarded as a reactive phenomenon; a preceding upper respiratory syndrome is present in many patients. In about 15% to 20% of cases, Sweet's syndrome is associated with malignancy.

SKIN FINDINGS

- There is a sudden onset of painful, round, often coalescing, red to plum, juicy plaques with a subtle yellowish central coloration that may be targetlike or pseudovesicular.
- Lesions are often clustered and coalesce within the areas of involvement.
- This syndrome appears on the head, neck, legs, arms, dorsal hands, and fingers.
- Occasionally, there is pain or burning within skin lesions.
- Systemic symptoms include fever higher than 38° C (50% of cases), malaise, arthralgias or arthritis (62%), eye involvement (conjunctivitis, episcleritis, iridocyclitis) (33%), and oral aphthae (13%).
- Rarely, neutrophilic infiltrates occur within the upper respiratory tract, lungs, liver, and kidneys. There are case reports of central nervous system involvement.

LABORATORY

- The white blood cell count is higher than 8000 cells/mm^3 with more than 70% polymorphonucleocytes.
- The sedimentation rate is elevated.
- Alkaline phosphatase levels may be elevated in 40% of cases.
- Skin biopsy reveals massive neutrophilic infiltration in the papillary and reticular dermis with marked subepidermal edema. Leukocytoclasis and swelling of vascular endothelium are common. Vasculitis is not present.

DIFFERENTIAL DIAGNOSIS

- Erythema multiforme
- Erythema nodosum
- Adverse drug reaction
- Urticaria

TREATMENT

- This disease clears spontaneously in some patients.
- Systemic corticosteroids (prednisone, 0.5 to 1.5 mg/kg/day) produce rapid improvement. The fever, white blood cell count, and eruption improve within 72 hours. Skin lesions clear within 3 to 9 days. The drug is tapered and discontinued over 2 to 6 weeks.
- Minocycline, 100 mg twice a day, or doxycycline, 100 mg twice a day, may be effective.
- Oral potassium iodide, 15 mg/kg/day, inhibits neutrophil chemotaxis in peripheral blood and may be as effective as corticosteroids.
- Other alternatives to corticosteroid treatment include colchicine, dapsone, clofazimine, nonsteroidal antiinflammatory agents, and cyclosporine.

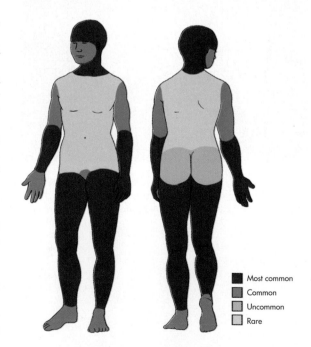

Most common
Common
Uncommon
Rare

DISCUSSION

- Lesions respond well to oral corticosteroids, although recurrence is frequent. A minority of patients (≈15%) have chronic relapsing disease for several years.
- Most cases are idiopathic, but some are parainflammatory or paraneoplastic. Upper respiratory infection, gastrointestinal tract infection, and vaccination can be causes. Inflammatory bowel disease, and autoimmune conditions such as Hashimoto's thyroiditis and Sjögren's syndrome have been associated with Sweet's syndrome. Hemoproliferative disorders such as myelodysplastic syndrome, nonlymphocytic leukemia, and solid tumors can be found.
- Many consider Sweet's syndrome and pyoderma gangrenosum related disorders.

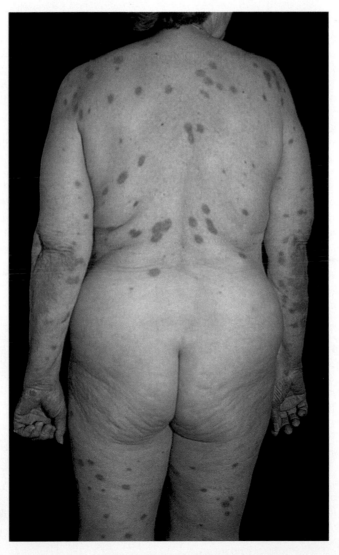

Acute, tender, erythematous plaques, nodes, pseudovesicles, and occasionally, blisters with an annular or arciform pattern occur. The trunk is sometimes involved in extensive cases.

15

Light-Related Diseases and Disorders of Pigmentation

■ SUN-DAMAGED SKIN

DESCRIPTION

- Sun-damaged skin has recognizable, morphologic changes as a result of years of accumulated exposure to ultraviolet radiation.

HISTORY

- Currently, men appear to be affected more often than women, although there is no known innate gender difference in susceptibility. Presumably, traditional occupational differences are responsible for this difference in incidence.
- Persons with fair complexions (skin types I and II) are at greatest risk.
- Sign of photoaging are apparent by age 40.

SKIN FINDINGS

- The face, lateral neck, and dorsa of the hands are the most severely affected areas.
- The posterior neck is equally involved in male patients.
- The skin appears older than its chronological age.
- All skin components are affected.
- The epidermis is thinned and dry.
- Localized areas of erythema and scaling suggest actinic keratoses.
- The pigmentation is uneven and blotchy.
- Distinct solar lentigines are present.
- Fine wrinkles form lateral to the eyes, and deep furrows form on the forehead, at the angles of the mouth, and on the posterior neck.
- The skin appears loose and without resilience.
- The blood vessels become telangiectatic.

- The skin of the dorsa of the hands and the arms bruises with minimal trauma.
- Pilosebaceous units are prominent and dilated with retained keratin (solar comedones).
- Poikiloderma describes the combination of epidermal atrophy, hyperpigmentation and hypopigmentation, and telangiectasia.
- Poikilodermatous change is seen on sun-exposed areas of the face and lateral neck.
- The skin beneath the chin is unaffected.

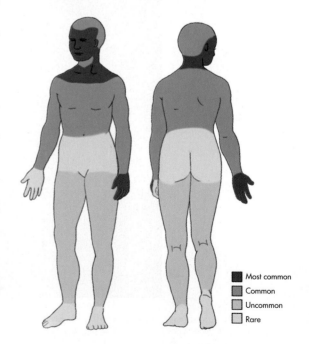

Most common
Common
Uncommon
Rare

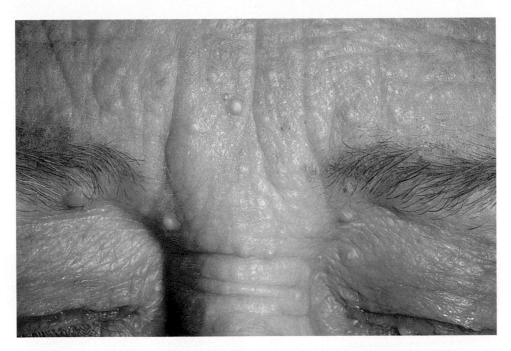

Photoaging. Wrinkling becomes coarse and deep rather than fine, and the skin is thickened. These wrinkles do not disappear by stretching.

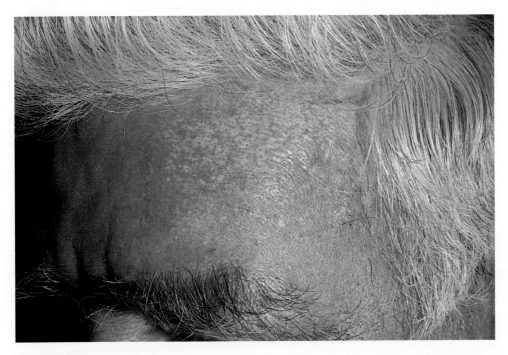

Solar elastosis is a sign highly characteristic of severe sun damage. There is a coarsening and yellow discoloration of the skin.

LABORATORY

- Hyperkeratosis of the stratum corneum, flattened rete ridges, keratinocyte atypia and dyskeratosis, dermal elastosis, and dilated cutaneous vessels occur.

COURSE AND PROGNOSIS

- Progressive damage from years of sun exposure continues even after proper sun avoidance.
- Some changes are reversible, however; actinic keratoses may regress completely with sun protection.

DISCUSSION

- A distinction is made between intrinsic aging of the skin and photoaging of the skin.

DIFFERENTIAL DIAGNOSIS

- Radiation dermatitis

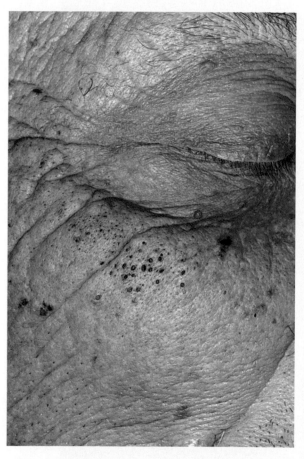

Coarse, deep wrinkles radiate from the lateral margin of the eye. Degraded collagen cannot support hair follicles. The follicles expand, accumulate sebum, and form comedones.

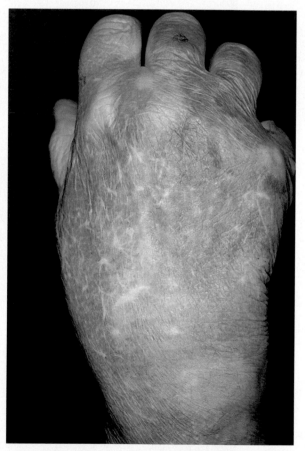

Bleeding occurs with the slightest trauma to the sun-damaged surfaces of the forearms and hands. The fragile skin tears easily and heals with crisscrossed scars.

TREATMENT

- Topical tretinoin reverses some photoaging over several months. Epidermal hyperkeratosis decreases. Pigmentation becomes more uniform and lighter. New collagen and new blood vessels form within the papillary dermis. Improvement is dose dependent and persists as long as the tretinoin is continued.
- Various peeling agents can also improve the texture and appearance of sun-damaged skin.
- Alpha-hydroxy acids reduce hyperkeratosis and promote epidermal hyperplasia.

- New collagen formation in the papillary dermis also occurs.
- Deeper peeling agents such as trichloroacetic acid and phenol cause full-thickness epidermal damage with intentional wounding of the papillary dermis. This wounding causes a thin zone of scar formation (new collagen) in the papillary dermis and effectively reduces wrinkles.
- Laser resurfacing has a similar effect.
- Broad-spectrum ultraviolet A– and ultraviolet B–blocking sunscreens, especially those containing avobenzone (Parsol 1789) and titanium dioxide, should be worn. Protective clothing is more effective.

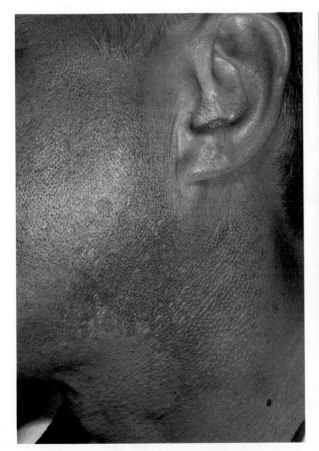

Poikiloderma of Civatte. Chronic sun exposure may cause red-brown pigmentation with telangiectasia and atrophy on the sides of the neck in predisposed individuals. The shaded area under the chin is spared.

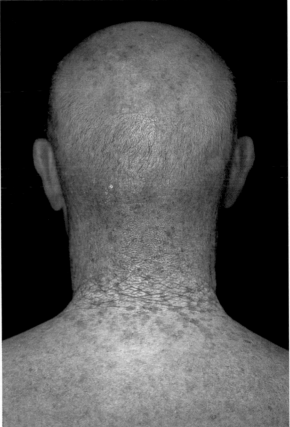

Sun-induced wrinkling on the back of the neck shows a series of crisscrossed lines. Reactive hyperplasia of melanocytes causes lentigines. Diffuse persistent erythema is prominent in fair-skinned people.

◼ POLYMORPHOUS LIGHT ERUPTION

DESCRIPTION

- Polymorphous light eruption is an idiopathic, recurrent photodermatitis that comes on acutely, usually in the spring.
- It is commonly referred to as *sun poisoning* or *sun allergy*.

HISTORY

- Polymorphous light eruption occurs in all races and at any age but is most common in young female patients.
- The incidence is as high as 10% of the population.
- It occurs in northern climates, where sun intensity increases in spring.
- It occurs during winter vacations when the patient visits southern, sunny spots, appearing 2 hours to 5 days after sun exposure.
- Symptoms include pruritus, malaise, chills, headache, and nausea. They vary over the years.
- Rash and pruritus develop hours after exposure.
- Patients develop the same clinical type each year.
- The rash first occurs in limited areas and becomes more extensive during subsequent summers.
- Most patients have exacerbations each summer for many years.
- Ultraviolet A is the trigger in most cases.
- The amount of light needed to trigger this condition varies.
- The rash persists for 7 to 10 days.
- Light sensitivity decreases with repeated sun exposure.
- Hereditary polymorphous light eruption occurs in the Inuit and Native Americans.
- It has an autosomal dominant transmission with incomplete penetrance and variable expressivity.

SKIN FINDINGS

- The initial symptoms are burning, itching, and erythema on exposed skin.
- A V on the chest, the backs of the hands, the extensor aspects of the forearms, and the lower legs are involved.
- The face tends to be spared (except in the hereditary form).
- There are several clinical types of polymorphous light eruption.
  - In the papular type (most common), small papules are disseminated or densely aggregated on a patchy erythema.
  - In the plaque type (second most common), superficial or urticarial plaques appear.
  - The papulovesicular type (least common) begins with urticarial plaques from which groups of vesicles arise.

LABORATORY

- The findings from the history and physical examination determine the diagnosis.
- Histopathologic changes are not specific.
- The findings from antinuclear antibody titers, anti-Ro/anti-La antibody titer, and direct and indirect immunofluorescence differentiate polymorphous light eruption from lupus.

DIFFERENTIAL DIAGNOSIS

- Systemic and discoid lupus erythematosus
- Atopic dermatitis (which the papular form resembles)
- Photodrug eruption

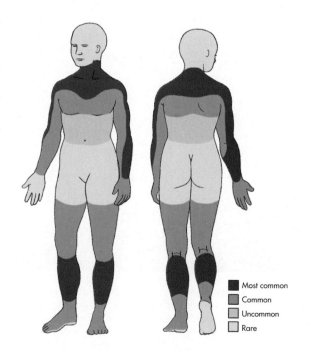

Most common
Common
Uncommon
Rare

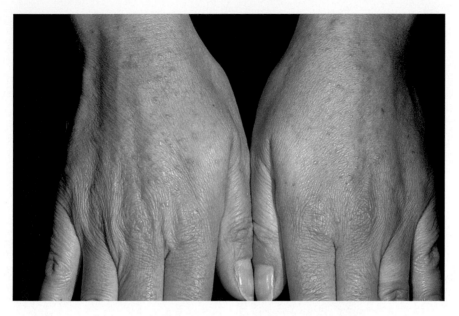

The papular type is the most common form. Small papules are densely aggregated. The back of the hands is a common site.

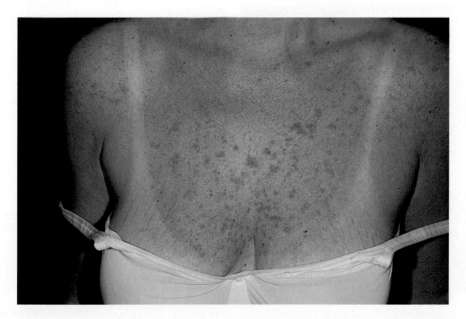

The papulovesicular type begins with urticarial plaques from which groups of vesicles arise.

TREATMENT

- Sun-protective clothing should be worn. Special protective clothing is available from Sun Precautions, 2815 Wetmore Avenue, Everett, WA 98201, 1-800-882-7860, www.sunprecautions.com.
- Sun exposure should be minimized (especially between 10 AM and 3 PM).
- Broad-spectrum, ultraviolet A–blocking sunscreens, especially those containing avobenzone (Parsol 1789) and titanium dioxide, should be worn.

- Groups II through V topical steroids should be prescribed for 3 to 14 days.
- A 2-week taper of oral steroids is useful in severe cases.
- Controlled, gradual exposure to sunlight or ultraviolet B or A can harden the skin and increase tolerance.
- Hydroxychloroquine, 400 mg/day for the first month and 200 mg/day thereafter, is administered for difficult cases.

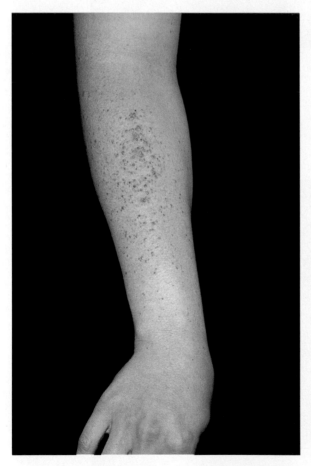

Small papules are disseminated or densely aggregated on a patchy erythema.

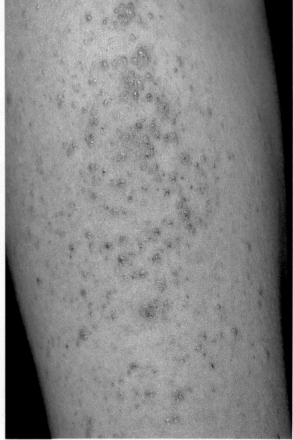

The papulovesicular type occurs primarily on the arms, lower limbs, and V area of the chest.

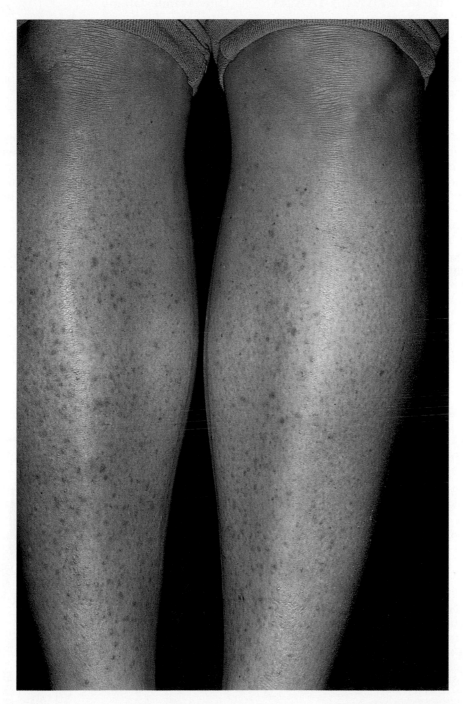

The most commonly involved areas are the V of the chest, the backs of the hands, the extensor aspects of the forearms, and the lower legs of women.

■ PORPHYRIA CUTANEA TARDA

DESCRIPTION

- The porphyrias represent abnormalities in the pathway for heme synthesis. Enzyme deficiencies along this pathway result in increased formation of metabolic intermediaries (porphyrinogens) just before the specific enzyme defect.
- Each type of porphyria is characterized by a specific enzyme deficiency and distinct clinical characteristics.
- The porphyrias are divided into disorders of bone marrow heme synthesis (the erythropoietic porphyrias) and disorders of hepatic heme synthesis (the hepatic porphyrias).
- Porphyria cutanea tarda (PCT) is the most common form of porphyria.
  - It results from a deficiency of hepatic uroporphyrinogen decarboxylase activity.
  - Both acquired and familial forms exist.
  - It occurs when the heme biosynthetic pathway is compromised by an exogenous agent.
- The acquired ("sporadic") form occurs as a complication of hepatic dysfunction or is induced by alcohol, drugs, or hormones.
- Specific cutaneous changes occur in sun-exposed areas.

HISTORY

- PCT occurs in middle-aged patients and in younger women on oral contraceptives.
- There is an autosomal dominant transmission in familial PCT.
- "Sporadic" PCT may be an autosomal recessive trait.
- The estimated prevalence is 1 in 25,000 in North America.
- Alcohol and estrogens are associated with more than 80% of cases.

SKIN FINDINGS

Early Changes

- Erythema, edema, pruritus, and blisters appear.
- Blisters occur in sun-exposed areas (face, dorsa of the hands, forearms, neck).
- Blisters rupture, leaving erosions and ulcers that heal with scarring.
- Milia form in previously blistered sites on the hand.

Later Manifestations

- Periorbital and temporal hypertrichosis occur.
- Hyperpigmentation appears on the face, neck, and hands.
- Sclerotic changes and increased skin fragility on the cheeks, posterior neck, ears, and fingers produce a sclerodermoid pattern.

NONSKIN FINDINGS

- Liver disease occurs in association with ethanol; estrogens; aromatic hydrocarbons; benign, malignant, or metastatic tumors; chronic renal failure during dialysis; sarcoidosis; and infection with the hepatitis C or B and human immunodeficiency viruses.

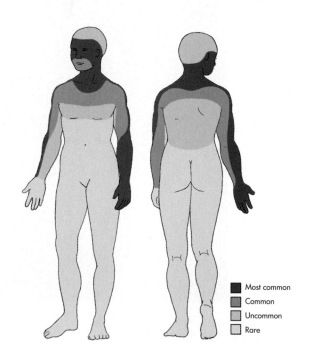

- Most common
- Common
- Uncommon
- Rare

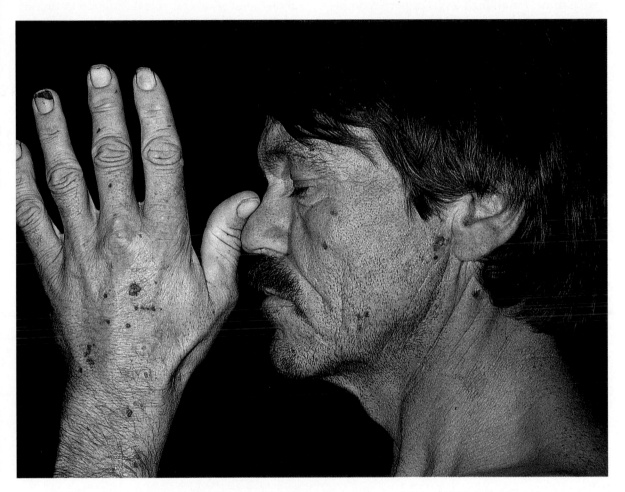

The clinical features in order of frequency are blistering in sun-exposed areas, facial hypertrichosis, hyperpigmentation, and sclerodermoid changes.

LABORATORY

- Quantitative assays of fecal, urine, and red blood cell porphyrins are ordered.
- A 24-hour urine collection contains uroporphyrin in a ratio of about 4:1 to the coproporphyrin fraction.
- Urine may have a red-brown discoloration ("port-wine urine") from high levels of porphyrin pigments. It may show a bright pink fluorescence under a Wood's light.
- Histopathologic testing reveals subepidermal split and thickening of the superficial dermal vascular endothelium.
- Direct immunofluorescence shows the deposition of immunoglobulins G and M and complement C3 around the blood vessels in the papillary dermis.
- Fecal analysis shows elevated coproporphyrins.
- Tests for hepatitis B and C and human immunodeficiency virus should be ordered.
- Liver function tests, iron studies, and renal function tests should also be ordered.
- Ultrasound of the liver allows the clinician to look for tumors.

DIFFERENTIAL DIAGNOSIS

- Pseudo-PCT
- Variegate porphyria
- Epidermolysis bullosa acquisita
- Other forms of porphyria
- Other bullous diseases
- Porphyria variegata (The cutaneous signs of PCT coexist with the abdominal pain and neuropsychiatric symptoms of acute intermittent porphyria. Skin manifestations are absent in acute intermittent porphyria. There are protoporphyrin and coproporphyrin in the feces. Elevated urinary levels of gamma-aminolevulinic acid and porphobilinogen occur during attacks.)

TREATMENT

- Complete elimination of alcohol and exposure to other hepatotoxins results in complete clinical clearing of bullae and skin fragility in 2 months to 2 years.
- Iron removal by phlebotomy is the treatment of choice. It reduces hepatic iron stores and produces remissions of several years' duration. A unit of blood should be removed every 2 to 4 weeks until the hemoglobin level drops to 10 gm/dl or until the serum iron level drops to 50 mg/dl. The average number of units required for remission varies between 8 and 14.
- Measuring plasma uroporphyrin is an effective way to monitor the progress of patients with PCT. Treatment should continue until plasma uroporphyrin levels drops under 10 mmol/L.
- Chloroquine in very low dosages may also be used. This medication causes the release of hepatic tissue–bound uroporphyrin, and subsequently, it is rapidly eliminated by the plasma and excreted by the urine. A too-rapid release of porphyrins might severely affect liver function. Complete clinical and biochemical response has occurred with the use of chloroquine, 125 mg twice a week for 8 to 18 months. Remission in most patients lasts more than 4 years.
- Combined treatment with repeated bleeding and chloroquine results in remission in an average of 3.5 months. The time necessary for remission with chloroquine alone is 10.2 months. The time for remission with phlebotomy alone is 12.5 months.
- Sunscreens that contain Parsol 1789 (e.g., Ombrelle) that block ultraviolet A light should be used. Physical sun-blockers that contain titanium dioxide are moderately effective.

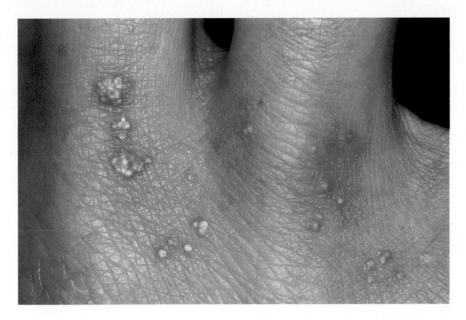

White milia form during the healing process and are permanent.

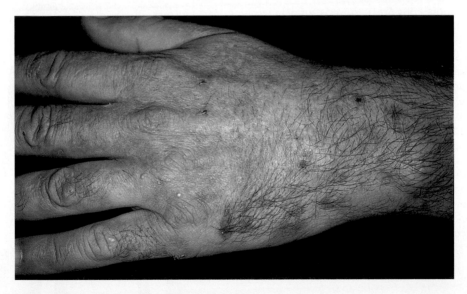

Blistering, erosions, and atrophic scars on the back of the hands are the classic signs of porphyria cutanea tarda.

■ VITILIGO

DESCRIPTION

- Vitiligo is a disfiguring disease of unknown origin that causes destruction of melanocytes.

HISTORY

- There is a positive family history in 30% of patients.
- Both sexes are affected equally.
- Some 1% of the population affected.
- Half of cases begin before age 20 years.
- Patients may state that the first onset occurs after emotional stress, illness, or trauma (e.g., sunburn).
- Initially, the disease is limited.
- It progresses slowly over the years in a highly variable course.
- Some patients have very stable disease; in others, vitiligo progresses at a alarming rate.
- Segmental vitiligo develops quickly and then stabilizes, rarely spreading.
- This condition may be associated with autoimmune thyroid disease.
- Childhood vitiligo is distinct, with an increased incidence of segmental vitiligo, autoimmune and endocrine disease, premature graying, organ-specific antibodies, and a poor prognosis.
- New patches appear throughout life.

SKIN FINDINGS

- In type A (most common), there is a fairly symmetric pattern of white macules (5 mm to 5 cm or more) with well-defined borders.
- Type B is segmental vitiligo, which is limited to one segment of the body (e.g., the extremities). It is more common in childhood.
- The borders may have a red halo (inflammatory vitiligo) or a rim of hyperpigmentation.
- Loss of pigmentation is not as apparent in fair-skinned individuals but is disfiguring in African-Americans.
- Common sites include the dorsa of the hands, face, body folds, axillae, and genitalia.
- It is common around body openings (e.g., eyes, nostrils, mouth, nipples, umbilicus, anus).
- Vitiligo occurs at sites of trauma (Koebner's phenomenon).

LABORATORY

- Wood's light accentuates the hypopigmented areas.
- Skin biopsy reveals an absence of melanocytes.
- Thyroid disease is possible.

DIFFERENTIAL DIAGNOSIS

- Lupus erythematosus
- Pityriasis alba
- Piebaldism
- Pityriasis versicolor (tinea versicolor)
- Chemical leukoderma
- Leprosy
- Nevus depigmentosus
- Nevus anemicus
- Tuberous sclerosus
- Postinflammatory leukoderma
- Postmelanoma leukoderma

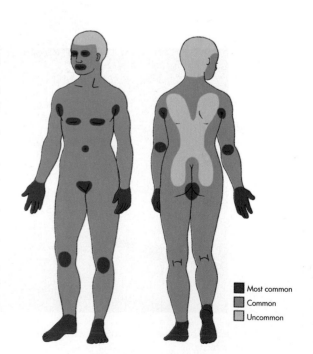

Most common
Common
Uncommon

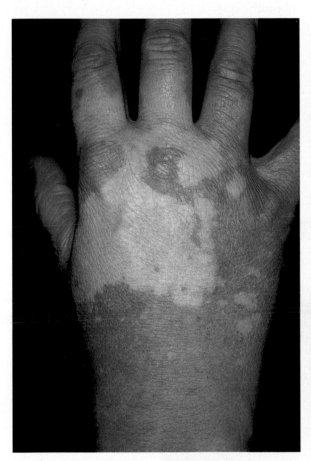

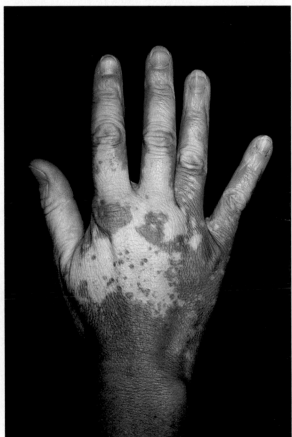

The margins of the lesions may become more hyperpigmented. The borders are sharply defined.

The backs of the hands are commonly affected and are most resistant to treatment.

TREATMENT

Sun Protection

- The patient should use broad-spectrum sunscreens that contain avobenzone (Parsol 1789) (e.g., Ombrelle, PreSun Ultra), titanium dioxide, or both products.
- The patient should also wear sun-protective clothing. Such clothing is available from Sun Precautions, 2815 Wetmore Avenue, Everett, WA 98201, 1-800-882-7860, www.sunprecautions.com.

Cosmetic Treatment

- Concealing and camouflaging agents (e.g., Dermablend, Covermark, Elizabeth Arden Concealing Cream) can be used.
- Topical dyes (e.g., Dy-O-Derm, VitaDye) require less regular use.
- Sunless self-tanning lotions darken the skin by staining; Elizabeth Arden Self Tanning Lotion and Estée Lauder Self-Action Tanning Cream work best on skin phototypes II and III.
- The major problem is color blending and matching.

Topical Steroids

- Group I or II topical steroid ointment is safe and effective for limited disease.
- It is applied twice a day for 6 weeks and then stopped for 2 weeks; this regimen is repeated for two more cycles if there are no side effects.
- The face and neck respond better than other areas.

Phototherapy

- Topical or systemic photochemotherapy with psoralens and ultraviolet A (PUVA) is somewhat effective, but the potential side effects, expense, and inconvenience limit its usefulness.
- Narrow-band ultraviolet B treatment may be effective.

Depigmentation

- Patients with more than 40% involvement may choose to remove the remaining normal pigment with 20% monobenzone (Benoquin cream).
- Monobenzone is applied twice a day for 6 to 18 months to chemically destroy all melanocytes in the skin.
- It creates permanent removal and thus requires that patient be informed about it and pay close attention to sun protection.

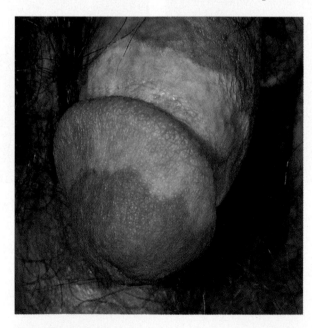

The genitalia, axillae, and anal areas may be the first or only areas affected. These sites should be examined in all patients suspected of having vitiligo.

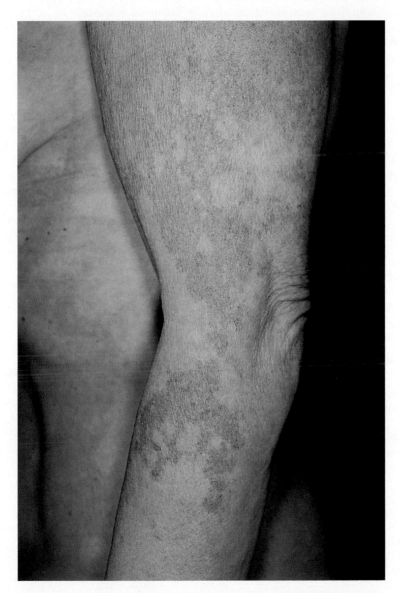

Loss of pigment may be partial or complete. Complex patterns are typical.

■ IDIOPATHIC GUTTATE HYPOMELANOSIS

DESCRIPTION

- Idiopathic guttate hypomelanosis (senile depigmented spots), a common dermatosis of unknown etiology, consists of small, white macules on the exposed upper and lower extremities.

HISTORY

- Reassurance, explanation, and no treatment are usually adequate.
- Idiopathic guttate hypomelanosis occurs in middle-aged and older Caucasians.
- It occurs more often in women than in men.
- There is a higher prevalence in family members; genetic predisposition is likely.
- It occurs in 50% to 70% of people over age 50.
- This condition is asymptomatic.

SKIN FINDINGS

- Hypopigmented and white, 2- to 5-mm macules with regular borders appear on the skin. They are smooth to scaling.
- The macules are scattered on the exposed upper and lower extremities.
- Patients have signs of early aging and sun exposure, including seborrheic keratoses, lentigines, and xerosis in the same areas.

LABORATORY

- Epithelial atrophy, a patchy absence of melanocytes, and melanin are found.

COURSE AND PROGNOSIS

- The number of lesions increases with age.
- Lesions are benign.

DISCUSSION

- The appearance and potential for malignancy are the major reasons for patients' concern.
- Actinic damage has been incriminated as the major cause of this condition, but a senile degenerative phenomenon may play a role.

DIFFERENTIAL DIAGNOSIS

- Vitiligo
- Tinea versicolor
- Chemically induced hypomelanosis
- Tuberous sclerosis
- Pityriasis alba

TREATMENT

- White macules can be camouflaged with tinted makeup such as Covermark or Dermablend. Self-tanning creams that contain dihydroxyacetone darken the lesions, but the appearance is speckled and not pleasing.
- A light spray with liquid nitrogen may partially fade the lesions.
- A very small quantity of triamcinolone, 2.5 mg/ml, is infiltrated into individual lesions. Partial repigmentation may result.
- Sun protection with clothing should be encouraged. Sunscreens are less effective than clothing.

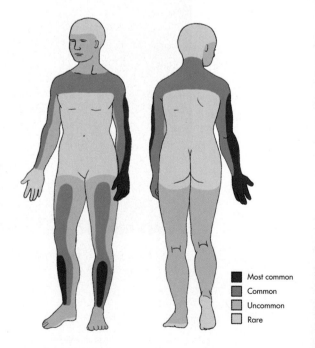

Most common
Common
Uncommon
Rare

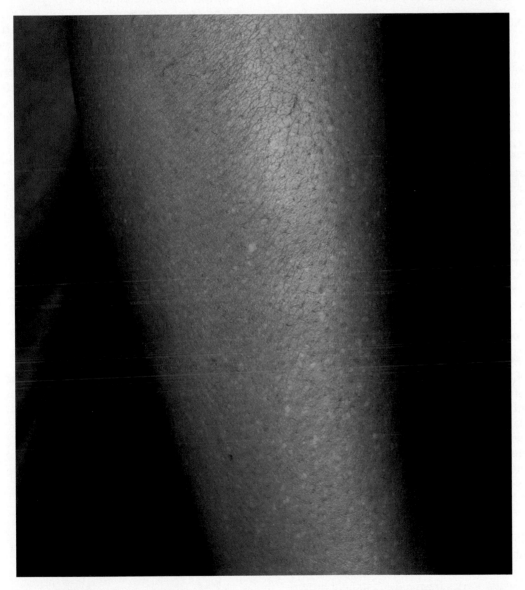

Idiopathic guttate hypomelanosis is characterized by 2- to 5-mm white spots with sharply demarcated borders. They are a sign of photodamage.

■ LENTIGO

DESCRIPTION

- Lentigo is a common condition in which benign, brown macules occur in Caucasians.

HISTORY

- Three lesions of localized hyperpigmentation occur in Caucasians: freckles or ephelides, juvenile lentigo, and solar lentigo.
- All share some similarity in size, distribution, and clinical appearance but differ in age of onset, clinical course, and relationship to sun exposure.
- Freckles appear in childhood and occur as an autosomal dominant trait.
  - They are usually confined to the face, arms, and upper trunk.
  - They increase in number and darken in color in response to sun exposure.
  - They lighten in color without sun exposure.
  - They often fade completely in the winter.
- Lentigines are extremely common to universal in Caucasian skin.
  - Juvenile lentigines appear in childhood.
  - Prepubertal children have a mean number of 30 lentigines.
  - These lesions do not increase in number or size or darken in color in response to sunlight.
  - Juvenile lentigines do not fade in the absence of sunlight.
  - Juvenile lentigines also occur as a characteristic feature of certain hereditary syndromes.
- Solar lentigines commonly occur on sun-exposed Caucasian skin.
  - They increase in number and size with advancing age.
  - Roughly 75% of Caucasians over the age of 60 have one or more lesion.
  - As the name implies, solar lentigines develop in response to actinic damage.

SKIN FINDINGS

- Freckles are 1- to 2-mm, sharply defined macules with uniform color.
  - The color varies from red-tan to light brown.
  - The number varies from a few sparse lesions over the nose and malar cheeks to hundreds with near confluence on sun-exposed skin.
  - Freckles are usually limited to the face, arms, and upper trunk.

- Juvenile lentigines are round to oval macules 2 to 10 mm in diameter.
  - They are usually darker than freckles and uniformly tan to brown to black.
  - The color is uniform, although the pigment may have a lacy or finely-grained pattern.
  - A drop of mineral oil applied to the lesion reduces surface glare and allows for the evaluation of the junctional pigmentation pattern.
- Solar lentigines tend to be larger (2 to 20 mm), oval to geometric macules.
  - The color is most often uniform, although pigment may appear as fine grains.
  - Lentigines may appear blotchy.
  - The surrounding skin shows actinic damage.
  - The borders should be sharply defined.

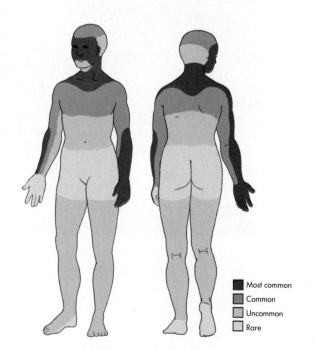

■	Most common
■	Common
□	Uncommon
□	Rare

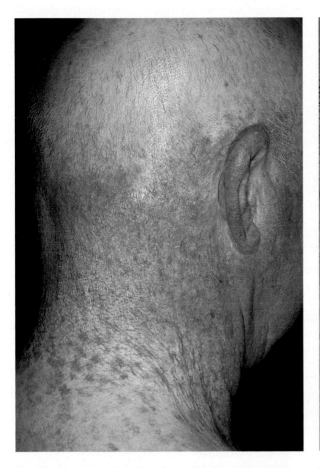

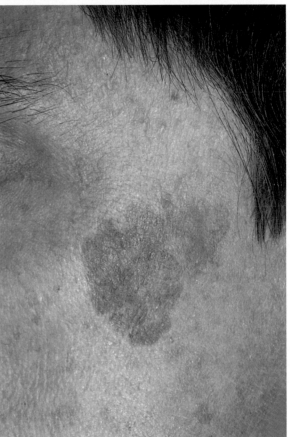

Reactive hyperplasia of melanocytes causes persistent pigmentation in the form of lentigines on the neck and upper back. These permanent lesions may occur after one bad sunburn.

The lesions vary in size from 0.2 to 2 cm and become more numerous with advancing age. The lesion should be carefully examined. Seborrheic keratosis and melanoma have a similar appearance.

NONSKIN FINDINGS

- Lentigines are a feature of rare autosomal dominant syndromes.
- Peutz-Jeghers syndrome consists of multiple lentigines of the oral mucosa with associated intestinal polyposis.
- The LEOPARD syndrome consists of multiple *l*entigines, *e*lectrocardiographic abnormalities, *o*cular disorders, *p*ulmonary stenosis, *a*bnormalities of the genitalia, *r*etardation of growth, and *d*eafness.
- A third syndrome described by Carney is known as *LAMB* or *NAME syndrome.* This syndrome consists of lentigines, atrial and/or mucocutaneous myxomas, myxoid neurofibromas, ephelides, and blue nevi.

LABORATORY

- Freckles show increased melanin within basal layer keratinocytes.
  - The rete ridges are not elongated.
  - Junctional melanocytes are larger but not increased in number.
- Juvenile lentigines have an increased number of nonnested melanocytes along the dermoepidermal junction.
  - The rete ridges are elongated.
  - Melanin is increased within basal-layer keratinocytes.
- Solar lentigines also show irregular elongation of rete ridges, basal-layer keratinocyte hyperpigmentation, and increased numbers of junctional melanocytes.
  - Melanophages may be present in the papillary dermis.
  - Histologically similar lesions occur on the lower mucosal lip and in the nailbed.

COURSE AND PROGNOSIS

- Freckles appear in early summer and usually fade by early winter.
- Juvenile lentigo persists year-round with little change over the years and may spontaneously resolve.
- Solar lentigo is usually persistent; additional lesions may appear elsewhere on sun-exposed skin.
- Lesions are symptomatic, but they may be of cosmetic concern to the patient.

DIFFERENTIAL DIAGNOSIS

- Solar lentigo
- Flat seborrheic keratosis
- Spreading pigmented actinic keratosis
- Lentigo maligna

DISCUSSION

- It is difficult to distinguish between freckles and similar juvenile lentigines. Freckles are darker and then fade with the seasons, but lentigines do not.
- Junctional nevi of similar size are also similar in appearance.
- Skin biopsy confirms melanocyte nesting along the dermoepidermal junction in a junctional nevus.
- Seborrheic keratoses and spreading pigmented actinic keratoses usually show some epidermal hyperkeratosis.
- The distinction of solar lentigo from lentigo maligna depends on skin biopsy and careful histologic review.
- Any lentigo that develops a localized area of hyperpigmentation or hypopigmentation, an irregular outline, or localized thickening should be biopsied.
- When numerous lentigines are present, the possibility of an associated syndrome such as Peutz-Jeghers, LEOPARD, NAME, or LAMB must be considered.

TREATMENT

- Freckles do not require treatment and fade in the winter.
- Broad-spectrum sunscreens appear to prevent the appearance of new freckles and seasonal darkening.
- Juvenile lentigines do not require treatment.
- Solar lentigines are best prevented with sun-protective measures, including sun avoidance, sun-protecting clothing, and sunscreens.
- Existing lesions should be monitored at regular intervals for change.
- Stable lesions do not require treatment, although it may be requested for cosmetic reasons.
- Hydroquinone solutions, azelaic acid cream, and glycolic acid peels and creams are all of value in reducing hyperpigmentation over weeks to months.
- Cryosurgery is also effective.

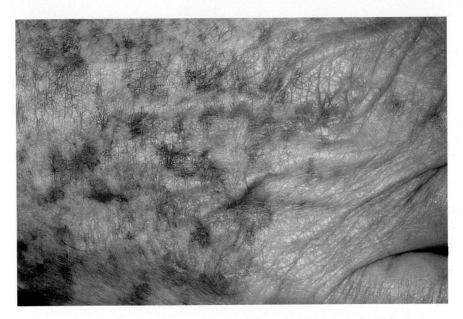

Lentigo, or liver spot, occurs in sun-exposed areas of the face, arms, and hands.

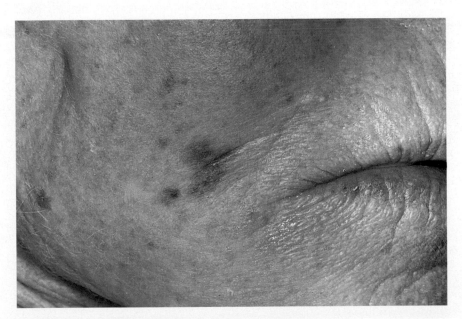

A biopsy should be taken from any lentigo that develops a highly irregular border, localized increase in pigmentation, or localized thickening to rule out lentigo maligna melanoma.

■ MELASMA

DESCRIPTION

- Melasma is an acquired brown hyperpigmentation involving the face and neck.
- It occurs in genetically predisposed women.

HISTORY

- Melasma is a common complaint in women with darker skin tones.
- Some 10% of cases occur in men.
- The forehead, malar eminences, upper lip, and chin are most frequently affected.
- The pigmentation develops slowly and may be faint or dark.
- It is more prevalent after sunlight exposure.
- It occurs during the second or third trimester of pregnancy.
- It occurs in some women taking oral contraceptives.
- Usually after pregnancy or with discontinuation of contraceptives, the pigment fades slowly over months.

SKIN FINDINGS

- A symmetric macular or patch eruption of brown hyperpigmentation appears.
- The intensity of the color varies.
- It is darker in darker-skinned individuals.
- The color is usually uniform but may be variable.
- The edges of the lesions can be irregular.
- There are no signs of inflammation.

DIFFERENTIAL DIAGNOSIS

- Postinflammatory hyperpigmentation
- Lentigo

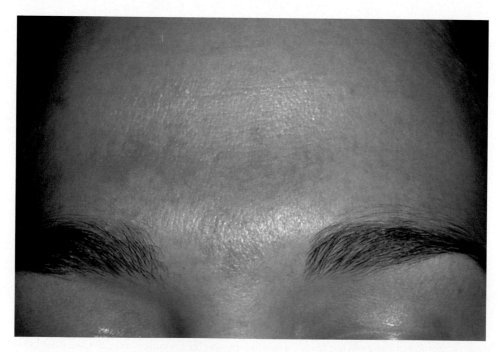

The pigmentation develops slowly without signs of inflammation and may be faint or dark.

TREATMENT

- Sun exposure should be minimized.
- Broad-spectrum sunscreens that block both ultraviolet A and B (e.g., PreSun Ultra, Ombrelle) should be used.
- Depigmentation with bleaching creams that contain hydroquinone should be applied twice a day.
  - Over-the-counter 2% concentrations (Porcelana)
  - Prescription 3% concentrations (Melanex) and 4% concentrations (Lustra, Eldoquin Forte, Eldopaque Forte, Viquin Forte and Solaquin Forte, and generic formulations)

- Hydroquinone can be an irritant and a sensitizer. It must be used for months but results in gradual depigmentation.
- Tretinoin cream 0.025%, 0.05%, and 0.1% (Retin-A) or tretinoin emollient cream 0.05% (Renova) enhances hydroquinone's effectiveness. Tretinoin is also effective as a monotherapy.
- Azelaic acid (Azelex cream) with or without tretinoin is effective.
- Superficial peels with glycolic acid hasten the effects of tretinoin and hydroquinone.

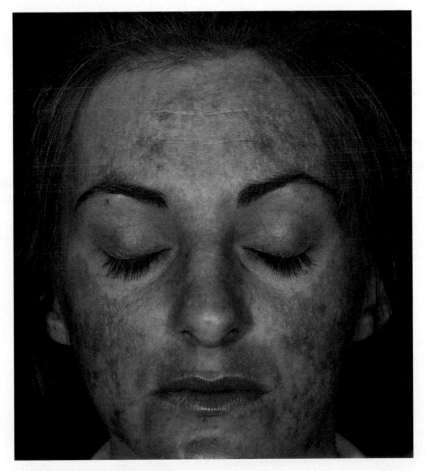

The forehead, malar eminences, upper lip, and chin are most frequently affected.

16

Benign Skin Tumors

■ SEBORRHEIC KERATOSIS

DESCRIPTION

- Seborrheic keratosis is a common, benign, persistent epidermal lesion with variable clinical appearance.

HISTORY

- Seborrheic keratoses are unusual before age 30.
- Most people develop at least one seborrheic keratosis in their lifetime.
- Male and female patients are equally affected.
- There is no racial predilection, although specific patterns are more common in specific racial groups.
- The tendency toward multiple seborrheic keratoses may be inherited.
- This condition is usually asymptomatic, and sometimes, it is cosmetically bothersome.
- Depending on the location, the lesion can be subject to irritation.

SKIN FINDINGS

- There are usually multiple lesions, which can arise at any site except the palms and soles.
- The size and surface appearance of the lesions vary considerably.
- Most are 0.2 to 2.0 cm, although larger lesions are common.
- Lesions may be flat or raised.
- The surface may be smooth, velvety, or verrucous.
- Retained keratin cysts may be seen just under the surface within clefts in smooth lesions.
- The color of lesions varies from white to pink to jet black, and the color may vary within a single lesion.

- Lesions tend to be sharply demarcated, oval, and often oriented along skin cleavage lines.
- Most have a stuck-on appearance and waxy texture.
- The surface tends to crumble when picked.
- Dermatosis papulosa nigra describes the seborrheic keratoses more commonly found on African-Americans.
  - The incidence is estimated at 35%.
  - There are numerous 1- to 2-mm, dark brown keratotic papules concentrated around the eyes and on the malar cheeks.

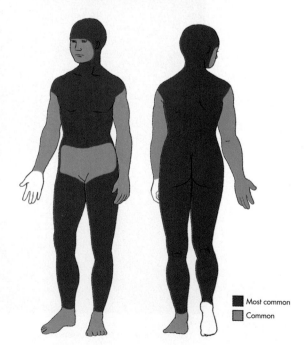

Most common
Common

- Stucco keratoses describe the seborrheic keratoses more commonly found on the lower legs of older Caucasians.
  - Numerous white-gray, barely raised, dry, 1- to 10-mm keratotic papules are concentrated on the dorsa of the feet, the ankles, and the dorsa of the hands.
- Irritated seborrheic keratoses do not differ in appearance from nonirritated seborrheic keratoses. This descriptive term is used for histologic purposes only.
- Inflamed seborrheic keratosis is a clinical description for a seborrheic keratosis with clinically obvious inflammation. A red halo is seen around an otherwise typical seborrheic keratosis. Trauma is usually the inciting event. With time, the lesion becomes edematous and intensely itchy.

Nonskin Findings

- The sign of Leser-Trélat (see p. 459) is the sudden explosive onset of numerous seborrheic keratoses in association with internal malignancy.

Laboratory

- Several histologic subtypes of seborrheic keratosis are recognized.
- Acanthosis, hyperkeratosis, and papillomatosis are universal features.
- The degree to which these features develop varies considerably within individual lesions and among subtypes.
- Two types of keratinocyte are present: basaloid and squamous.
- Horn cysts and pseudohorn cysts are usually present.
- The degree of melanin pigment varies from almost none (stucco keratosis) to extreme (melano-acanthoma).
- In irritated or activated seborrheic keratosis, squamous cells outnumber basaloid cells.
  - Whirls or eddies of eosinophilic squamous cells are found throughout the lesion.
  - Minimal dermal inflammation is present.
- Inflamed seborrheic keratoses show marked dermal inflammation.
  - The overlying acanthotic epidermis is often edematous.

Course and Prognosis

- Unless disturbed, seborrheic keratoses tend to persist and grow slowly.

Discussion

- Raised or pedunculated seborrheic keratoses may be indistinguishable from skin tags and compound melanocytic nevi.
- Flat seborrheic keratoses may mimic spreading pigmented actinic keratosis or superficial spreading melanoma. If doubt exists, a skin biopsy should be performed.
- Although seborrheic keratoses have no malignant potential, there are rare reports of melanoma and squamous cell carcinoma developing within a seborrheic keratosis.

Treatment

- Treatment is indicated for symptomatic lesions. Lesions are generally symptomatic because they are located in an area of friction and frequent trauma.
- Removal is often requested for cosmetic reasons.
- Patients should be informed that cosmetic removal of seborrheic keratoses is not usually covered by medical insurance.
- An appropriate fee for the service should be agreed on before the procedure.
- Cryosurgery is effective for flat to minimally raised lesions. Hypopigmentation or hyperpigmentation are possible side effects.
- Thicker lesions are best removed by curettage or scissors excision under local anesthesia.
- Residual scarring, if any, is minimal. Applying gentle pressure to the surrounding skin often provides enough tension to allow for easy curettage of lesions.

ROUGH SURFACE KERATOSES

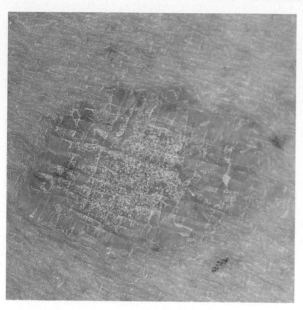 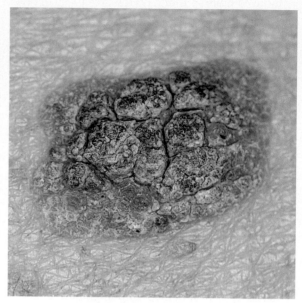

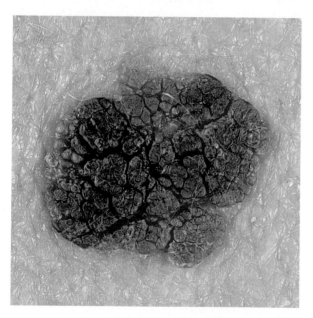 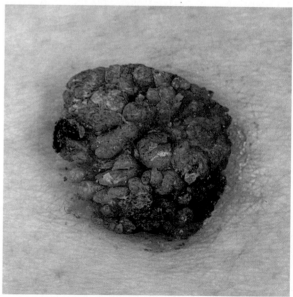

Rough surfaced. The rough-surfaced seborrheic keratoses are the most common benign skin tumor. They are oval to round, flattened domes with a granular or irregular surface that crumbles when picked. Lesions on the extremities are flatter.

Smooth Surface Keratoses

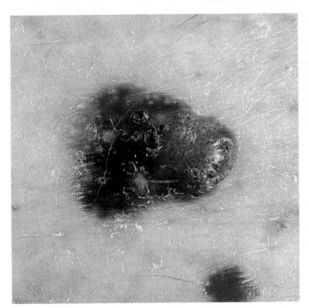
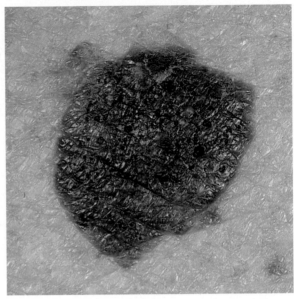
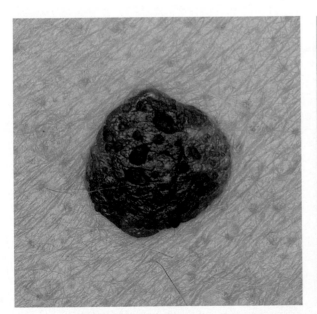
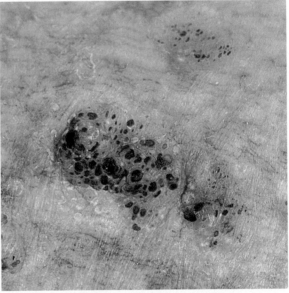

Smooth surfaced. Smooth-surfaced, dome-shaped tumors have white or black pearls of keratin, 1 mm in diameter, embedded in the surface. These horn pearls are easily seen with a hand lens.

KERATOSES MIMICKING MELANOMA

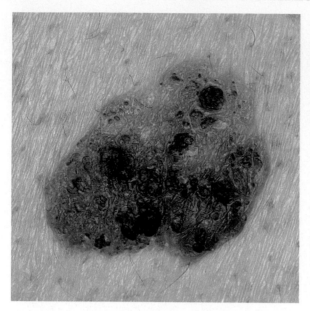

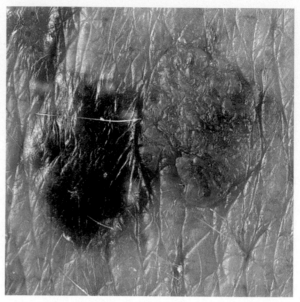

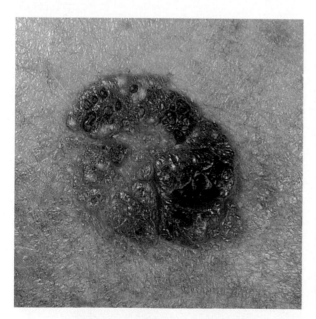

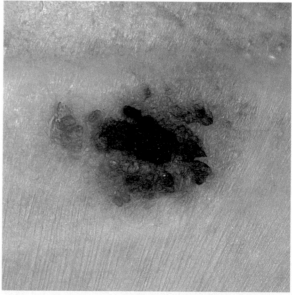

Seborrheic keratosis (mimicking melanoma). These lesions have many of the features of superficial spreading and nodular melanoma. The colors are variable, and the white areas look like areas of tumor regression. A magnified view shows several horn cysts that are typically found in seborrheic keratoses and rarely present in melanoma.

IRRITATED SEBORRHEIC KERATOSES

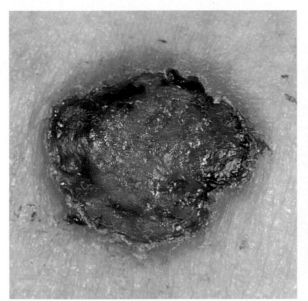
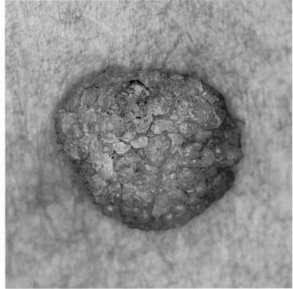

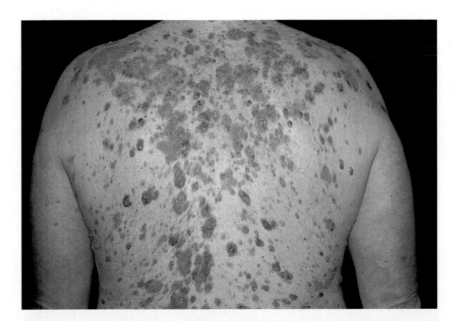

Irritated seborrheic keratoses become slightly swollen and develop an irregular, red flare in the surrounding skin. They may develop into a bright red, oozing mass with a friable surface that resembles an advanced melanoma or a pyogenic granuloma.

SEBORRHEIC KERATOSES

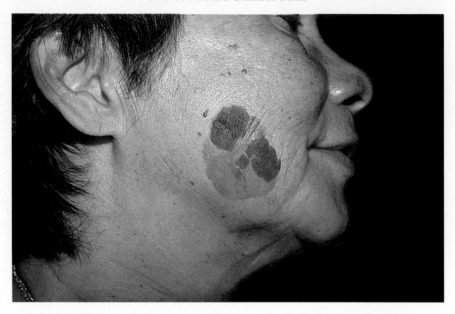

Lesions can become very large and disfiguring and resemble melanoma.

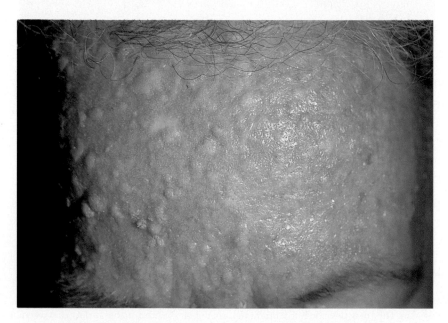

Numerous lesions may appear on the face in predisposed individuals.

SEBORRHEIC KERATOSES

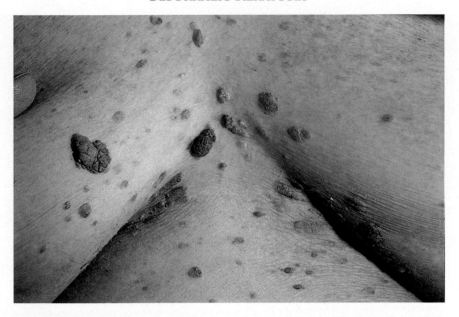

Lesions are often concentrated in the presternal area and under the breasts. Chafing from clothing or from maceration in this intertriginous area can start irritation.

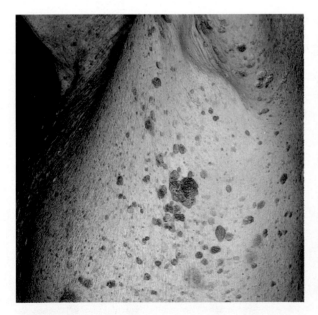

The number varies from less than 20 in most individuals to numerous lesions on the face or trunk.

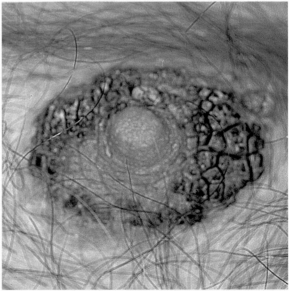

Lesions may be localized to the areola in both males and females.

STUCCO KERATOSES

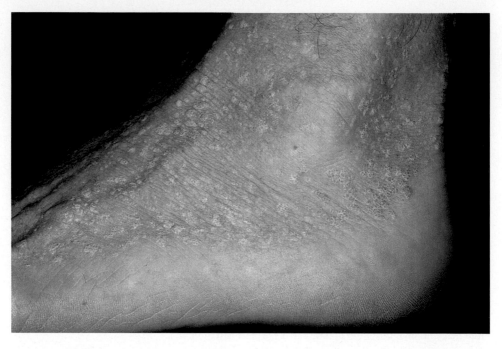

Stucco keratoses are papular, warty lesions occurring on the lower legs, especially around the Achilles tendon area, and the dorsum of the foot. The 1- to 10-mm, round, very dry, stuck-on lesions are considered by most patients to be simply manifestations of dry skin. The dry surface scale is easily picked intact from the skin without bleeding, but it recurs shortly thereafter.

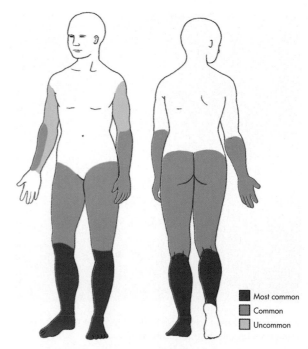

■ Most common
■ Common
□ Uncommon

STUCCO KERATOSES

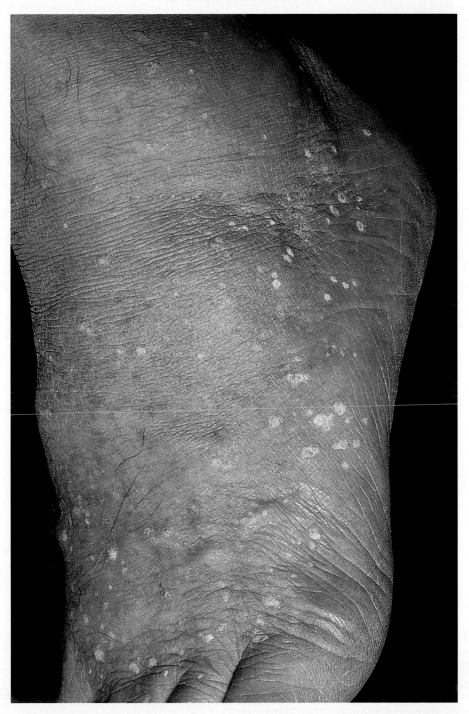

■ SKIN TAGS

DESCRIPTION

- Skin tags are common, benign fleshy papules occurring on the neck and in skinfold areas.

HISTORY

- Females are affected more often than males.
- Skin tags are uncommon before age 30 and common thereafter.
- Roughly 25% of adults have at least one skin tag.
- The majority of patients with skin tags have only a few such lesions.
- They are more common in overweight persons.
- Inheritance has not been reported, although there may be a familial tendency toward multiple skin tags.
- Undisturbed lesions are usually asymptomatic.
- As a result of location, skin tags may become irritated by jewelry or clothing.
- They may become tender when traumatized, twisted, torn, or thrombosed.

SKIN FINDINGS

- A skin tag is a skin-colored to brown, 1- to 10-mm papule.
- Papules may be flat or filiform, although most are soft, fleshy, and pedunculated on a thin stalk.
- The axillae are the most common location, followed by the neck.
- Lesions also occur on the eyelids as well as in other intertriginous areas such as the inframammary and inguinal creases.

NONSKIN FINDINGS

- An early reported association between skin tags and colonic polyps has not been confirmed in later studies.

LABORATORY

- Skin biopsy confirms a papule with a thinned epidermis and a loosely arranged fibrous stroma with capillaries.

COURSE AND PROGNOSIS

- Left undisturbed, skin tags persist indefinitely.
- With torsion, skin tags may become thrombosed and tender.
- With this acute change, patients usually seek care because they are concerned about skin malignancy.
- Thrombosed skin tags often appear black, hemorrhagic, or both.

- Any delay in seeking care allows the residual skin tag time to fall off on its own; thus no residual lesion is seen.

DIFFERENTIAL DIAGNOSIS

- Wart
- Nevus

TREATMENT

- Asymptomatic skin tags do not require treatment.
- Patients often request removal for cosmetic reasons.
- Patients should be informed that cosmetic removal of skin tags is not covered by medical insurance.
- An appropriate fee for the service should be agreed on before removal.
- Skin tags are best treated by scissors-snip removal with or without local anesthesia.
  - Aluminum chloride or electrocautery is used to obtain hemostasis.
  - EMLA Cream improves comfort when a large number of lesions are removed from a localized area.
- Electrocautery and cryosurgery are also used.
- The need to submit all skin tags for histologic review has been a topic of debate in recent years.
  - Many dermatologists feel that histologic confirmation is usually not necessary.

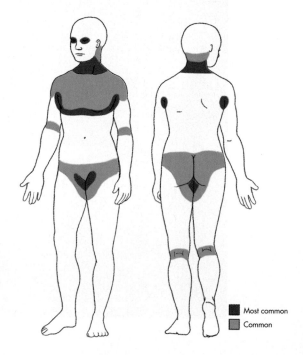

Most common

Common

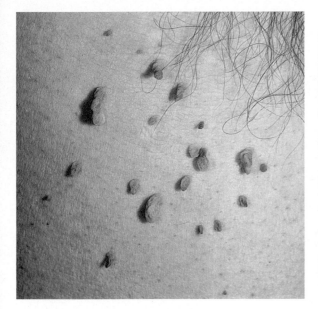

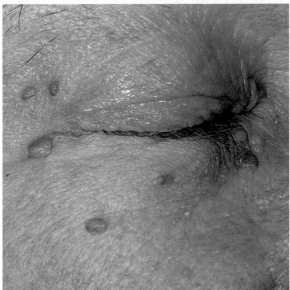

Skin tags begin as a tiny, brown or skin-colored, oval excrescence attached by a short, broad-to-narrow stalk.

Skin tags occur around the eyes and may resemble warts.

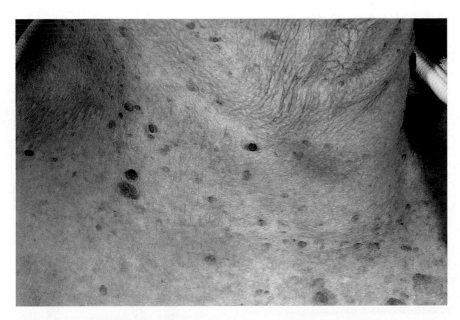

Patients complain that when they wear clothing or jewelry, these tumors are annoying.

■ DERMATOFIBROMA

DESCRIPTION

- Dermatofibroma is a common, benign, indolent, firm, dermal papule most commonly occurring on the legs of adults.

HISTORY

- The common dermal lesions arise spontaneously in adults and occasionally in children.
- Most are asymptomatic, but itching and tenderness are fairly common.
- Dermatofibromas may occur more often in women.
- Lesions on the legs of women are subject to repeated trauma from shaving and can be annoying.
- The etiology is unknown.
  - Controversy exists as to whether the lesion represents benign neoplasia or reactive hyperplasia in response to injury.
  - Most patients do not recall a specific trauma to the area.
  - Some patients note itching when the lesion is first noted and attribute this to an insect bite.
- Dermatofibromas tend to persist indefinitely while remaining stable in size and appearance.

SKIN FINDINGS

- Discrete firm dermal papules are usually smaller than 0.7 cm in diameter, although lesions as large as 3.0 cm are occasionally seen.
- Most dermatofibromas are dome shaped, although some are depressed below the surrounding skin surface.
- The lesion is fixed within the skin, but movable over the underlying subcutaneous fat.
- On palpation, the lesion feels like a button.
- Pinching a dome-shaped dermatofibroma between two fingers causes the lesion to dimple below the level of the now-elevated surrounding skin.
- Dermatofibromas are typically flesh colored to pink with a poorly defined rim of tan to brown pigmentation.
  - Rarely, lesions may be blue to black in color as a result of hemosiderin deposition deep within the tumor.
  - Such lesions may suggest melanoma clinically.
  - The surface may be smooth and shiny to scaly or excoriated.
- Although dermatofibromas may arise on any cutaneous surface, most are found randomly distributed on the extremities.

- Lesions may be solitary; typically, a few lesions are present.
- Lesions rarely occur on the palms or the soles.

LABORATORY

- Skin biopsy confirms a localized unencapsulated proliferation of spindle-shaped cells resembling fibroblasts, histiocytes, and collagen.

COURSE AND PROGNOSIS

- Dermatofibromas attain their maximum size over months to years and then persist indefinitely.
- Spontaneous involution is rare.
- Depending on location, lesions may be subject to repeated trauma from shaving or friction from boots.

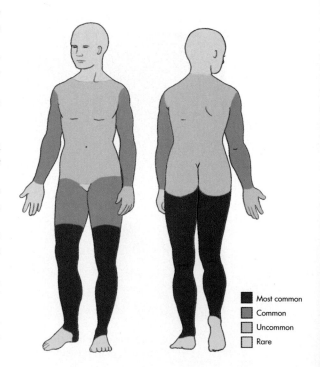

Most common
Common
Uncommon
Rare

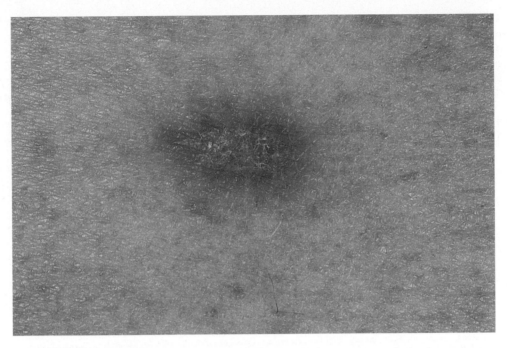

Dermatofibromas appear as 3- to 10-mm, slightly raised, pink, sometimes scaly, hard growths.

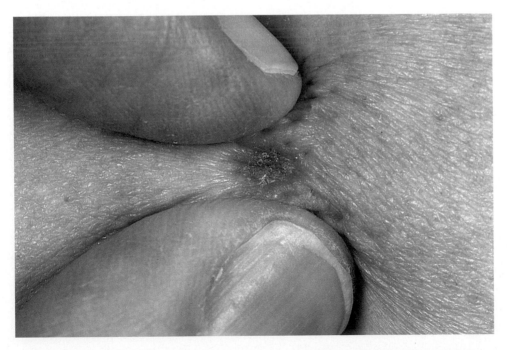

Dermatofibromas retract beneath the skin surface during attempts to compress and elevate them.

DISCUSSION

- Lesions with large amounts of hemosiderin deep within the tumor may be blue to black in color and suggestive of nodular melanoma or pigmented dermatofibrosarcoma protuberans. Biopsy is warranted in such cases.
- Dermatofibroma can clinically mimic melanoma with a central pink nodule and surrounding pigmentation.
- When doubt exists, a biopsy should be performed.

- Dermatofibrosarcoma protuberans resembles dermatofibroma histologically and, less commonly, clinically.
- This insidious malignancy usually occurs on the trunk and presents as a slow-growing, often recurrent, poorly defined, red-purple nodule or plaque.
- Overall, the histologic findings are similar to those of dermatofibroma, so a superficial biopsy may be falsely reassuring.
- Deep punch or excisional biopsy that includes subcutaneous fat confirms that dermatofibrosarcoma protuberans is more cellular than most dermatofibromas.
- Malignant cells extend into the subcutaneous fat.

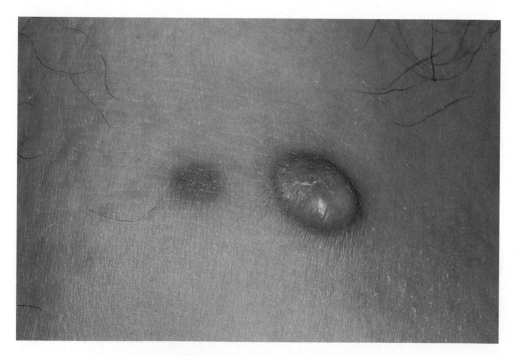

Dermatofibromas may be dome shaped.

TREATMENT

- Dermatofibromas are benign skin tumors that do not require treatment unless they are symptomatic, repeatedly traumatized, or cosmetically bothersome. The patient should be assured that the lesion is benign.
- Surgical excision with primary closure is the treatment of choice for symptomatic lesions.
  - Excision may not be technically feasible for larger lesions, especially in the pretibial area where scars tend to widen over time.
  - The final appearance may be less cosmetically acceptable than the original lesion.
- Shave excision with healing via secondary intention or cryosurgery may be acceptable alternatives for such lesions. It is important to realize that the lesion is not completely removed.
- The patient should be warned of possible recurrence.
- Intralesional corticosteroid injection has been used to flatten elevated lesions. This form of treatment produces unpredictable results and is generally not recommended.

CAVEAT

- Dermatofibromas should be stable in size, appearance, and minimally, if at all, symptomatic.

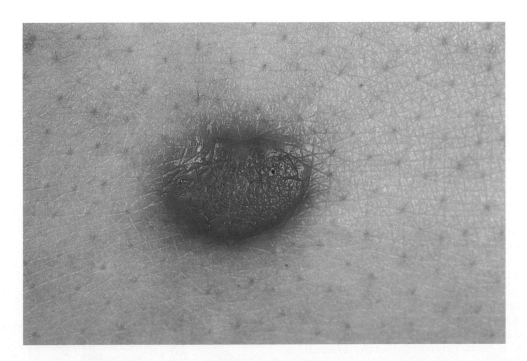

Dermatofibromas develop a pink-brown border and a lighter center as they age.

■ KELOIDS AND HYPERTROPHIC SCARS

DESCRIPTION

- A keloid or hypertrophic scar is an inappropriately exuberant healing response to trauma occurring in a predisposed person.

HISTORY

- Males and females are affected with equal frequency.
- Keloids can occur at any age but tend to occur before age 30.
- They are more common in African-Americans than Caucasians.
- Hypertrophic scars and keloids can arise at any skin site. Most occur on the anterior chest, shoulder, and neck. Another frequent site is the earlobe after ear piercing.
- Lesions occur at the site of injury, including that resulting from surgery, or the site of inflammation (e.g., acne).

SKIN FINDINGS

- Early scars are usually red and firm during the initial weeks of healing.
- Hypertrophic scars have a similar color and a firm texture but are apparent for a longer period of time, lasting months.
  - They are larger and more raised than the scars expected for the injury.
  - The overlying skin appears shiny and stretched with prominent vessels.
  - The surface is smooth and dome shaped.
  - One portion of a scar may appear normal, and another portion appears to be hypertrophied.
  - Unlike keloid scars, hypertrophic scars remain confined to the site of injury.
  - Itching and tenderness on palpation are common.
- Keloid scars are even larger, are more raised, and are often quite tender.
  - Keloids extend beyond and often distort the original site of injury.
  - Keloids are usually hyperpigmented in African-Americans and red to purple in Caucasians.
  - Depending on the type of original injury, the lesion may be linear or nodular.
  - The surface is often irregular, with strands of fibrous tissue extending into the adjacent normal skin.

LABORATORY

- A skin biopsy is usually not needed and should be performed with caution.
- Biopsy can induce further scarring.
- Hypertrophic scars contain randomly dispersed fibroblasts and whorled bundles of new collagen.
- Keloids extend beyond the wound margins and contain thick bands of eosinophilic collagen with fewer fibroblasts.

COURSE AND PROGNOSIS

- Hypertrophic scars tend to regress even without treatment, although it may take several years to reach a final outcome.
- Keloid scars show no tendency toward regression and tend to enlarge over time.

DIFFERENTIAL DIAGNOSIS

- Keloid scars
  - Dermatofibrosarcoma protuberans
  - Sarcoidosis, especially for facial keloids
  - Recurrence of tumor for keloids arising in surgical scars from excision of malignancy

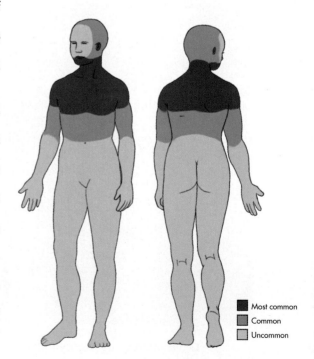

Most common
Common
Uncommon

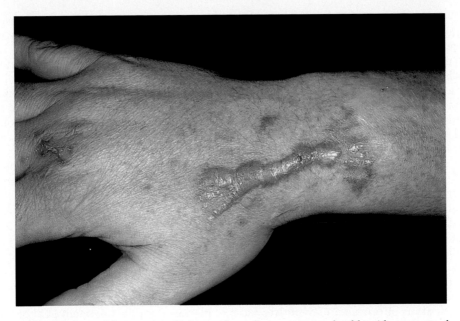

A keloid extends beyond the margins of injury and usually is constant and stable without any tendency to subside.

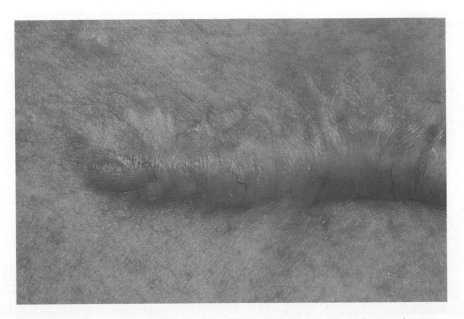

A hypertrophic scar is inappropriately large but remains confined to the wound site and in time regresses.

DISCUSSION

- The diagnosis of hypertrophic scar is usually straightforward.
- There is a history of localized trauma, and the injury site is intact.
- There is no history of prior injury in dermatofibrosarcoma protuberans.
- If doubt exists, biopsy is warranted.
- Injury and scar appears to be a nidus for skin involvement in sarcoidosis.

TREATMENT

- People with a history of hypertrophic or keloid scars should be discouraged from having cosmetic procedures.
- This is best explained as unpredictable scarring.
- Patients who require surgical procedures in areas at increased risk of abnormal scarring should be advised of this possibility in advance and should be reminded at the time of suture removal.
- Despite meticulous surgical care, hypertrophic and keloid scars do occur.
- The parents of a child who has had a procedure that resulted in hypertrophic scarring need reassurance and a management plan.

- Early abnormal scarring typically responds better than older, less active scarring; early intervention is advised.
- In general, early active scars respond to treatment better than older scars.
- Intralesional corticosteroid injection is probably the treatment of choice.
  - Triamcinolone (Kenalog) injection at concentrations of 10 to 40 mg/ml are given at 2- to 4-week intervals.
  - Close follow-up is needed at higher concentrations to minimize the risk of overtreatment and permanent atrophy.
- Radiation therapy and more recently pulse-dye laser therapy have been used for keloid scars. These modalities are not widely tested or available today.
- Compression therapy and silastic sheeting are helpful but inconvenient.
- Newer topical silicon-containing gels have been marketed for the treatment of hypertrophic scars, although little data on efficacy are available.
- Surgical correction of hypertrophic scars and keloids requires experience and careful monitoring.
- A referral to a dermatologist or plastic surgeon should be considered.

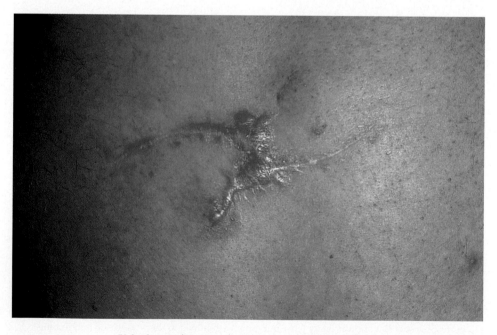

Keloids are often very disfiguring and difficult to treat.

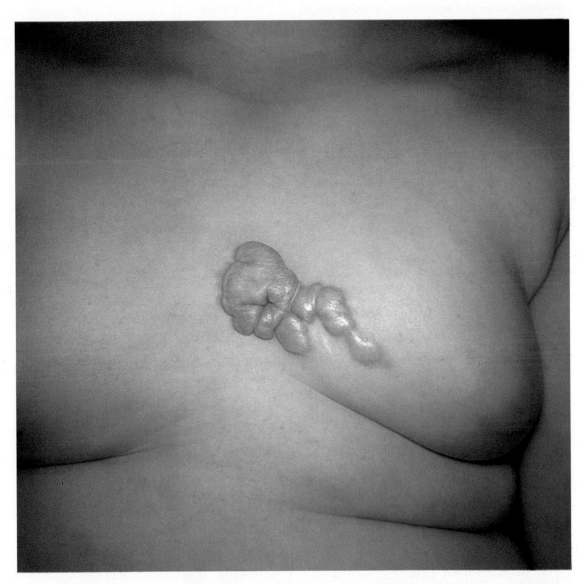

Keloids are most common on the shoulders and chest.

■ KERATOACANTHOMA

DESCRIPTION

- Keratoacanthoma is a common, rapidly growing skin lesion with a distinctive appearance and clinical course; it is best regarded as a low-grade or abortive squamous cell carcinoma.

HISTORY

- Keratoacanthoma is rare before age 40; the peak incidence is between ages 50 and 69 years.
- The incidence is essentially equal to that of squamous cell carcinoma at any latitude.
- Caucasians with fair complexions (skin types I and II) are more often affected.
- Typical locations include the face, neck, and sun-exposed extremities.
- It occurs in the dorsa of the hands more often in men.
- It occurs on the legs more often in women.
- Keratoacanthoma does not occur on the palms or soles.
- The lesion is often quite tender during the proliferative phase.
  - Chemical exposure and human papillomavirus have been implicated in animal models, although their role in humans is controversial.

SKIN FINDINGS

- A solitary skin-colored to dull red, usually solitary, 0.5- to 2.0-cm beehive-shaped nodule appears.
- A central keratotic plug or cutaneous horn conceals a deep keratinous cavity.
- The nodule is firm in texture, feels superficial, and is tender to palpation or pressure.
- Keratoacanthoma nearly always appears on sun-damaged skin.
- Three growth phases are described:
  - In the proliferative phase, a solitary papule appears suddenly and then rapidly grows to its maximum size over 2 to 4 weeks.
  - In the mature phase, the lesion is stable in size and appearance for weeks to months; it may appear crateriform if the core has been partially removed.
  - In the resolving phase, the base becomes indurated, the central core is expelled, and the base resorbs, leaving a pitted scar over several months.

NONSKIN FINDINGS

- Rare cases of multiple keratoacanthomas have been reported, both as an eruptive (Grzybowski) form and as a familial adolescent (Ferguson-Smith) form.
- Patients with Muir-Torre syndrome develop sebaceous adenomas, at times with keratoacanthoma architecture. Such patients should be evaluated for occult gastrointestinal malignancy.
- Keratoacanthoma occurring in a child or adolescent should raise the possibility of xeroderma pigmentosum, an inherited disorder of defective DNA repair.
- Patients on immunosuppressive therapy after organ transplant are at increased risk of developing keratoacanthomas and invasive squamous cell carcinoma.

LABORATORY

- The pathologist may have difficulty distinguishing a keratoacanthoma from a squamous cell carcinoma.
- The epidermis is expanded with atypical keratinocytes.
- The keratin core is composed of eosinophilic, glassy-appearing, prematurely keratinized cells.

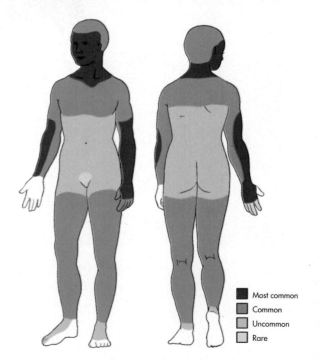

Most common
Common
Uncommon
Rare

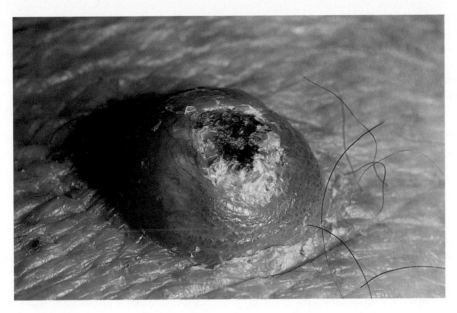

Keratoacanthoma begins as a smooth, dome-shaped, red papule that may rapidly develop a central keratin-filled crater.

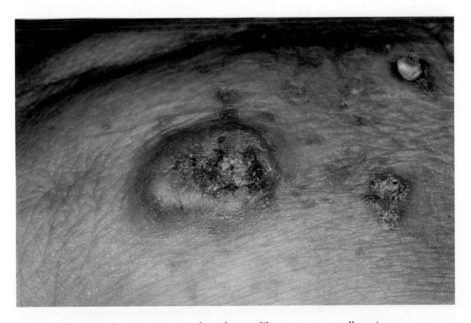

The growth retains its smooth surface, unlike a squamous cell carcinoma.

COURSE AND PROGNOSIS

- Left undisturbed, keratoacanthomas may resolve spontaneously or progress into invasive squamous cell carcinoma.
- Depending on location, the resultant pitted scar may be cosmetically unacceptable.
- Rarely keratoacanthomas will attain a size of up to 9 cm and are locally destructive.
- Subungual keratoacanthomas are especially painful and locally destructive.
- There are no data regarding the risk of developing more keratoacanthomas or other skin malignancies.

DIFFERENTIAL DIAGNOSIS

- Invasive squamous cell carcinoma
- Molluscum contagiosum
- Wart
- Opportunistic infection in patients with disease caused by the human immunodeficiency virus

DISCUSSION

- Keratoacanthoma cannot be reliably discriminated from invasive squamous cell carcinoma clinically or histologically.

TREATMENT

- It is best to presume a diagnosis of squamous cell carcinoma pending biopsy results and clinical follow-up.
- An excisional biopsy or shave biopsy should be performed.
- It is important to biopsy deep enough to evaluate the dermis for possible invasion.
- Pending histologic review, electrodesiccation and curettage may result in a more cosmetically acceptable scar than would be obtained by allowing the lesion to involute on its own.
- Follow-up is mandatory and should be scheduled for within 2 weeks of biopsy.
- If the histology is consistent with keratoacanthoma and the area appears to be healing, then continued follow-up may be all that is necessary.
- If the histology is more consistent with squamous cell carcinoma or the lesion is not healing, then excision should be performed without delay.

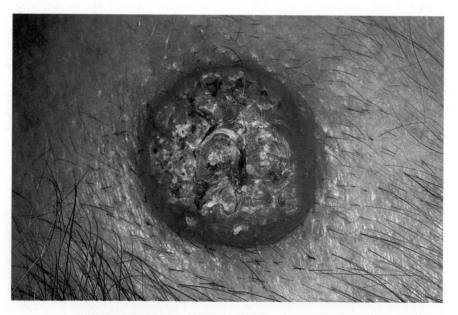

The central keratin-filled crater is a most characteristic feature.

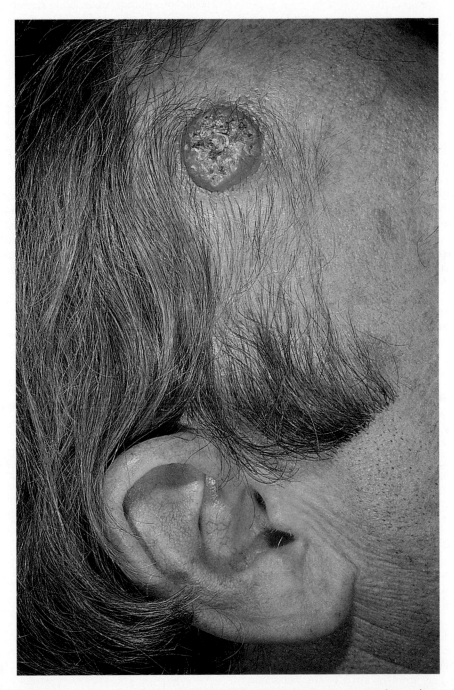

The limbs are the most common site but keratoacanthoma may occur on any skin surface.

■ NEVUS SEBACEUS

DESCRIPTION

- Nevus sebaceus is a distinctive congenital lesion composed of skin and appendageal components.

HISTORY

- Nearly all lesions are present at birth or appear in early childhood.
- Lesions change clinically and histologically with age.

SKIN FINDINGS

- Nevus sebaceus occurs most commonly on the scalp, forehead, or postauricular areas.
- Usually, only a single lesion is present.
- A linear to oval plaque usually measuring 1 to 3 cm in diameter appears.
- The lesion evolves in three stages corresponding to sebaceous gland maturation through childhood, puberty, and adulthood.
  - In childhood, the plaque is barely raised and has a velvety surface, is hairless, is pink to tan, and is asymptomatic.
  - Around puberty, the plaque tends to thicken, become larger and more verrucous, and has a yellow-white and pink speckled appearance. Lesions at this stage are easily traumatized and may be tender.
  - The third stage of evolution occurs during adulthood. Approximately 20% of lesions undergo neoplastic change and may develop either benign or malignant tumors of the skin. Such change appears as a new nodule or erosion developing within a previously stable nevus sebaceus.
  - The malignancies are low grade and show little tendency to become invasive.

NONSKIN FINDINGS

- A triad of nevus sebaceus, epilepsy, and mental retardation is very rare.
- This appears to overlap clinically with the linear epidermal nevus syndrome.

LABORATORY

- The histopathologic characteristics vary depending on the age of the patient at the time of biopsy.
- In the first few months of life, the sebaceous glands are well developed as a result of maternal hormonal stimulation, although surrounding hair structures are incompletely differentiated.

- Thereafter and through the rest of childhood, the sebaceous glands are small in size and number; incompletely developed hair structures may be seen.
- With puberty, hormonal influences bring about diagnostic changes.
  - Sebaceous glands mature and increase in size and density.
  - Hair structures remain undifferentiated, and papillomatous epidermal hyperplasia develops. Ectopic apocrine glands may also be found deep within the underlying dermis.
- Appendageal tumors may develop later in life within nevus sebaceus. Each such tumor has its own histologic pattern.
  - The most common tumor is syringocystadenoma papilliferum, a benign apocrine tumor seen in up to 20% of lesions.
  - Basal cell carcinoma is the second most common tumor and most common malignancy that develops in nevus sebaceus; it occurs in roughly 7% of lesions.
  - Squamous cell carcinoma and melanoma rarely develop within nevus sebaceus.

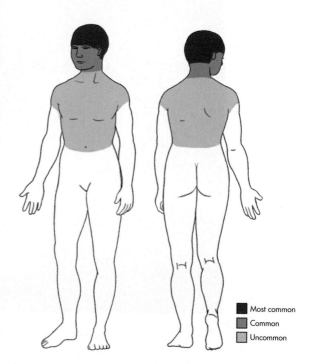

Most common
Common
Uncommon

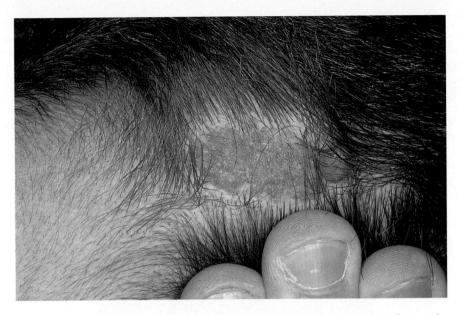

Lesions are oval to linear, smooth to gently papillated, waxy, hairless thickenings in infants and children.

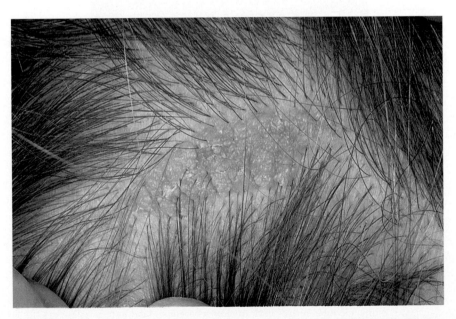

Nevus sebaceus is most commonly found on the scalp, followed by the forehead and retroauricular region.

COURSE AND PROGNOSIS

- Nevus sebaceus remains stable throughout childhood and undergoes predictable change at puberty.
- Depending on location, nevus sebaceus can be disfiguring.
- Verrucous lesions are more difficult to excise than immature lesions.
- Neoplastic change occurs during adulthood with enough frequency to warrant prophylactic excision.

DIFFERENTIAL DIAGNOSIS

- Linear epidermal nevus, which may share some histologic features with nevus sebaceus

TREATMENT

- Excision of the entire lesion is recommended.
- Excision is best performed just before puberty, when the lesion is still small and the patient is old enough to understand and tolerate the procedure.

CAVEAT

- A larger lesion may be excised in stages without any concern of inducing malignant change.

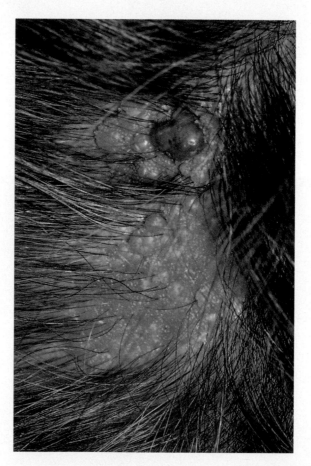

White, globular surface indicative of sebaceous gland hyperplasia that occurs after puberty.

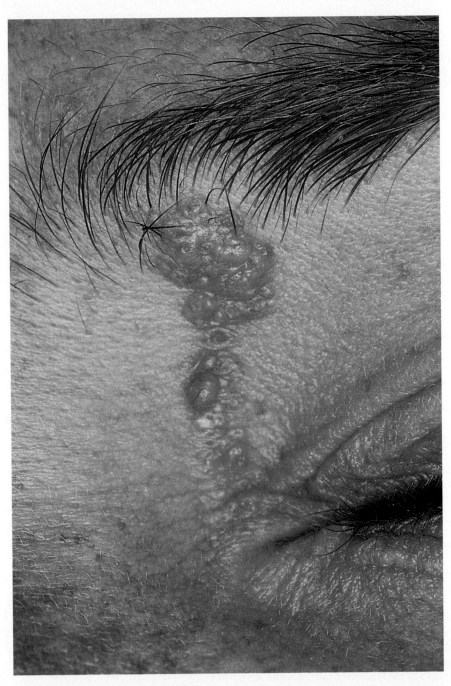

During puberty, there is a massive development of sebaceous glands, and they develop a verrucous irregularity of the surface covered with numerous, closely aggregated, yellow to dark brown papules.

■ CHONDRODERMATITIS NODULARIS HELICIS

DESCRIPTION

- Chondrodermatitis nodularis helicis is an uncommon, exquisitely tender, persistent papule usually found on the lateral edge of the helix.

HISTORY

- This painful lesion occurs in Caucasians over the age of 40.
- Men are affected more often than women.
- The lesion varies clinically between men and women.
  - The helix is involved more commonly in men.
  - Lesions on the antihelix are more common in women.
  - Women with chondrodermatitis nodularis helicis tend to be older than men with it.
  - These variations may relate in part to historical differences among men and women in sun exposure patterns, occupation, recreational activities, and hair styles.
  - Gender differences in ear structure may also play a role.
- The incidence increases with age.
- As a rule, most patients are in the habit of sleeping on the side, with the affected area in a dependent position.
- The universal symptom is pain described as stabbing and sharp.
- This condition is less symptomatic during the daytime.
- Pressure from resting on a pillow causes pain, forcing the patient to alter sleeping position and affecting the ability to sleep comfortably.

SKIN FINDINGS

- The primary lesion is a firm, dull red, 2- to 4-mm indurated, poorly defined papule with a central depression.
- The depression has firm, adherent, transparent scaling or crusting.
- The surrounding skin shows actinic damage with atrophy and often telangiectasias.
- Occasionally, there is more than one lesion.
- Papules are quite tender to palpation.
- This condition is classically found on the most prominent, firmest portion of the pinna.
  - In male patients, this is most often the lateral edge of the helix.

- In female patients, the antihelix is often the more prominent part of the pinna, and lesions are found there.

LABORATORY

- Skin biopsy reveals both acute and chronic inflammation.
- The epidermis is thinned, with compacted parakeratotic scaling, and often shows central ulceration.
- There is dermal necrosis with surrounding granulation tissue.
- A deep biopsy may contain underlying degenerated cartilage.

COURSE AND PROGNOSIS

- The etiology of chondrodermatitis nodularis helicis is unclear, although is believed to be related to focal dermal necrosis.
- Over many years, dermal injury may result from actinic damage, physical pressure, or a combination thereof.
- The vascular supply to this tissue is tenuous, and damage is slow to heal.
- Inflammation and granulation tissue reflect attempts at healing the damaged collagen.
- Without treatment, the lesions persist indefinitely.
- Recurrences are common, even after aggressive therapy.

DIFFERENTIAL DIAGNOSIS

- Sun-related primary skin malignancy, namely basal cell carcinoma and squamous cell carcinoma

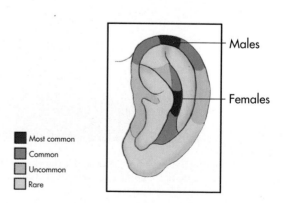

Most common
Common
Uncommon
Rare

DISCUSSION

- Chondrodermatitis nodularis helicis tends to be dull red in appearance with less well-defined, gently sloping borders than keratoacanthomas.
- Basal cell carcinomas tend to produce well-defined borders and have a translucent appearance.
- Squamous cell carcinomas as a rule tend to be larger and more necrotic.
- Skin biopsy should be performed and is diagnostic.

TREATMENT

- Any therapy must include efforts to relieve pressure on the affected area to allow for healing.
- Patients who are able to sleep on the back should be encouraged to do so.
- Pillows should be positioned to minimize pressure on the ear.
- Topical therapy is rarely successful but worth trying in conjunction with pressure relief.

- Class I corticosteroids should be applied to the lesion twice a day for 2 weeks.
- Intralesional steroids are more effective and are given at 2-week intervals.
- Patients should expect some residual discomfort after injection.
- Lesional therapy involves surgical removal of the necrotic, inflamed tissue.
- Scissors or shave excision is directed at removing all the inflamed tissue, thus exposing the underlying cartilage.
- Curettage and light electrodesiccation of the base is performed, and the wound is allowed to heal by secondary intention.
- Definitive therapy involves surgical resection of the involved portion of the pinna.
- Plastic surgery consultation should be considered.
- Recurrences are common after any therapy.

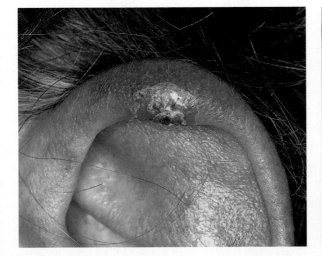

During the active stage, the base may become red and swollen; pain is constant.

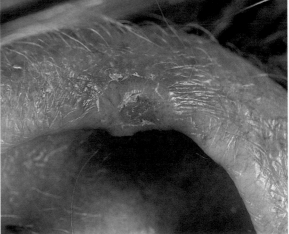

The central scale lacks the keratinous plug of a keratoacanthoma. Removal of the scale reveals a small central erosion.

■ EPIDERMAL CYST

DESCRIPTION

- An epidermal cyst is a firm, mobile, subcutaneous, keratin-filled cyst originating from true epidermis, most often from a hair follicle infundibulum.

HISTORY

- Epidermal cysts arise spontaneously, usually after puberty.
- They occur most commonly on the face, in the postauricular fold, on the posterior neck, and on the trunk.
- Cysts frequently develop in areas of friction.
- Lesions are usually solitary, although there may be multiple cysts.
- Most epidermal cysts are found in hair-bearing areas and arise from the squamous epithelium of the follicle.
- Cysts occasionally develop on the palms or soles as a result of penetrating trauma. These are true epidermal inclusion cysts.
- Unlike pilar cysts, the cyst wall is fairly delicate and thus prone to rupture.
- Rupture is followed by a foreign body reaction to keratin extruded into the dermis and acute inflammation. Such lesions appear to be infected.
- Although bacteria can at times be isolated from the cysts, they usually contain normal skin flora with little pathogenicity.

SKIN FINDINGS

- The firm, dome-shaped, pale intradermal or subcutaneous cystic nodules range from 0.5 to 5.0 cm in size.
- Cysts are somewhat mobile but are tethered to the overlying skin through a small punctum that often appears as a comedo (blackhead).
- This punctum represents the follicle from which the cyst developed.
- Inflamed epidermal cysts are red, hot, and boggy and tender on palpation. Furuncles have the same appearance.
  - Sterile, purulent material and keratin debris often point and drain to the surface.
  - If the inflammatory response is brisk enough to destroy the cyst wall, then the cyst will not recur.
  - More often, the inflammation subsides, and the cyst recurs.
  - Scarring often follows, which makes the cyst more difficult to remove.

NONSKIN FINDINGS

- Multiple epidermal cysts occurring on the face, scalp, and back should raise suspicion of Gardner's syndrome. This autosomal dominant condition is associated with colonic polyposis and early malignant degeneration into adenocarcinoma of the colon.

LABORATORY

- The epidermal cyst is lined with squamous epithelium that appears thinned and flattened.
- The cyst cavity is filled with layers of cornified lamellated keratin.

COURSE AND PROGNOSIS

- Epidermal cysts grow slowly to a maximum size and tend to persist indefinitely.
- Depending on location, epidermal cysts may be subject to repeated external trauma and rupture.

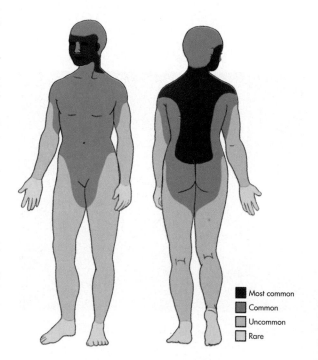

Most common
Common
Uncommon
Rare

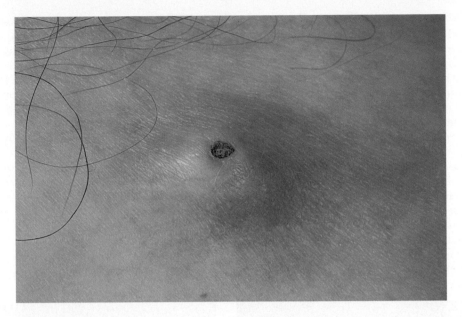

The cyst communicates with the surface through a narrow channel, and the surface opening appears as a small, round, sometimes imperceptible, keratin-filled orifice (i.e., a blackhead).

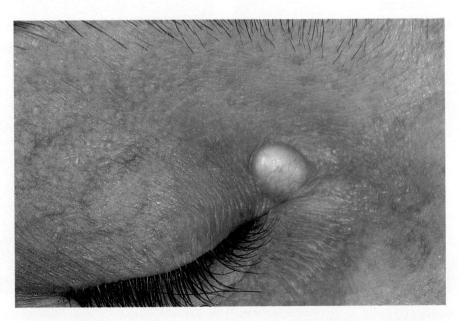

The cyst occurs primarily on the face, back or base of the ears, chest, and back or on almost any skin surface.

TREATMENT

- Epidermal cysts on the face should be removed electively to reduce the risk of rupture and scarring.
- Such lesions are far more difficult to remove once they have ruptured.
- Asymptomatic epidermal cysts occurring elsewhere do not require treatment.
- Symptomatic or recurrent epidermal cysts should be removed.
- Ruptured acutely inflamed epidermal cysts should be incised and drained under local anesthesia.
  - Attempts should be made to remove the cyst lining either by curettage or blunt dissection.
  - The cyst cavity may then be packed with a wick to aid in further drainage.
- Epidermal cysts that have not previously ruptured are easily and completely removed under local anesthesia.
- Tumescence from anesthesia external to the cyst wall aids in separating the delicate cyst wall from the surrounding connective tissue.
- A small incision is carefully made over the cyst.
- The cyst wall is identified and further separated from the connective tissue by blunt dissection.
- The cyst wall is then incised and the cheesy cyst contents removed.
- Gentle traction allows complete removal of the remaining intact cyst wall.
- Recurrent epidermal cysts that have previously ruptured and scarred are best excised along with the surrounding scar once the inflammation has subsided.

CAVEAT

- Inflammation after rupture of an epidermal cyst is often misdiagnosed as infection.

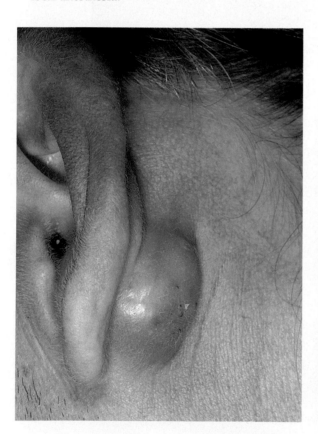

Spontaneous rupture of the wall results in discharge of the soft, yellow keratin into the dermis. A tremendous inflammatory response ensues.

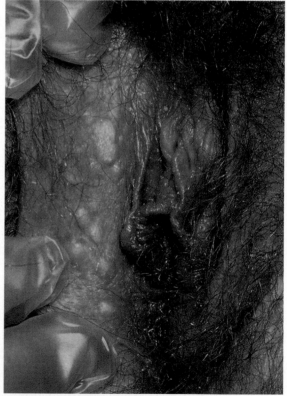

Epidermal cysts occur in areas where sebaceous glands are large and numerous, such as on the labia.

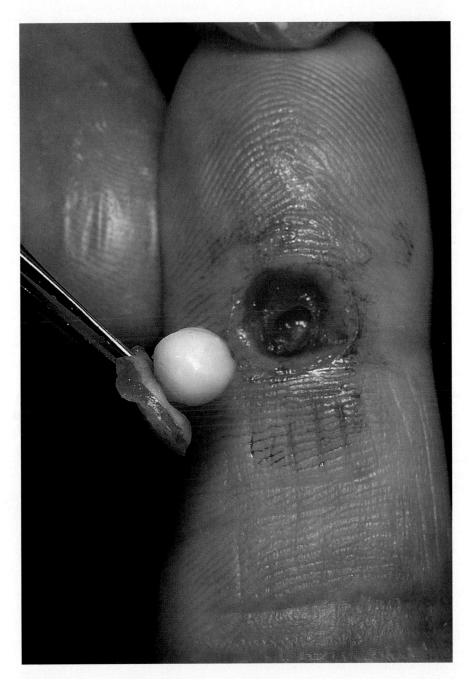

The round, smooth-surfaced mass varies in size from a few millimeters to several centimeters.

■ PILAR CYST (WEN)

DESCRIPTION

- A pilar, or trichilemmal, cyst is a firm, mobile subcutaneous, keratin-filled cyst originating from the outer root sheath; it is most commonly found on the scalp.

HISTORY

- Pilar cysts are less common than, but otherwise similar to, epidermal cysts.
- Roughly 90% of pilar cysts are found on the scalp, with the remaining 10% occurring within hair-bearing skin, including the face, neck, back, and scrotum.
- Pilar cysts develop from epithelial cells of the outer root sheath of the hair follicle.
- This epithelium undergoes a different form of keratinization than surface epithelium.
- Patients develop pilar cysts, almost always after puberty.
- The tendency to develop pilar cysts often has an autosomal dominant inheritance within families.
- Pilar cysts are usually multiple: 70% of patients possess more than 1 cyst, and 10% have more than 10.
- Pilar cysts persist indefinitely and slowly grow to a stable size unless they rupture.
- Pilar cysts rupture less frequently than epidermal cysts, presumably because the pilar cyst possesses a thicker wall.
- Rupture usually results from an external blow to the head, thus releasing cyst contents into the surrounding dermis.
- A brisk foreign body inflammatory reaction follows and can be quite painful and resembles a furuncle.

SKIN FINDINGS

- Pilar cysts are clinically indistinguishable from epidermal cysts, differing only in their distribution.
- Both present as a firm, mobile subcutaneous nodule ranging from 0.5 to 5.0 cm.
- No central punctum is seen over a pilar cyst, as is found over an epidermal cyst.
- When such a cyst is surgically dissected, the pilar cyst possesses a tough, white-gray wall that is more resistant to tearing than the wall of an epidermal cyst.
- The pilar cyst wall separates easily and cleanly from the surrounding dermis.

- After rupture of a pilar cyst, the cyst wall is no longer discretely palpable.
- The area is acutely inflamed, red, and tender and boggy on palpation.

LABORATORY

- The histologic characteristics of the pilar cyst are distinct from those of the epidermal cyst.
- The cyst contains concentric layers of homogeneous eosinophilic keratin.

DISCUSSION

- Large cysts may be cosmetically objectionable.
- Acute inflammation after rupture is often misdiagnosed as infection.
- Antibiotics are of little value in such cases.
- Incision and drainage under local anesthesia improve comfort and limit scarring.
- Elective excision before rupture prevents this complication.

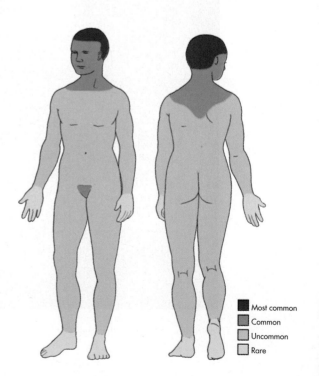

Most common
Common
Uncommon
Rare

TREATMENT

- Pilar cysts are easily removed under local anesthesia.
- The overlying hair is trimmed away, and the area is prepared.
- An incision is made over the cyst, exposing the cyst's glossy white external surface.
- The cyst wall is freed easily from the surrounding connective tissue by blunt dissection.
- At this stage, smaller cysts may be expressed intact up through the incision by steady, firm pressure on each side of the incision.
- Larger cysts, which cannot be expressed in this manner, should be incised and their contents removed by curettage.
- The incised cyst wall is then grasped with an Allis clamp, and through a combination of gentle traction and pressure on each side of the incision, the now smaller, partially emptied cyst is delivered through the incision.
- If sutures are needed, they are placed and removed in 7 to 10 days.

CAVEAT

- The term *sebaceous cyst* has been incorrectly applied to these common lesions.

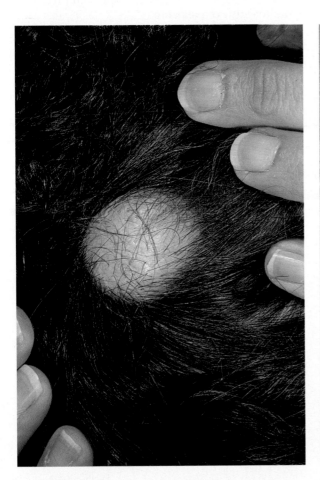

Pilar cysts occur in the scalp and are freely movable.

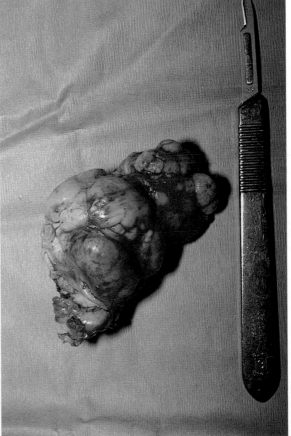

Pilar cysts are frequently multiple and may become large masses.

■ SEBACEOUS HYPERPLASIA

DESCRIPTION

- Sebaceous hyperplasia is a common benign condition consisting of scattered, prominently enlarged, sebaceous glands on the face.

HISTORY

- Sebaceous hyperplasia occurs in both men and women.
- Papules rarely appear before age 30 but become increasingly more common with advancing age.
- Perhaps 80% of patients over age 70 have at least one such lesion.
- Most lesions represent a single, hypertrophied sebaceous gland with multiple lobules arranged around a central enlarged sebaceous duct.
- Lesions occur in all skin types but are more easily seen in lighter skin.
- The etiology of sebaceous hyperplasia is unknown, although it is likely multifactorial.
  - There is almost certainly some heritable tendency toward developing the lesions.
- Sun damage has been suggested as a contributing factor.
- The lesions are entirely asymptomatic but persistent.
- Papules may be of cosmetic concern.
- Older patients are typically concerned that the lesions represent basal cell carcinoma.

SKIN FINDINGS

- The lesion begins as a 1- or 2-mm, soft, pale yellow to skin-colored, minimally elevated papule.
- With time, the lesion attains a maximum size of no more than 3 mm and develops a central umbilication.
- Mature papules possess a distinctly yellow color and are more sharply defined from the surrounding skin.
- The appearance of a mature papule is suggestive of a doughnut.
- Papules may be solitary but are more commonly multiple and scattered randomly on the forehead, eyelids, nose, and malar cheeks.
- Papules remain soft and, with pressure, may yield sebum from the central umbilication.
- An orderly array of fine telangiectasias may radiate outward from the umbilication toward the periphery of the papule.

LABORATORY

- Skin biopsy confirms the presence of multiple sebaceous lobules of a single sebaceous gland arranged around a central sebaceous duct.
- This duct corresponds to the central umbilication seen clinically.

DISCUSSION

- Individual lesions may be confused with basal cell carcinoma.
- Lesions of sebaceous hyperplasia have an orderly radial arrangement of telangiectasias in contrast to the haphazard distribution of telangiectasias on the surface of a basal cell carcinoma.
- Other lesions that might be confused with sebaceous hyperplasia include herpes simplex and molluscum contagiosum.
  - A small keratoacanthoma may resemble sebaceous hyperplasia with a central crater.

TREATMENT

- Treatment is not required for sebaceous hyperplasia, although it may be requested for cosmetic reasons.
- Cryosurgery, carbon dioxide laser, electrodesiccation and curettage, and trichloroacetic acid are all effective in ablating individual lesions.

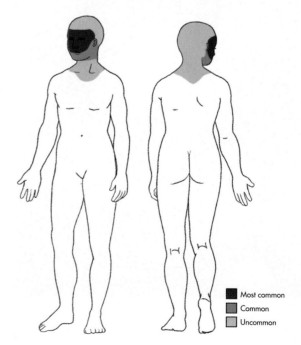

Most common
Common
Uncommon

- The sebaceous lobules located within the superficial dermis must be destroyed for the treatment to be successful.
- Care must be taken to avoid overtreatment so as to minimize the risk of permanent scarring.
- Reassurance is often all that is needed for the patient with sebaceous hyperplasia.

CAVEAT

- The orderly arrangement of telangiectasias is a valuable clue to discerning sebaceous hyperplasia from basal cell carcinoma.

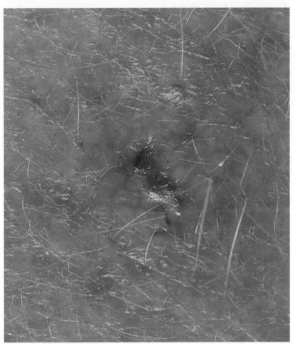

Close examination of the surface shows vessels in the valleys between the small, yellow lobules.

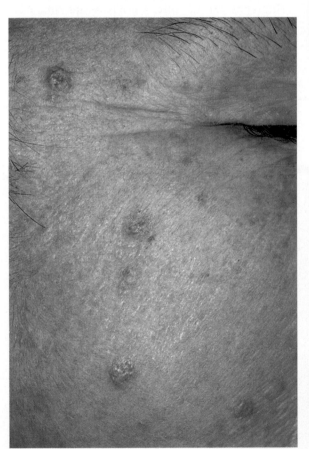

Senile sebaceous hyperplasia begins as pale yellow, slightly elevated papules, that are commonly found on the forehead, cheeks, lower lid, and nose.

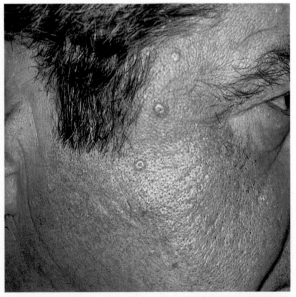

With time, they become yellow, dome shaped, and umbilicated.

■ SYRINGOMA

DESCRIPTION

- Syringomas are multiple small, firm, skin-colored papules occurring most commonly in women after puberty; these lesions can be found around the eyelids, on the upper chest, and on the vulva.

HISTORY

- Syringomas are the most common tumor of the intraepidermal eccrine sweat glands.
- Small, benign, appendageal tumors develop after puberty and increase in number throughout young adulthood.
- Women are affected more often than men.
- Although sometimes solitary, syringomas most commonly present as multiple small papules around the eyes.
- Lesions are asymptomatic, stable in size and appearance, and persistent.
- The autosomal dominant inheritance of multiple syringomas is well established.
- Syringomas occur with increased frequency in individuals with Down syndrome or trisomy 21.
- Facial lesions are of cosmetic concern, and most patients request removal.
- The patient may be concerned that the lesions are cancerous.
- Women seeking evaluation of vulvar lesions may be concerned that the lesions are genital warts.

SKIN FINDINGS

- The skin-colored to yellow, 1- to 2-mm papule is not umbilicated.
- Usually, multiple papules are symmetrically distributed.
- Papules are most commonly found on the lower eyelids.
- They also occur on the malar cheeks, axillae, anterior chest, abdomen, umbilicus, and vulva.

LABORATORY

- Increased numbers of dilated, epithelium-lined eccrine ducts are encased in a fibrous stroma.

COURSE AND PROGNOSIS

- Syringomas persist indefinitely and remain small.
- This lesion has no potential for malignancy.

DIFFERENTIAL DIAGNOSIS

- Other appendageal tumors, including trichoepithelioma
- Sebaceous hyperplasia
- Warts
- Xanthelasma
- Sarcoidosis

DISCUSSION

- Trichoepithelioma is a benign appendageal tumor with differentiation toward hair.
- Like syringomas, trichoepitheliomas also appear after puberty and occur most commonly on the face.
- Multiple lesions can be inherited in autosomal dominant fashion.
- The appearance of trichoepitheliomas and syringomas can be quite similar; biopsy may be needed to distinguish one from the other.
  - Trichoepitheliomas do not occur as frequently on the eyelid skin as syringoma.
  - Trichoepithelioma can be a solitary lesion that may become quite large and sclerotic; syringomas remain small.

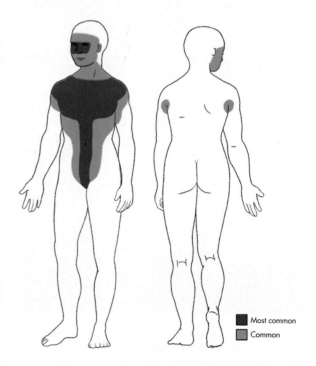

Most common
Common

- Sebaceous hyperplasia tends to be scattered on the face rather than grouped around the eyes.
  - Often, the lesions are umbilicated and are more yellow than syringomas.
- Flat warts also occur on the face as small, flat, skin-colored to pink papules.
  - Flat warts can be notoriously difficult to clear and thus are persistent.
  - Flat warts are rarely as symmetrically distributed as syringomas.
  - Flat warts favor the perioral skin, chin, and cheeks.
  - Condylomata might similarly be confused with vulvar syringomas.
  - If doubt exists, biopsy should be performed.
- Xanthelasma occurs on eyelid skin and represents cholesterol deposition within dermal macrophages.
- Cutaneous sarcoidosis may also present on the skin around the eyes.

TREATMENT

- Syringomas may be removed for cosmetic purposes.
- Electrodesiccation and curettage, laser surgery, and trichloracetic acid may be used with success.
- Cryosurgery is not recommended.
- Sharp dissection of lesions is easily performed under local anesthesia.
- The firm papule may be gently elevated from the softer surrounding skin with forceps and removed with iris scissors.

CAVEAT

- The dense stroma of syringomas allows for sharp dissection of the tumor from the surrounding skin.

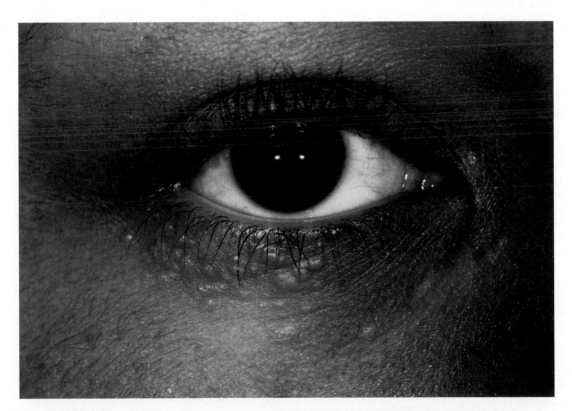

Syringomas are small, firm, flesh-colored dermal papules that occur on the lower lids and less commonly, on the forehead, chest, and abdomen.

17

Premalignant and Malignant Nonmelanoma Skin Tumors

■ BASAL CELL CARCINOMA

DESCRIPTION

- Basal cell carcinoma is the most common form of primary cutaneous malignancy.
- It is locally destructive, slow growing, and relentless.

HISTORY

- It may occur at any age but is more common after age 40.
- The highest incidence occurs in people with skin types I and II; it is less common in Asian-Americans and is rare in African-Americans.
- Cumulative sun exposure and prior ionizing radiation therapy are important risk factors.
- Tumors occur most commonly on the face, scalp, ears, and neck; less often on sun-exposed areas of the trunk and extremities; and rarely on the dorsal hands.
- Several clinical variants of basal cell carcinoma are recognized; these include nodular basal cell carcinoma, pigmented basal cell carcinoma, superficial basal cell carcinoma, micronodular basal cell carcinoma, and morpheaform basal cell carcinoma. Each varies slightly in terms of clinical appearance and aggressiveness.

SKIN FINDINGS

Nodular basal cell carcinoma

- Nodular basal cell carcinoma is the most commonly occurring variant.
- A pearl white, dome-shaped papule with overlying random telangiectasias appears.

- The papule enlarges slowly and has a flattened center and a raised, rolled translucent border.
- Tumors frequently ulcerate in the center, bleed, and become crusted.
- Curettage demonstrates the characteristic soft texture of the tumor as compared to the surrounding normal skin.

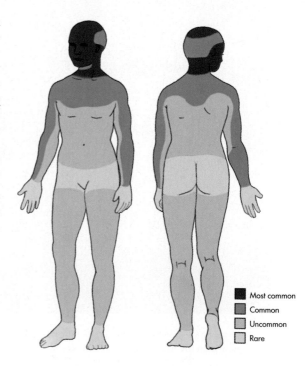

- Most common
- Common
- Uncommon
- Rare

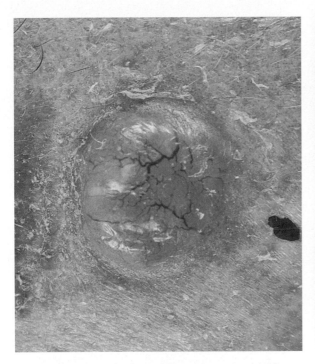

Nodular basal cell carcinoma. The lesion begins as a pearly white or pink, dome-shaped papule.

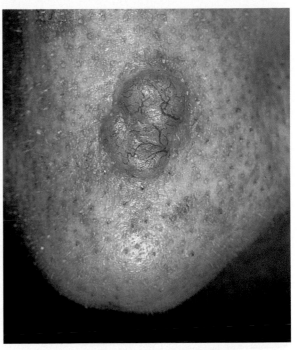

Nodular basal cell carcinoma. Telangiectatic vessels become prominent as the lesion enlarges. The growth pattern is irregular, forming an oval mass whereby the surface may become multilobular.

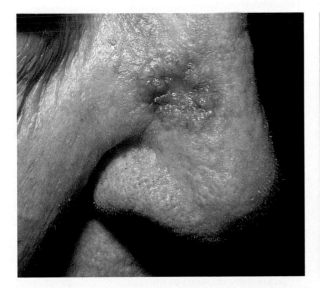

Nodular basal cell carcinoma. The center frequently ulcerates and bleeds and subsequently accumulates crust and scale.

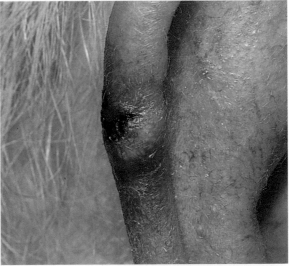

Nodular basal cell carcinoma may present as a papule or nodule on the ear and resembles squamous cell carcinoma.

Pigmented basal cell carcinoma
- Pigmented basal cell carcinoma is equivalent to nodular basal cell carcinoma, except that there is also melanin pigment.
- It may resemble melanoma.

Superficial basal cell carcinoma
- Superficial basal cell carcinoma is the least aggressive form; it is found more commonly on the trunk or extremities.
- The lesions are flatter and not as deeply invasive as the lesions of nodular basal cell carcinoma. The borders are less distinct but have the same pearly quality.

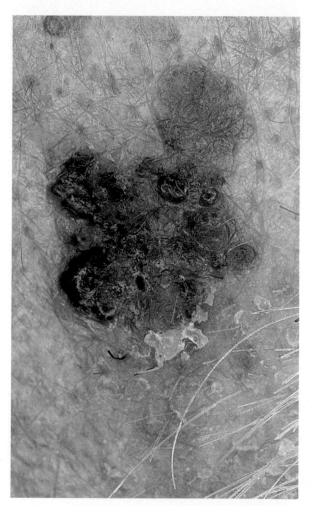

Basal cell carcinomas may contain melanin that imparts a brown, black, or blue color through all or part of the lesion.

- Areas within tumor may show healing with scarring.
- This form may resemble psoriasis or Bowen's disease (squamous cell carcinoma in situ).

Micronodular basal cell carcinoma
- Micronodular basal cell carcinoma resembles nodular basal cell carcinoma clinically, but there are microscopic islands of tumor cells extending beyond the clinical margins.

Morpheaform (sclerosing) basal cell carcinoma
- Morpheaform basal cell carcinoma is the most subtle and least common variant; it is also the most difficult to eradicate.
- The lesions resemble scar tissue; they are pale white to yellow and waxy on palpation.
- Because of this form's innocuous appearance, biopsy and diagnosis are often delayed.
- The margins are indistinct, and tumor cells may extend more than 7 mm from the clinical lesion.

Nonskin Findings

- Basal cell nevus syndrome is an autosomal dominant condition with multiple possible associated anomalies of the skeleton, skin, and central nervous system.
  - Possible skeletal anomalies include frontal bossing, hypertelorism, odontogenic cysts, bifid ribs, kyphoscoliosis, and shortened fourth metacarpals.
  - Possible skin anomalies include multiple basal cell carcinomas appearing in childhood and palmoplantar pitting.
  - Possible central nervous system anomalies include calcification of the falx cerebri and medulloblastoma.

Laboratory

- Basaloid tumor cells are in close approximation to a distinctive stroma.
- The size of tumor islands, the relative proportion of tumor cells to stroma, and the depth of tumor invasion indicate a tumor's aggressiveness.
- Superficial basal cell carcinomas appear as multifocal extensions of the basal layer of the epidermis into the superficial dermis.
- In nodular basal cell carcinomas, there are larger islands of tumor cells within the dermis; tumor islands may be solid or contain cystic cavities.

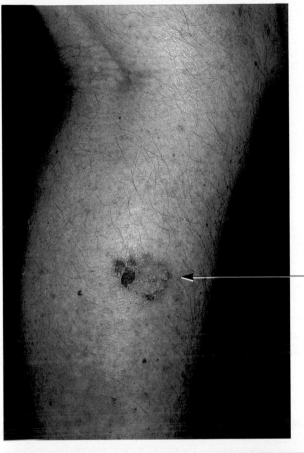

Superficial basal cell carcinoma. The circumscribed, round to oval, red, scaling plaque resembles a plaque of eczema, psoriasis, extramammary Paget's disease, or Bowen's disease. The superficial basal cell carcinoma spreads peripherally, sometimes for several centimeters, and invades after considerable time.

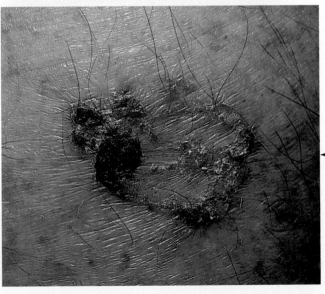

- Pigmented basal cell carcinoma is similar to nodular basal cell carcinoma; tumor islands contain melanin pigment.
- In micronodular basal cell carcinomas and infiltrative basal cell carcinomas, there are numerous islands and strands of tumor cells with increased stroma extending deeply into the dermis.
- In sclerosing or morpheaform basal cell carcinomas, there are innumerable scattered fine strands of tumor cells embedded within a fibrous stroma.

COURSE AND PROGNOSIS

- Without treatment, basal cell carcinomas persist, enlarge, and invade and destroy the surrounding structures.
- In large lesions, focal areas of healing, always with scarring, may appear.
- Inadequately treated basal cell carcinomas persist, often under scarring, when detection is delayed.
- In patients who develop one basal cell carcinoma, the annual risk of developing another basal cell carcinoma is 5% to 8%.

DISCUSSION

- Basal cell carcinomas are rarely, if ever, life threatening; metastases virtually never occur.
- Depending on tumor location, local destruction of normal tissue by the tumor can result in significant impairment.

TREATMENT

- The goal of treatment is eradication of the tumor and return of normal anatomic form and function.
- The treatment of basal cell carcinoma is determined by the site of the tumor and its clinical aggressiveness.
- Clinical aggressiveness correlates with histologic pattern.
- Electrosurgery involves electrodesiccation and curettage of obvious tumor.
  - It is usually performed for well-defined, small nodular basal cell carcinomas and superficial basal cell carcinomas.
  - The 5-year cure rates can approach 92% for primary tumors and 60% for recurrent tumors.
- Office excision is preferred for well-defined nodular, infiltrative, most micronodular, and recurrent basal cell carcinomas.
  - Office excision allows confirmation of surgical margins and depending on anatomic site, may

result in a more acceptable scar than one from electrosurgery.
  - The 5-year cure rates approach 90% for primary tumors and 83% for recurrent tumors.
- Mohs' micrographic surgery is a highly specialized method of excision used for difficult tumors with contiguous growth, including basal cell carcinomas.
  - Obvious tumor is debulked, and then excision is performed in stages. Excision is guided by sequential frozen-section mapping in three dimensions.
  - This allows for histologically confirmed removal of the tumor with the smallest of surgical margins and surgical defect.
  - The 5-year cure rates approach 99% for primary tumors and 96% for recurrent tumors.
  - Mohs' micrographic surgery is useful when tissue sparing is required because of anatomic location, recurrent tumors and tumors with a high risk of recurrence.
  - It is the treatment of choice for morpheaform basal cell carcinoma.
- Nonsurgical options are limited but include radiation therapy and photodynamic therapy.
  - Radiation therapy may be useful for tumors that are difficult to treat surgically and for patients who are unwilling or unable to tolerate surgery.
  - Improvements in computerized treatment models now allow the radiation oncologist to precisely treat a localized tumor with high-dose radiation in fractional doses over several weeks.
  - The 5-year cure rates are roughly 90% for both primary and recurrent tumors.
  - Cosmesis can be excellent, although expected long-term radiation changes in the treated skin may limit the use of this modality to older patients.
  - Photodynamic therapy is an evolving chemotherapeutic modality that is not widely available but may be useful in the future.
- All patients with basal cell carcinomas require follow-up to monitor for recurrence at the treated site and for the development of new tumors.

CAVEAT

- The patient needs to know that basal cell carcinomas are neither life threatening nor trivial.
- The importance of adequate treatment and close follow-up cannot be overstated.

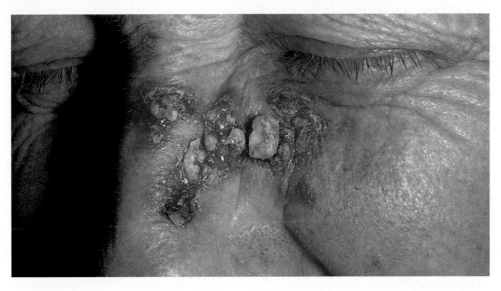

The cycle of growth, ulceration, and healing continues as the mass extends peripherally, and deeper masses of enormous size may be attained.

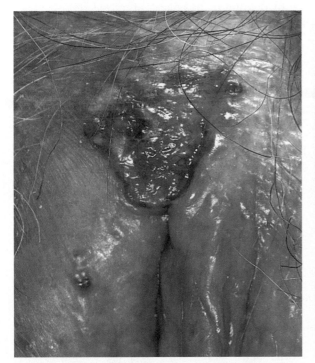

Basal cell carcinomas may present as nonhealing ulcers and may appear on any body surface, including the vulva.

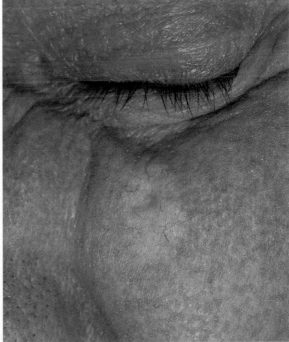

Morpheaform basal cell carcinoma is waxy, firm, flat to slightly raised, and either pale white or yellowish, and it resembles localized scleroderma.

■ ACTINIC KERATOSIS

DESCRIPTION

- Actinic keratoses are common, persistent, keratotic lesions with malignant potential.
- Multiple lesions are most commonly found in sun-exposed areas of older patients with fair skin types.

HISTORY

- Years of cumulative sun exposure and keratinocyte damage may lead to the formation of actinic keratoses.
- Lesions become progressively more common after age 40, and multiple lesions are often present.
- Patients with skin types I and II tend to develop the most lesions.
- The slight variation in the distribution of lesions among men and women may relate to differences in hairstyle because the ears, neck, and balding scalp are more affected in men.
- If symptomatic, lesions usually burn or sting.
- Spontaneous regression is reported, although most lesions persist without treatment.
- Depending on the site, a small percentage of these lesions progress to invasive squamous cell carcinoma over several years.

SKIN FINDINGS

- Actinic keratoses are found among other signs of sun exposure, such as uneven pigmentation, atrophy, and telangiectasias (see p. 298).
- Lesions are found predominantly on the head, neck, and dorsal hands.
- Actinic keratoses initially present as a poorly defined area of hyperemia.
- Over time, the lesion becomes more defined and develops a thin, adherent transparent scale. At this stage, lesions are sometimes easier to detect by palpation than by observation. One finds a discrete change in skin texture associated with slight erythema.
- With time, the adherent scale becomes progressively thicker and yellow in color.
- Retained scale may form a cutaneous horn.
- Such advanced lesions may be difficult to distinguish from invasive squamous cell carcinoma without skin biopsy.
- Spreading pigmented actinic keratosis (SPAK) describes actinic keratoses with fine reticulated pigmentation and thinner scaling.
  - This distinct clinical presentation is a variant of the more classic actinic keratosis with similar malignant potential and treatment options.
  - The importance of recognizing this pattern lies in the fact that SPAK lesions can be difficult to distinguish clinically from lentigo maligna or melanoma in situ.
  - Lentigo maligna also occurs most frequently on sun-damaged skin. Skin biopsy usually establishes the correct diagnosis.
- Actinic cheilitis is a sun-induced keratinocyte atypia and atrophy involving the lower lip.
  - The lower lip shows focal crusting and scaling along with blurring of the vermilion border.
  - Actinic lesions in this location can be quite subtle clinically and behave aggressively.

LABORATORY

- Biopsy is often helpful for distinguishing advanced actinic keratoses and actinic cheilitis from invasive squamous cell carcinoma.
- The histologic hallmark is a disordered epidermis with keratinocyte atypia.
- By definition, invasion of atypical keratinocytes is not seen.
- SPAK lesions similarly show keratinocyte atypia, whereas atypical melanocytes are seen in lentigo maligna.

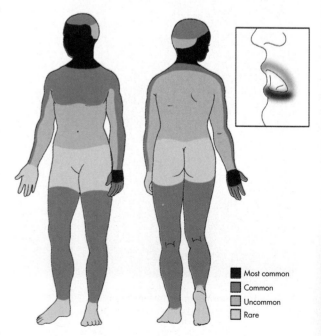

■ Most common
■ Common
■ Uncommon
□ Rare

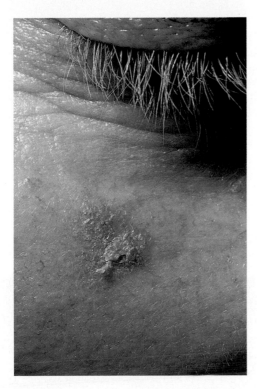

Adherent yellow crust forms, the removal of which may cause bleeding.

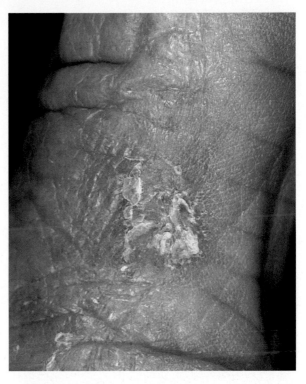

Individual lesions vary in size from 3 to 6 mm or larger.

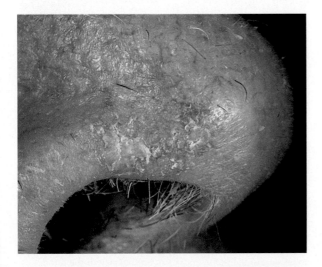

A broad-based lesion on the nose.

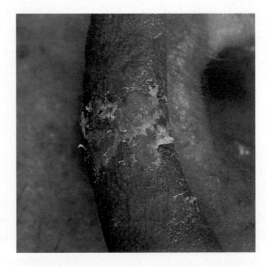

Actinic keratosis are frequently found on the ears.

COURSE AND PROGNOSIS

- As a rule, untreated actinic keratoses persist and grow slowly.
- A small percentage of lesions spontaneously regress with continued sun protection, and a smaller percentage progress to squamous cell carcinoma.
- The behavior of an individual lesion cannot be predicted.
- It has been estimated that one in five patients with multiple actinic keratoses develops squamous cell carcinoma in one or more lesions.
- Squamous cell carcinomas that develop on the ear or at the vermilion border are more likely to metastasize than squamous cell carcinomas that develop at other skin sites.

DISCUSSION

- Inflammatory disorders involving the head and neck, such as seborrheic dermatitis and rosacea, can limit detection of actinic keratoses. Adequate control of these disorders helps in the prompt recognition and treatment of actinic keratoses.

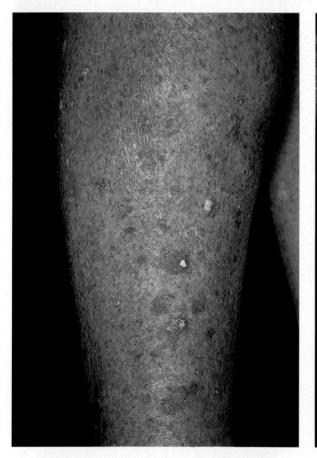

Actinic keratoses of the lower legs are frequently multiple, hyperkeratotic, and distributed over a large area.

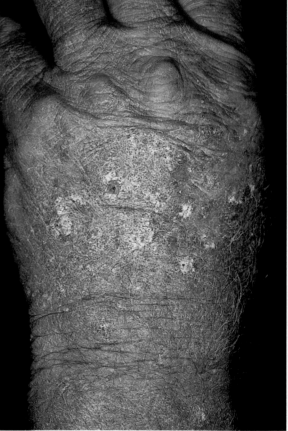

Numerous lesions may form on the back of the hand.

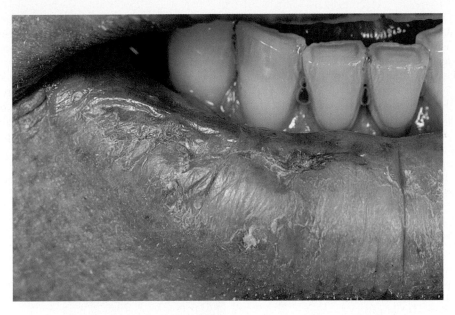

Actinic cheilitis. Scale and crust can be easily removed but will recur.

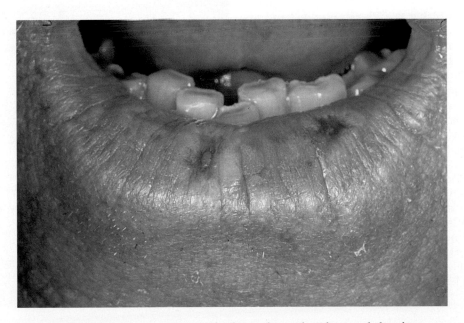

Actinic cheilitis. The lower lip is pink-white and smooth with an eroded surface.

TREATMENT

- The patient with multiple actinic keratoses requires at least annual follow-up.
- Detectable lesions represent a fraction of the total number of atypical keratinocytes such patients possess.
- Most of the atypia is scattered within sun-damaged skin and below the level of clinical detection.
- The patient will almost certainly develop more clinically apparent lesions.
- Adequate sun protection with sun-protective clothing and sunscreens should be encouraged to limit further damage.
- Topical 5-fluorouracil (5-FU) cream or solution is useful in reducing the effects of atypical keratinocytes.
  - Although effective, treatment should be individualized for specific areas of the skin, both in terms of concentration of the cream, applications per day, and duration.
  - The patient should be advised of what to expect during and after treatment.
  - Although treatment of all sun-damaged areas may be appropriate, it is rarely practical to treat large areas at one time. It may instead be convenient to treat limited areas on a rotating basis.
  - 5-FU is available as a 1% (Fluoroplex) and 5% (Efudex) cream and a 1% (Fluoroplex) and 2% (Efudex) solution. The stronger concentrations are often required to treat the nonfacial lesions.
  - Treatment with 5-FU involves application of medication twice a day for 3 to 5 weeks or longer.
  - Erythema appears. This is followed by burning and oozing. Treatment is stopped when intense inflammation or crusting appears.
  - Patients should be evaluated every 2 weeks during the treatment period.
  - Some physicians use Group V to VII topical steroids during the treatment period to suppress inflammation. This may make it difficult to determine when therapy should be stopped.
- Cryosurgery with liquid nitrogen is effective for superficial lesions.
  - Thicker lesions should be débrided of scale before cryosurgery.

- Electrodesiccation and curettage are also effective. Carbon dioxide laser vermilionectomy is the preferred treatment for extensive actinic cheilitis.
- All destructive methods ablate the epidermis with minimal effect on the dermis. All have some risk of post-procedure dyspigmentation, especially in patients with darker skin. This should be clearly explained to the patient before treatment.

CAVEAT

- Invasive squamous cell carcinoma can occur, especially with thicker lesions, lesions not responding to treatment, and lesions of the lower lip. A biopsy should be considered.

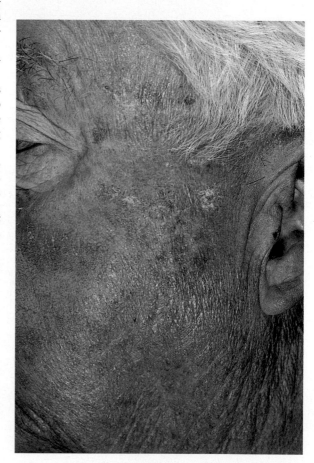

Numerous superficial lesions on the face.

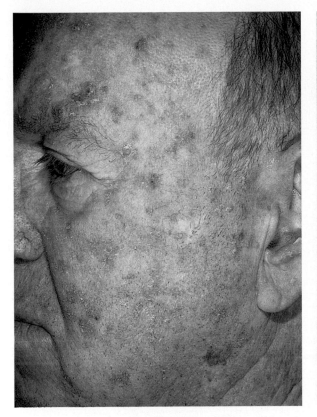

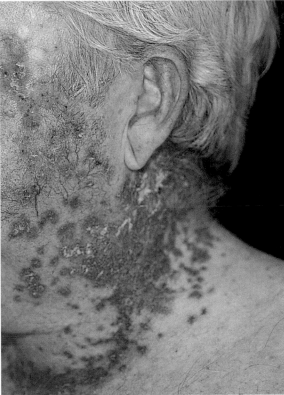

Topical chemotherapy with 5-fluorouracil. Lesions become inflamed during the first week of treatment.

Topical chemotherapy with 5-fluorouracil. Intense Inflammation is induced. Thick, indurated lesions become inflamed.

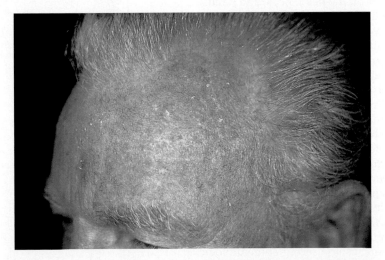

The extent of disease varies from a single lesion to involvement of the entire forehead, balding scalp, or temples.

■ SQUAMOUS CELL CARCINOMA

DESCRIPTION

- Squamous cell carcinoma is an invasive, primary cutaneous malignancy arising from keratinocytes of the skin or mucosal surfaces.
- It is most commonly found on the head, neck, or hands of older patients.
- Lesions may develop from precursor actinic keratoses or may arise de novo.

HISTORY

- Squamous cell carcinoma is the second most common form of skin cancer.
- It comprises 20% of all primary cutaneous malignancies.
- The lifetime risk of developing a cutaneous squamous cell carcinoma is estimated to be between 4% and 14%.
- More than 100,000 new cases of primary cutaneous squamous cell carcinoma are diagnosed in the United States each year.
- Approximately 2500 deaths occur annually from squamous cell carcinoma arising in the skin.
- The incidence of squamous cell carcinoma doubles with each 8° to 10° decline in latitude.
- Primary cutaneous squamous cell carcinomas usually occur on sun-exposed skin from years of accumulated actinic damage.
  - Nearly 90% of cutaneous squamous cell carcinomas in men and nearly 80% of such tumors in women occur on the head, neck, and hands.
  - Squamous cell carcinoma on the leg occurs more often in women than in men.
  - Caucasians with fair complexions (skin types I and II) are at greatest risk.
- Although the majority of squamous cell carcinomas are caused by ultraviolet light exposure, other extrinsic factors can play a causal role.
  - Such factors include other forms of radiation, chemicals such as hydrocarbons and arsenic, tobacco, chronic infection such as osteomyelitis, chronic inflammation, burns (Marjolin's ulcer), and human papillomavirus infection.
  - Historically, squamous cell carcinoma has been considered a low-grade tumor with a metastatic rate of less than 1%.
  - With the current epidemic of all primary cutaneous malignancies and recent epidemiologic attention, it is clear that squamous cell carcinoma is far more aggressive than previously believed.

- Squamous cell carcinomas spread within the skin first by local invasion and expansion of the skin.
  - On reaching the deeper tissue planes, the tumor spreads laterally along the path of least resistance.
- *Conduit spread* refers to perivascular or perineural extension of tumor cells.
- Ultimately, tumors may metastasize, usually via the lymphatics, to local lymph nodes.

SKIN FINDINGS

- As with actinic keratoses, squamous cell carcinomas typically occur on sun-exposed areas.
- Tumors are found within a background of sun-damaged skin with atrophy, telangiectasias, and blotchy hyperpigmentation.
- Actinic keratoses (see p. 366) are aggregates of atypical keratinocytes contained within the epidermis.
  - At the very least, actinic keratoses represent squamous atypia, if not carcinoma in situ.
  - Unlike Bowen's disease, actinic keratoses are not full-thickness lesions.
  - Actinic keratoses progress toward invasive squamous cell carcinoma more slowly.

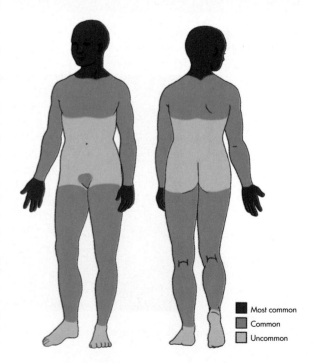

Most common
Common
Uncommon

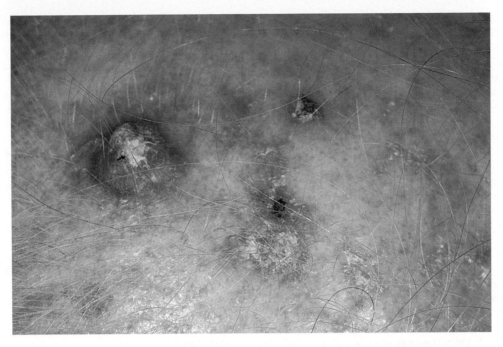

Many lesions may appear on the sun-exposed bald scalp.

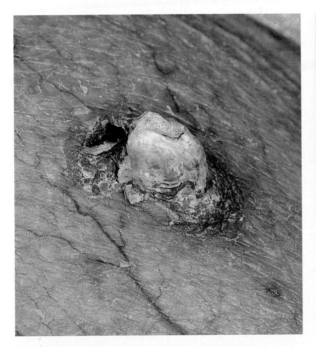

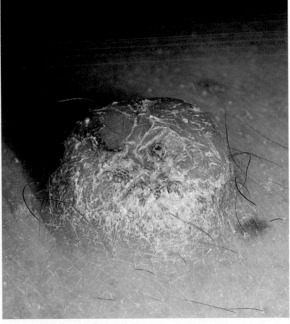

Squamous cell carcinomas arising from actinic keratosis may have a thick, adherent scale.

The tumor is soft and freely movable and may have a red, inflamed base.

- Early invasive squamous cell carcinoma may have the appearance of a hypertrophic actinic keratosis.
  - The lesion has a red, poorly defined base and an adherent yellow-white cutaneous horn.
  - Invasion is seen, and the diagnosis is made by skin biopsy.
  - The untreated lesion becomes larger and more raised, developing into a firm, red nodule with a necrotic crusted center.
- Squamous cell carcinoma may arise de novo, appearing as a sharply defined, smooth, dull red, firm, dome-shaped nodule with a crusted center.
  - Removal of the crust reveals a central cavity filled with necrotic keratin debris, often with a foul odor.
- Keratoacanthoma (see p. 340) cannot be reliably distinguished from invasive squamous cell carcinoma on clinical grounds.
  - Most authors consider keratoacanthoma to be a low-grade squamous cell carcinoma.
  - Diagnosis is based on histologic studies and ultimately on follow-up.
- Bowen's disease (see p. 378) represents full-thickness squamous cell carcinoma in situ.
  - A slowly growing, barely raised, red plaque with adherent dry scaling appears.
  - Untreated, invasion ultimately occurs within a lesion of Bowen's disease.
  - When this occurs, the area of invasion develops the dull red, nodular thickening of squamous cell carcinoma.
  - Similarly, erythroplasia of Queyrat (squamous cell carcinoma in situ of the penis) may also become invasive.
  - Nodular or ulcerated areas should suggest invasion and warrant biopsy.

NONSKIN FINDINGS

- As previously discussed, squamous cell carcinomas have metastatic potential.
- Metastases are usually to the regional lymph nodes and are detected within 2 to 3 years.
- Palpable regional lymph nodes suggest metastatic disease.

LABORATORY

- Skin biopsy should be performed for all suspected squamous cell carcinomas.
- Biopsy should include the dermis so that invasion can be assessed.
- Malignant keratinocytes are confined to the epidermis in both actinic keratoses and Bowen's disease.
- In actinic keratoses, malignant cells are usually few in number, are well demarcated, and possess overlying parakeratosis.
- In Bowen's disease, malignant cells are greater in number, are found at all levels of the epidermis, and extend into the epithelium of adnexal structures.
- In invasive squamous cell carcinomas, malignant cells breach the dermoepidermal junction and invade the dermis.
- Tumor cells vary in their degree of differentiation.
- The surgical margins of excised lesions should be examined carefully to ensure complete excision.
- Lesions should be graded as to their degree of differentiation, their depth of invasion, and the presence of perineural invasion.

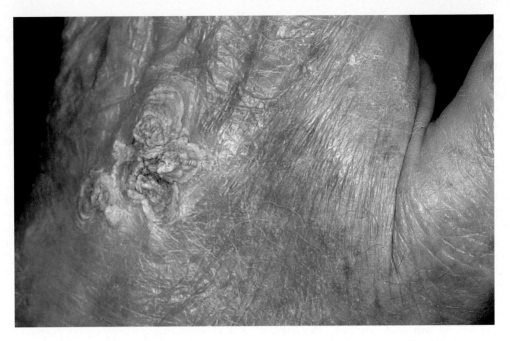

Actinic keratosis may become thick, indicating degeneration into squamous cell carcinoma.

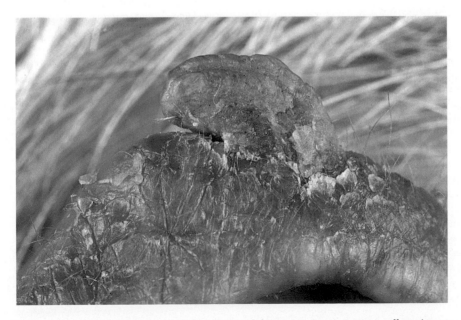

Cutaneous horns may begin as actinic keratosis and degenerate into squamous cell carcinoma.

COURSE AND PROGNOSIS

- The long-term prognosis for surgically treated, nonmetastatic squamous cell carcinoma of the skin is excellent.
- Such patients are at increased risk of developing additional primary skin malignancies, so periodic follow-up is advised.
- The metastasis rate of squamous cell carcinomas arising on sun-exposed skin is now estimated to be between 2% and 6%.
  - Unlike melanoma, squamous cell carcinoma metastasizes first to the regional lymph nodes in more than 80% of cases, usually within the first 2 to 3 years.
  - Risk factors for metastasis include:
    - Tumor larger than 2.0 cm in diameter, invasion deeper than 0.4 cm, or both factors
    - Decreased degree of differentiation of tumor cells
    - Prior treatment with recurrence
    - Perineural invasion
    - Adenoid or mucin-producing variant of squamous cell carcinoma
    - Immunosuppressed host
    - Tumor arising in a scar or a chronic wound
- The risk of metastases is also higher for tumors at specific anatomic sites.
  - The metastatic rate for squamous cell carcinomas arising on the lip or ear is estimated at 10% to 20%.
  - The 5-year mortality rate is similar to that of other head and neck tumors.
  - Half of such patients ultimately die as a result of metastatic disease.
  - Tumors arising within scar tissue have a metastatic rate as high as 30%.

COMPLICATIONS

- Patients on immunosuppressive therapy after organ transplantation are at higher risk for cutaneous malignancy, including squamous cell carcinoma.
- Tumors arise with increasing frequency between 5 and 10 years after transplantation.
- Such patients must be followed closely and their tumors treated aggressively.

TREATMENT

- The treatment of primary squamous cell carcinoma of the skin involves wide local excision with histologic confirmation of margins.
  - Mohs' micrographic excision may be useful for specific sites where tissue sparing is of importance.
  - Cure by Mohs' technique assumes contiguous tumor growth such as that seen in basal cell carcinoma.
  - Squamous cell carcinoma can have skip areas (noncontiguous growth), and this renders Mohs' technique somewhat less effective.
- Palpation of regional lymph nodes is mandatory for all invasive squamous cell carcinomas.
  - Lymph node biopsy is indicated for suspected nodal disease.
  - The role of elective node dissection for high-risk lesions is currently under investigation.
- Imaging studies may be warranted for high-risk tumors.
- Radiation therapy may be considered when surgical resection is not feasible.
- Careful follow-up at regular intervals is recommended for all squamous cell carcinomas. Follow-up should include the following:
  - Skin examination and biopsy of new lesions suspicious for malignancy
  - Visual inspection and palpation of the excision scar for nodularity and other evidence of skin recurrence
  - Careful examination of the regional lymph node with node biopsy, if indicated, to detect early metastatic disease
- Patients should be taught how to perform periodic skin self-examination and should be advised to seek care for any suspicious changes.

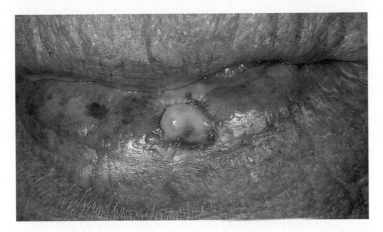

The sun-exposed lower lip is a common site. Palpation may reveal a deep nodular mass. Squamous cell carcinomas originating on the lip are aggressive and metastasize to the regional lymph nodes and beyond.

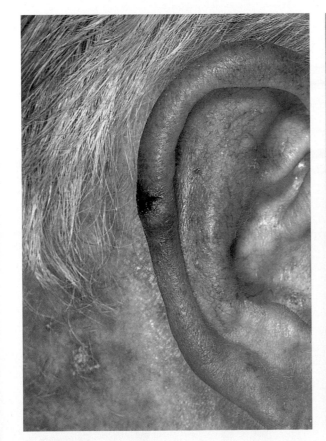

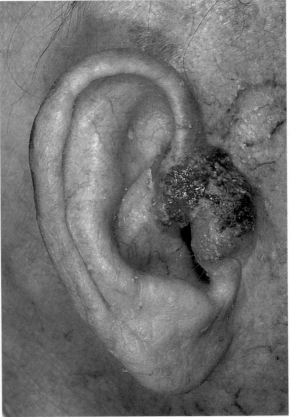

Squamous cell carcinomas arise in actinically damaged skin of the ear and may be aggressive.

This neglected tumor has attained a very large size and metastasized to regional lymph nodes.

■ BOWEN'S DISEASE

DESCRIPTION

- Bowen's disease is an intraepidermal (in situ), primary cutaneous malignancy arising from keratinocytes of the skin or mucosal surfaces.

HISTORY

- Bowen's disease is somewhat more common in male than female patients.
- It may arise in sun-exposed and relatively sun-protected areas.
- There are multiple etiologies, including ultraviolet light (actinic), other forms of radiation, chemicals, and human papillomavirus.
- Lesions within sun-protected areas suggest a past history of arsenic exposure.
- The onset is insidious; lesions are persistent and slowly enlarge over months to years. Slow progression ultimately leads to invasion.
- Lesions are minimally symptomatic, and patients often delay seeking care.

SKIN FINDINGS

- A solitary, barely raised, red plaque with adherent dry scaling appears.
- At first glance, the plaque suggests a single plaque of psoriasis with sharply defined borders.
- On closer inspection, the surface scaling is irregular, fissured, and adherent.
- Focal areas of pigmentation are often present and suggest superficial basal cell carcinoma.
- The border is not raised or rolled.
- Little if any inflammation is present.
- Lesions do not show a tendency for healing centrally.
- Untreated, the plaque extends laterally over many years eventually becoming invasive squamous cell carcinoma.
- Unlike actinic keratoses, Bowen's disease represents full-thickness replacement of the epidermis with tumor cells.
- Erythroplasia of Queyrat is also squamous cell carcinoma in situ occurring under the foreskin of the penis.
  - Plaques are also red and sharply defined, as in Bowen's disease.
  - Plaques lack scale and instead have a moist, glistening surface.
  - Analogous lesions occur on the vulva.

NONSKIN FINDINGS

- Patients with plaques in sun-protected areas may have a history of arsenic exposure.
- Those with a confirmed history of arsenic exposure are at increased risk of lymphoreticular and gastrointestinal malignancies.

LABORATORY

- There is epidermal thickening with disorder and parakeratosis.
- Malignant keratinocytes are seen at all levels within the epidermis in a "windblown" pattern.
- Atypical cells extend down along the adnexal epithelium well below the surface.
- Atypical cells do not breach the dermoepidermal junction.

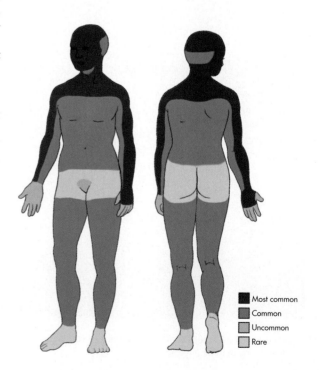

Most common
Common
Uncommon
Rare

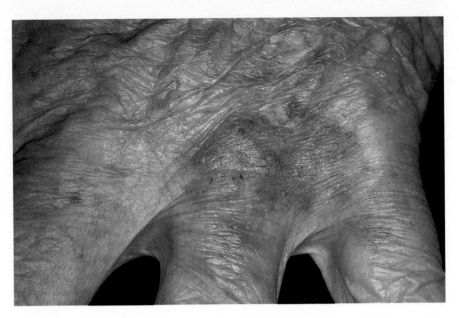

Bowen's disease lesions are slightly elevated, red, scaly plaques with surface fissures and foci of pigmentation.

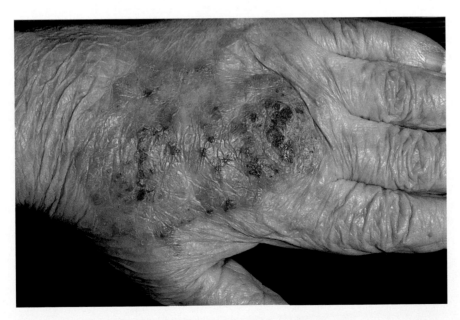

The plaque grows very slowly by lateral extension and may eventually, after several months or years, invade the dermis, producing induration and ulceration.

COURSE AND PROGNOSIS

- Bowen's disease is similar to actinic keratoses in that both are intraepidermal lesions containing malignant keratinocytes. However, Bowen's disease is a less common and more virulent lesion.
- Lesions are full-thickness, extend in continuity with epithelium of adnexal structures, and predictably become invasive.
- Erythroplasia of Queyrat has a greater tendency toward invasion and metastases, estimated at 10% to 30%.

DIFFERENTIAL DIAGNOSIS

- Clinical
  - Psoriasis
  - Localized chronic eczematous dermatitis
  - Superficial basal cell carcinoma
  - Seborrheic keratosis
- Histologic
  - Mammary and extramammary Paget's disease
  - Amelanotic melanoma

DISCUSSION

- Skin biopsy discerns among the clinical differential diagnoses.
- Special stains may be required to discriminate among the histologic differential diagnoses.

TREATMENT

- When feasible, the treatment of choice is excision with confirmation of margins.
- Other treatment modalities include electrodesiccation and curettage, cryosurgery, and topical 5-fluorouracil.
- These treatments are less effective because of the extension of tumor cells down into adnexal structures.
- Occlusion may augment the effectiveness of topical 5-fluorouracil.
- Close follow-up after any treatment is mandatory.
- Any areas suspicious for recurrence should be excised with confirmation of margins.

CAVEAT

- Bowen's disease should be treated as invasive squamous cell carcinoma until proved otherwise by skin biopsy.

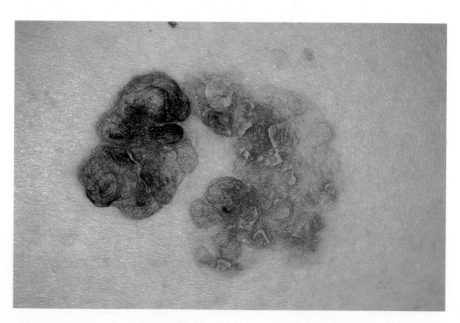

Bowen's disease. The borders are well defined, and lesions closely resemble psoriasis, chronic eczema and seborrheic keratosis.

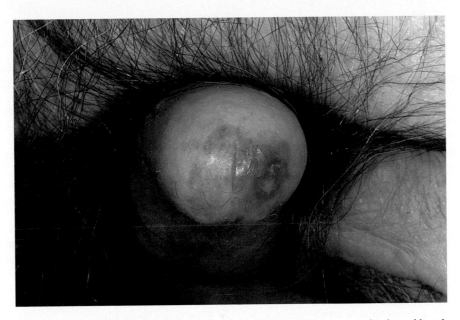

Analogous to Bowen's disease of the skin, erythroplasia of Queyrat grows very slowly and has the potential for degeneration into squamous cell carcinoma.

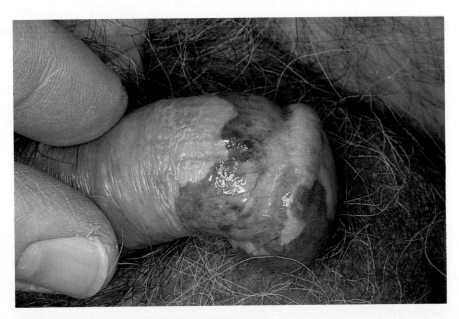

Bowen's disease of the penis (erythroplasia of Queyrat) is a moist, slightly raised, well-defined, red, smooth or velvety plaque.

■ LEUKOPLAKIA

DESCRIPTION

- *Leukoplakia* is a descriptive clinical term reserved for white patches or plaques occurring on the oral mucosa pending definitive diagnosis.

HISTORY

- Leukoplakia is a common chronic condition of the oral mucosa.
- It occurs more frequently in men than in women.
- It usually appears after age 40, and the prevalence approaches 8% after age 70.
- Most lesions are asymptomatic.

SKIN FINDINGS

- Leukoplakia begins as a single small, well-defined, translucent to white, slightly elevated papule.
- Individual lesions may resolve completely, recur, or progress.
- Multiple papules may coalesce into larger plaques over time.
- Uneven hyperkeratosis or small erosions may develop.
- Focal red areas termed *erythroplakia* may develop within plaques, giving a speckled appearance.
- Lesions may occur anywhere on the oral mucosa but are most commonly found on the buccal mucosa and lower lip.

LABORATORY

- The clinical appearance is often more striking than the histologic characteristics are.
- Varying degrees of hyperplasia and hyperkeratosis occur.
- There is a sparse, mixed inflammatory infiltrate in the submucosa.
- Epithelial dysplasia is seen in less than 25% of biopsies.
- If demonstrated by biopsy, malignancy establishes a diagnosis of squamous cell carcinoma in situ.

COURSE AND PROGNOSIS

- *Leukoplakia* is a descriptive clinical term, not a definitive diagnosis. The term is often misused to designate a premalignant condition. *Premalignant* implies epithelial dysplasia, which may be seen on biopsy.

- Thus *leukoplakia* is best used to describe a chronic oral lesion in which dysplasia has yet to be demonstrated by biopsy.
- There is a risk of malignant transformation with time, especially for lesions on the ventral tongue and floor of the mouth.
  - Factors that favor malignant transformation include tobacco, alcohol, ultraviolet light, and some human papilloma viruses.
  - More than 80% of patients with leukoplakia use some form of tobacco.
  - When malignant change is demonstrated, a definitive diagnosis of squamous cell carcinoma is made.
  - Invasive squamous cell carcinoma of mucosa has a much greater risk of metastasis than squamous cell carcinoma arising in skin.

DIFFERENTIAL DIAGNOSIS

- Candidiasis (thrush)
- Oral hairy leukoplakia
- Frictional hyperkeratosis
- Lichen planus
- White sponge nevus
- Squamous cell carcinoma

DISCUSSION

- Oral candidal lesions are less adherent; this diagnosis is confirmed by potassium hydroxide examination.
- The presence of *Candida* organisms does not exclude the possibility of an underlying condition.
- Oral hairy leukoplakia occurs in patients with advanced disease caused by the human immunodeficiency virus. Lesions occur most commonly on the lateral aspect of the tongue. Epstein-Barr virus is believed to be the causal agent.

■ Most common
■ Common

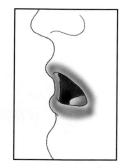

- Frictional hyperkeratosis results from surface trauma or from dental appliances or bite abnormalities.
- Lesion location correlates with the source of the trauma.

TREATMENT

- Patients who use tobacco products should be encouraged to stop.
- Clinical follow-up with oral biopsy at regular intervals is recommended.
- Any area of change, especially areas of erythroplakia, should be biopsied.
- Localized areas of demonstrated epithelial dysplasia may be treated by cryosurgery, electrosurgery, or topical 5-fluorouracil.
- Close clinical follow-up is required to guard against recurrence.
- Areas demonstrating squamous cell carcinoma, either in situ or invasive, are best treated by excision. Close clinical follow-up, including lymph node examination, is required.

CAVEAT

- One cannot overstate the importance of close clinical follow-up and oral biopsy.

The term *leukoplakia* implies that the results of the biopsy and the diagnosis are pending.

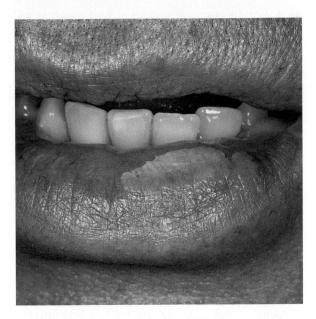

Leukoplakia. The patches are white, slightly elevated, usually well-defined plaques that show little tendency to extend peripherally.

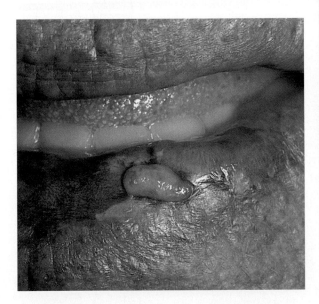

Leukoplakia may eventually degenerate and ulcerate.

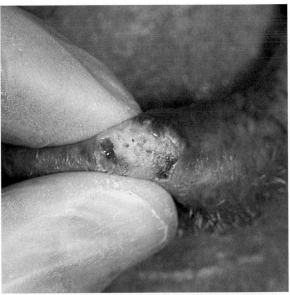

Degeneration to carcinoma develops in less than 20% of all patients with leukoplakia and takes 1 to 20 years. All lesions should be palpated; a firm mass indicates squamous cell carcinoma.

■ CUTANEOUS T-CELL LYMPHOMA
DESCRIPTION

- Cutaneous T-cell lymphoma, also known as *mycosis fungoides (MF)*, is a distinct helper T-cell lymphoma that in most cases presents in the skin.
- It may progress and involve the lymph nodes, peripheral blood, and viscera.
- Four phases characterize disease evolution: pre-MF, patch stage, plaque stage, and tumor stage. Some patients have only plaques and tumors. Lesions from the last three stages may be present simultaneously.
- Sézary syndrome is the leukemic form of MF; it occurs de novo or evolves from what appears to be chronic eczema.

HISTORY

- There are 0.42 cases per 100,000 people.
- Male patients are affected twice as often as female patients.
- African-Americans are affected twice as often as Caucasians.
- Most cases are diagnosed in the fifth and sixth decade of life, although all ages can be affected.

SKIN FINDINGS

- *Large-plaque parapsoriasis* is another name for the premycotic phase.
  - This stage persists for months or years and is suspected when inflammation persists and recurs after repeated courses of topical steroids.
  - Red, scaly, eczematous-like or psoriasis-like eruption and an atrophic, mottled, telangiectatic eruption occur.
- The eczematous form presents with persistent, nonspecific, flat, red, itchy, eczematous areas resembling asteatotic eczema or atopic dermatitis; lesions remain fixed in location and size, and margins are sharply delineated.
- In the patch and plaque stages, dusky red-to-brown, sometimes scaly areas may be elevated above the surrounding uninvolved skin.
  - Disease is often located on the "bathing-trunk" area—the buttocks, hip, and upper thighs. The inner aspects of the upper arms and legs are often involved early.
  - Plaque shape is variable; round, oval, arciform, or serpiginous patterns occur, occasionally with central clearing.
  - The extent varies from a few isolated areas to a major portion of the skin.

- In the tumor stage, lesions are variable in size and are within plaques or arise de novo. Red or violaceous nodules may ulcerate.
- In erythroderma, redness and scaling of the entire skin occur.
  - The palms and soles often have thick scaling.
  - Alopecia and ectropion may occur.
- Sézary syndrome often presents as erythroderma, peripheral node enlargement, and generalized pruritus.

NONSKIN FINDINGS

- The workup should include clinical evaluation for peripheral adenopathy.
- Baseline laboratory tests include complete blood count with smear review, liver function tests, blood urea nitrogen levels, creatinine level, and chest x-ray study. The results are usually normal in the patch and plaque stages.
- If there is palpable adenopathy or rapidly progressing disease or if the disease is at stage IIb or above, chest, abdominal and pelvic computed tomographic scans are performed.

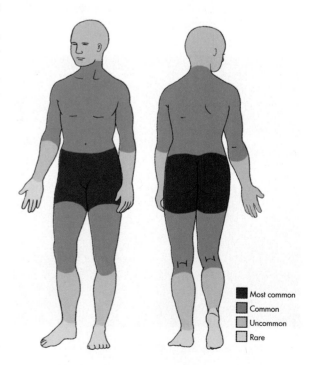

Most common
Common
Uncommon
Rare

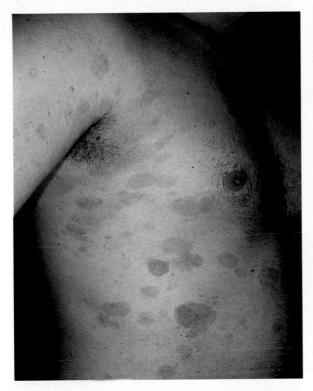

Lesions tend to remain fixed in location and size, and the margins are sharply delineated.

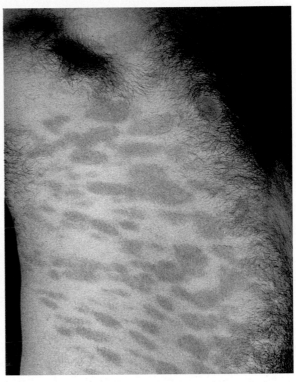

A red, psoriasis-like eruption and an atrophic, mottled, telangiectatic surface referred to as *large-patch parapsoriasis* or *poikiloderma vasculare atrophicans* occurs.

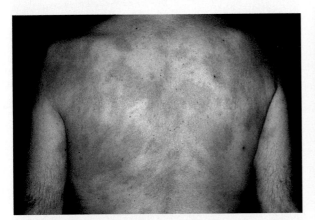

An eczematous form presents with persistent, nonspecific, flat, red, itchy, areas that resemble asteatotic eczema or atopic dermatitis, except that the lesions tend to remain fixed in location and size and the margins are sharply delineated.

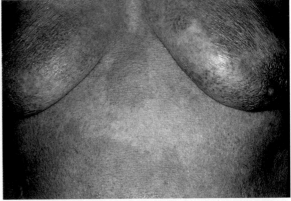

Infiltration of the entire skin produces a thickened, red hide with scale (exfoliative dermatitis) or without scale (erythroderma)

LABORATORY

- Despite new laboratory diagnostic methods, recognition of the physical signs of the disease by the clinician is still the most sensitive method of detection.
- Plaques exhibit a superficial and deep, bandlike and perivascular lymphocytic infiltrate with collections of lymphocytes (Pautrier's micro-abscesses) within a thickened, psoriasiform epidermis. The infiltrate becomes mixed (lymphocytes, eosinophils, and plasma cells) as the plaque stage progresses. Some lymphocytes are atypical, having a large, hyperconvoluted or cerebriform nucleus.
- Molecular studies may be diagnostically helpful in the early stages or in clinically atypical cases; polymerase chain reaction and Southern blotting may reveal T-cell receptor gene rearrangement, indicating the presence of a clonal population of cells.

DIFFERENTIAL DIAGNOSIS

- Atopic dermatitis
- Psoriasis or psoriasiform dermatitis
- Lymphomatoid drug eruption
- Lymphomatoid contact dermatitis

TREATMENT

- A referral to a dermatologist or oncologist is recommended for staging and treatment.
- Treatment is stage related.
  - In the patch and plaque stages, topical chemotherapy (nitrogen mustard, carmustine), psoralen plus ultraviolet A (PUVA), ultraviolet B, total-body electron beam therapy, and combination therapies (i.e., interferon with PUVA) are used.
  - In the tumor stage, spot radiation and interferon are used.
  - In erythroderma or Sézary syndrome: extracorporeal photopheresis, interferon, methotrexate, prednisone, and cyclophosphamide (Cytoxan) are used.

COURSE AND PROGNOSIS

- In general, the course and prognosis relate to the stage of the disease.
- The pre-MF and patch stages can last for many years without progression to tumor development, adenopathy, or visceral involvement.

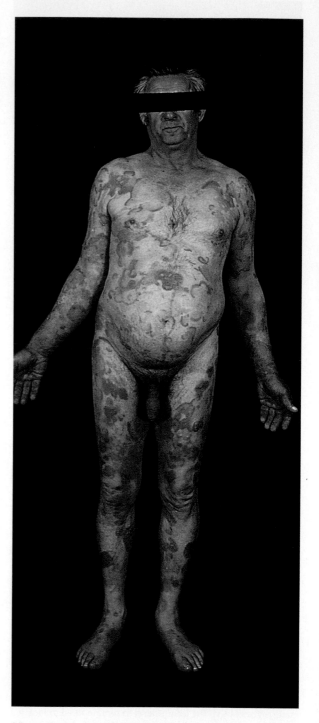

Necrosis and ulceration of plaques and tumors are common.

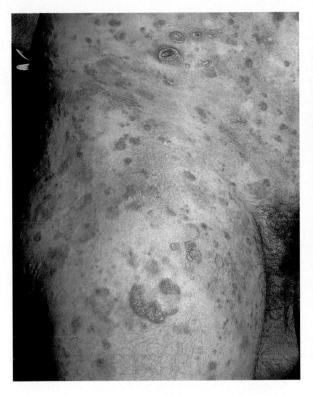

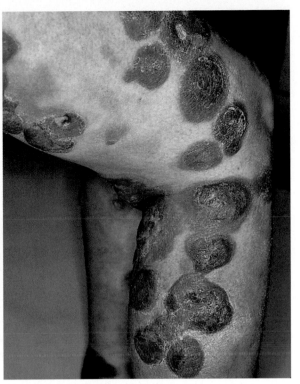

Tumors develop from preexisting plaques or erythroderma, or they may originate from red or normal skin.

Tumors vary in size, some becoming huge.

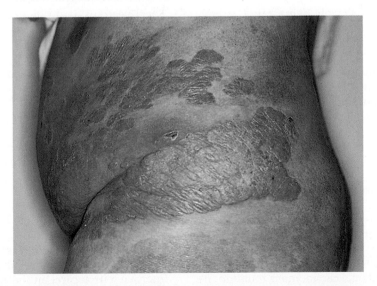

The plaques vary in shape, and the extent of involvement varies from a few isolated areas to a major portion of the skin.

■ PAGET'S DISEASE OF THE BREAST

DESCRIPTION

- Paget's disease of the breast is an uncommon, distinctive clinical presentation of intraductal carcinoma of the breast.

HISTORY

- Paget's disease is the most common cutaneous presentation of breast cancer.
- It represents less than 5% of all breast cancer cases.
- It occurs almost exclusively in women and is rare in men.
- The incidence increases with age, reflecting the incidence of breast cancer.
- It has an insidious onset, lasting months to years, usually in the fourth to sixth decades of life.
- It may be asymptomatic.
- When it is symptomatic, patients complain of localized itching, irritation, and discomfort.
- Patients report exudative staining of clothing.
- "Nipple eczema" that does not improve after the use of topical corticosteroids is suspicious for Paget's disease.
- Patient denial or delay in seeking care results in a delay in the biopsy and the diagnosis.

SKIN FINDINGS

- The lesion is a red, sharply demarcated, irregularly outlined papule or plaque.
- The nipple, areola, and surrounding skin may be involved.
- Most often, it is unilateral but can be bilateral.
- Thin, pinpoint, nonadherent scaling is seen over the entire surface of the plaque.
- Removal of the scale reveals a moist, oozing surface.
- Initially, induration is minimal.
- Over time, induration, infiltration, and nodularity develop.
- An underlying mass is palpable in roughly 50% of cases.
- Eventually, there is local destruction of the nipple and areola with retraction.

NONSKIN FINDINGS

- Underlying intraductal carcinoma is found in the ipsilateral breast.
- The contralateral breast should also be examined carefully.

- The risk of cancer in the second breast is increased in patients who already have cancer in one breast.
- The regional lymph nodes are rarely palpable unless a palpable breast mass or superficial ulceration is present.

LABORATORY

- Skin biopsy confirms the presence of Paget's cells, which are large, rounded, pale, mucin-producing cells within the epidermis.
- Paget's cells are scattered among the normal-appearing keratinocytes, often displacing cells along the basal layer.
- Unlike keratinocytes, Paget's cells lack intracellular bridges, are periodic acid-Schiff positive (mucin), and are carcinoembryonic antigen positive.
- Deep biopsy may show continuity with an underlying intraductal carcinoma of the ipsilateral breast.
- Special stains may be needed to distinguish mammary Paget's disease from melanoma or Bowen's disease.

COURSE AND PROGNOSIS

- Mammary Paget's disease is caused by the intraepidermal spread of malignant cells from an underlying ductal carcinoma of the breast.
- The prognosis is determined by breast cancer staging and therapy.
- The 5-year survival rate exceeds 90% when neither a breast mass nor regional lymph nodes are palpable.
- The 5-year survival rate is roughly 40% when an underlying breast mass is palpable.

DIFFERENTIAL DIAGNOSIS

- Erosive adenomatosis of the nipple
- Bowen's disease
- Superficial basal cell carcinoma
- Tinea and candidal infections
- Atopic and contact dermatitis

DISCUSSION

- Adenomatosis of the nipple is a benign condition best confirmed by biopsy.
- Yeast and fungal infections should be confirmed by potassium hydroxide examination and should improve with topical antifungal therapy.
- The presence of a yeast or a fungus does not exclude the possibility of Paget's disease.

- Eczematous dermatitis should respond to topical corticosteroids.
- Skin biopsy should be performed for lesions of the nipple and areola that do not respond to topical therapy.

TREATMENT

- Breast and nodal examination is indicated for all patients with possible Paget's disease of the breast.
- Skin biopsy should be performed to confirm the diagnosis.
- Mammography should be performed on both breasts.
- A referral to a qualified surgeon should be made for further evaluation of any palpable breast mass.
- For biopsy-confirmed breast carcinoma, treatment can include surgery, radiotherapy, chemotherapy, and hormonal therapy as indicated.

CAVEAT

- Skin biopsy should be performed for all dermatoses involving the nipple that do not respond to topical therapy or that persist for more than 1 month.

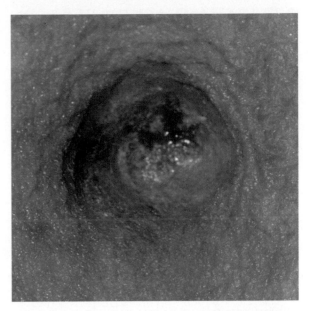

The disease begins insidiously in one breast, with a small area of erythema on the nipple that drains serous fluid and forms a crust.

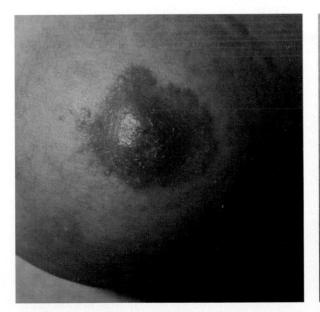

Malignant cells migrate through the epidermis, and the disease becomes initially apparent on the areola and at a much later date, on the surrounding skin.

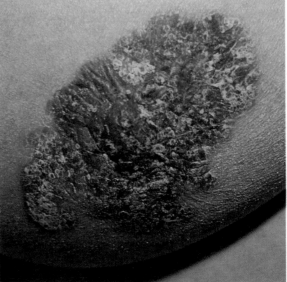

The process appears eczematous, but the plaque is indurated and has sharp margins, which remain relatively fixed for weeks.

■ EXTRAMAMMARY PAGET'S DISEASE

DESCRIPTION

- Extramammary Paget's disease is an uncommon, easily overlooked, intraepidermal malignancy involving the anogenital or axillary skin.

HISTORY

- Extramammary Paget's disease is adenocarcinoma within the epidermis.
- It occurs in areas where apocrine glands are found.
- It may be divided into two groups based on the source of the underlying primary adenocarcinoma.
- The majority of cases represent adenocarcinoma in situ with extension of primary adenocarcinoma in situ from adnexal structures.
- Apocrine gland carcinoma is the most common form of adnexal malignancy associated with extramammary Paget's disease (carcinoma in situ).
- The minority of cases reflect an intraepidermal spread of tumor cells from noncutaneous adenocarcinomas (local contiguous or lymphatic spread).
  - Urogenital and rectal carcinomas are the origins of noncutaneous adenocarcinoma cells associated with extramammary Paget's disease.
  - These include transitional cell cancer of the urethra and bladder as well as carcinomas of the cervix, vagina, Bartholin's glands, and prostate.
  - Local contiguous or regional lymphatic spread of these cancer cells to the epidermis and subsequent invasion lead to intraepidermal spread.
- Extramammary Paget's disease is rare before age 40.
- It occurs more often in women than in men.
- It most commonly occurs on the vulva and perineum in older women.
- It affects male genitalia less often; the scrotum, penis, and anal and perianal skin are most commonly affected.
- It may extend to involve the lower abdomen, inguinal folds, buttocks, and thighs. Other sites include the axillae, ears, and eyelids.
- The patient complains of itching and irritation but rarely pain.
- The lesion slowly and relentlessly increases in size.

SKIN FINDINGS

- A red to white-gray plaque with a velvety surface appears.
- The plaque is sharply demarcated and has irregular borders.
- The degree of scaling varies by site.
- The lesion may appear eczematous or lichenified.
- Pinpoint scaling and erosions, crusting, and serous exudate occur.
- There may be local induration.
- Unless located in the midline, it is rarely symmetric; it is usually unilateral.

NONSKIN FINDINGS

- Depending on site of origin, the noncutaneous primary adenocarcinoma may be visible and palpable.
- Regional lymph nodes are usually not palpable until later in the course with regional metastases.

LABORATORY

- The histologic features of extramammary Paget's disease are identical to those of mammary Paget's disease (see p. 388).
- Deep biopsy may reveal an underlying adnexal adenocarcinoma or Paget's cells within the lymphatics.

COURSE AND PROGNOSIS

- Unlike Bowen's disease, in extramammary Paget's disease, dermal invasion and regional metastases appear to occur earlier in the disease course.
- Therefore once the diagnosis is made, aggressive treatment and close follow-up are indicated.
- One-fourth of all patients ultimately die from extramammary Paget's disease or from the underlying malignancy.
- Less than 25% of all patients have an underlying noncutaneous malignancy. In this group, the 5-year mortality rate approaches 50%.
- Perianal disease is more likely to be associated with underlying noncutaneous adenocarcinoma (25% to 35%) than genital disease (4% to 7%).
- The most common sites of metastases are the inguinal and pelvic lymph nodes and then the liver, bone, the lungs, the brain, the bladder, the prostate, and the adrenal glands. Regional and widespread metastases may develop from any one of the primary sites.
- The prognosis depends on site of the primary adenocarcinoma, its clinical stage, and the therapy rendered.

DIFFERENTIAL DIAGNOSIS

- Clinical
  - Eczematous dermatitis
  - Lichen simplex chronicus
  - Intertrigo
  - Candidiasis
  - Tinea
  - Bowen's disease
  - Amelanotic melanoma
- Histologic
  - Bowen's disease
  - Melanoma

TREATMENT

- Wide local excision of involved areas is performed.
- Although the lesion appears to be sharply defined clinically, histologic confirmation of margins is vital.
- The surrounding, clinically normal-appearing skin may also be involved.
- There is a high recurrence rate, even after excision with apparently appropriate margins.
- There may be benefit from Mohs' micrographic excision.
- The dissection of palpable regional lymph nodes may be warranted.
- Radiotherapy might also be an option for difficult tumors.

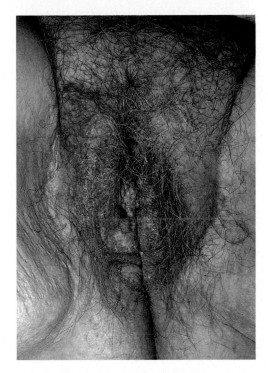

The disease appears as a white to red, scaling or macerated, infiltrated, eroded, or ulcerated plaque most frequently observed on the labia majora and scrotum.

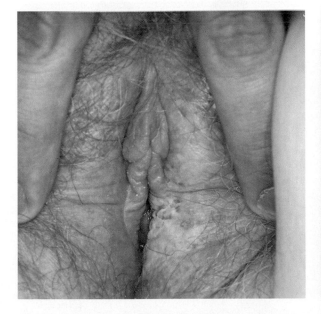

A white, eroded plaque with ill-defined borders on the labia.

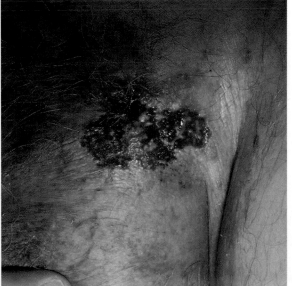

Three biopsies were taken before malignant cells were demonstrated at the periphery of this chronic ulcer at the base of the scrotum.

■ CUTANEOUS METASTASIS

DESCRIPTION

- Cutaneous metastasis is an uncommon, frequently overlooked sign of underlying malignancy.

HISTORY

- Cutaneous metastases occur in 0.7% to 9.0% of all cancer patients.
- Detection of cutaneous metastases may alter disease staging and therapy.
- Cutaneous metastases presenting as the first sign of underlying occult malignancy are uncommon but occur most frequently with tumors of the lung, kidney, and ovary.
- More commonly, cutaneous metastases are a sign of extranodal disease in patients with known underlying malignancy.
- Cutaneous metastases may herald recurrence in a patient with a prior history of malignancy.
- Excluding lymphomas, the sites of primary tumors metastasizing to skin reflect the underlying gender differences in the incidence of primary tumor.
  - For women with cutaneous metastases, the more common primary sites are breast (69%), colon (9%), skin (melanoma) (5%), lung (4%), ovary (4%), connective tissue (sarcoma) (2%), cervix (2%), pancreas (2%), oral cavity (squamous cell carcinoma) (1%), and bladder (1%).
  - In men with cutaneous metastases, the more common primary sites are the lung (24%), colon (19%), skin (melanoma) (13%), oral cavity (squamous cell carcinoma) (12%), kidney (6%), stomach (6%), esophagus (3%), connective tissue (sarcoma) (3%), pancreas (2%), bladder (2%), salivary glands (2%), breast (2%), prostate (1%), thyroid (1%), liver (1%), and skin (squamous cell carcinoma) (1%).
- Metastases appear in the skin via one of two mechanisms:
  - Direct extension to the skin from underlying metastases (often nodal)
  - Lymphatic or hematogenous spread

SKIN FINDINGS

- Some 75% of skin metastases in male patients occur on the head and neck, anterior chest, and abdomen.
- Some 75% of skin metastases in female patients occur on the anterior chest or abdomen.
- The abdominal wall is the most common site for tumors presenting as metastatic disease, usually lung cancer.
- Scalp metastases in men tend to be from the lung or kidney and present early in the disease.
- Scalp metastases in women tend to be from the breast and represent a late event.
- Facial metastases tend to be from oral squamous cell carcinoma, renal cells, the lungs, or the breast.
- Eyelid metastases tends to be from the breast or melanoma.
- Neck metastases are more often a direct extension from deep nodes from the lung, oral squamous cell carcinoma, or breast carcinoma.
- Most cutaneous metastases do not have a distinct clinical appearance.
- Most present as a cluster of discrete, firm, painless nodules.

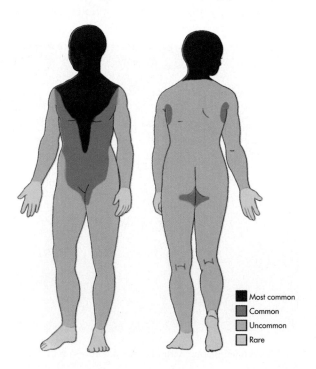

■ Most common
■ Common
■ Uncommon
■ Rare

Breast Cancer

- Some 69% of all cutaneous metastases in women are from breast cancer.
- Skin involvement occurs in 23.9% of breast cancer cases. It is the presenting sign in 3.5% of breast cancer cases.
- Several distinct clinical patterns are recognized:
  - Inflammatory metastatic carcinoma resembles erysipelas in the anterior chest but without fever or tenderness. It is caused by capillary congestion; there is no inflammatory infiltrate.
  - En cuirasse metastatic carcinoma is a diffuse morphea-like induration of skin ("encasement in armor") that begins as scattered, firm, lenticular papulonodules that coalesce. Local lymphatic spread is possible.
- In telangiectatic metastatic carcinoma, the violaceous papulovesicles resemble lymphangioma circumscriptum; there is local lymphatic spread. It may be pruritic and may resemble vasculitis.
- In nodular metastatic carcinoma, multiple firm papules or nodules appear on the anterior chest. They may be ulcerated and may suggest melanoma or pigmented basal cell carcinoma.
- Alopecia neoplastica has asymptomatic, noninflammatory, circular areas of alopecia. There is distant hematogenous spread.
- In Paget's disease, there is a sharply defined plaque of erythema and scaling on the breast. It is suggestive of eczema, but it is persistent. It is usually unilateral but may be bilateral. There is a direct spread from underlying breast cancer.

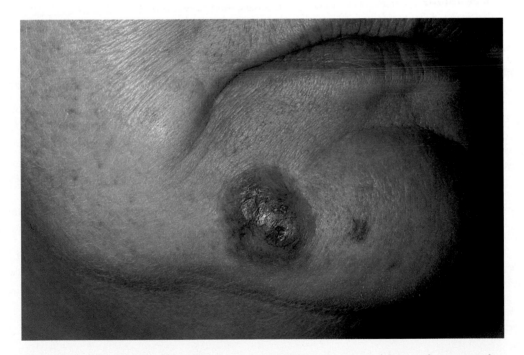

The most common representation of cutaneous metastasis is an aggregate of discrete, firm, nontender, skin-colored nodules that appear suddenly, grow rapidly, attain a certain size (often 2 cm), and remain stationary.

Lung Carcinoma

- Historically, lung carcinoma is more common in men than women.
- There is a localized cluster of cutaneous nodules, most often on the anterior chest or abdomen.

Colon and Rectal Carcinoma

- Colon and rectal carcinoma is the second most common source of skin metastases in both genders.
- It usually presents late in the disease course.
- The abdomen and perineum are the most common sites.
- It may present as inflammatory metastatic carcinoma of the inguinal folds or as a chronic cutaneous fistula.

Melanoma

- Melanoma is the third most common source of skin metastases.
- Skin is the most common primary site, followed by ocular and mucosal sites; primary tumor is not always identifiable.

Renal Cell Carcinoma

- Renal cell carcinoma comprises 6.8% of all cutaneous metastases.
- Cutaneous presentation, usually on the head and neck, is common.
- A well-circumscribed, bluish nodule with prominent vascularity appears.

Oral Squamous Cell Carcinoma

- Oral squamous cell carcinoma usually occurs in men with a known primary tumor.
- It presents as multiple nodules on the head and neck.
- It may be difficult to discern metastatic disease from primary squamous cell carcinoma of the skin.

Neuroblastoma

- Some 32% of patients with congenital neuroblastomas have subcutaneous metastases.
- "Blueberry muffin baby" presents as multiple firm, mobile, blue subcutaneous nodules that blanch when stroked.
- Periorbital ecchymosis suggests orbital metastases.

Lymphomas

- Cutaneous metastases occur in 6.6% of all patients with lymphoma.
- A skin lesion is the presenting sign in 5% of patients and the first sign of extranodal disease in 7.6% of patients.
- The firm, raised, smooth, red to violaceous nodules and plaques, may ulcerate.
- It may be difficult to discern primary lymphoma arising in skin from metastatic disease.

Leukemias

- Leukemia cutis appears as macules, papules, ecchymoses, palpable purpura, or ulcers.
- It often precedes or is concurrent with a diagnosis of systemic leukemia.
- Lesions are seen in 25% to 30% of infants with congenital leukemias and may precede other manifestations of leukemia by up to 4 months.
- Myeloblastomas may occur in acute myelocytic leukemia; the greenish color (chloromas) is due to myeloperoxidase within the lesions.
- Mucocutaneous involvement is more common in monocytic leukemias, with involvement ranging from papules to plum-colored nodules and gingival infiltrations.
- Adult T-cell leukemia involves the skin in 75% of patients.

Nonskin Findings

- The primary tumor site and potentially other noncutaneous metastases are usually detectable by imaging studies.

Laboratory

- Skin biopsy confirms malignant cells of primary tumor origin.
- Tissue-specific immunohistochemical stains may be of value in cases in which the primary site is not obvious (i.e., adenocarcinoma).
- Fresh, unfixed specimens are optimal for specialized immunohistochemistry and molecular studies.

COURSE AND PROGNOSIS

- The prognosis is determined by the tumor type, extent of disease, and available treatment options for the primary tumor.
- In general, metastatic disease has a poor prognosis.

DISCUSSION

- In some cases, excision of symptomatic or disfiguring skin metastases can significantly improve a patient's quality of life.

TREATMENT

- Therapy is directed by the underlying malignancy.

CAVEAT

- Biopsy should be performed for any new nodule in an old scar or any new nodule in a new scar if a malignancy was the reason for excision.

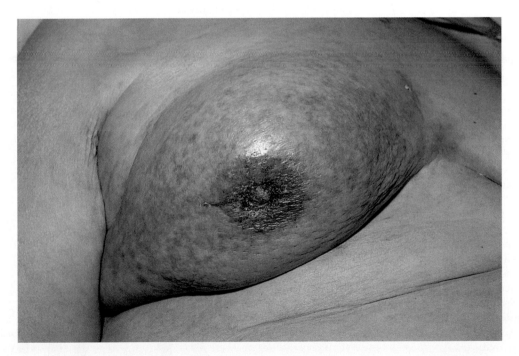

The second most common pattern of cutaneous metastasis is inflammation with erythema, edema, warmth, and tenderness.

18

Nevi and Malignant Melanoma

■ NEVI

DESCRIPTION

- Nevi are benign skin tumors composed of melanocyte-derived nevus cells; they are classified by the age at onset and the arrangement of nevus cells in the dermis.

HISTORY

- The term *nevus* refers to any inherited hamartomatous growth of normal cells or tissues.
- Such hamartomas may be vascular, adnexal, or soft tissue in origin.
- This discussion is limited to hamartomas of melanocyte-derived nevus cells commonly known as *melanocytic nevi, pigmented nevi,* or *common moles.*
- Melanocytic nevi are composed of organized clusters of nevus cells arranged at various levels in the skin. The majority have no malignant potential.
- Nevi are ubiquitous in humans and equally common among male and female patients.
- Those present at birth or appearing during infancy are termed *congenital nevi.* Roughly 1% of newborns have at least one melanocytic nevus. New nevi are acquired throughout childhood and into early adulthood.
- The incidence of acquired nevi reaches a peak incidence during adolescence, and fewer nevi are acquired after age 30. Nevi appearing or changing after age 30 should be regarded as suspicious.
- Sun exposure appears to be a stimulus for nevus cell growth.
- Most acquired nevi appear on sun-exposed skin. Acquired nevi appearing in sun-protected areas should be considered suspicious.

- Most adults have between 12 and 20 nevi; larger numbers may be a familial trait.
- Existing nevi may increase in size and become more heavily pigmented during puberty or during pregnancy.
- Nevi are usually asymptomatic, although they may on occasion be irritated by clothing or external trauma.

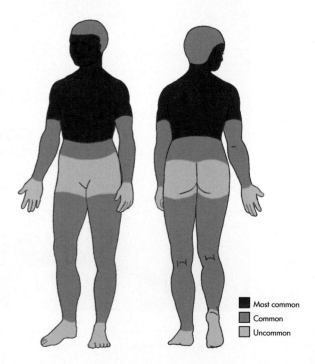

Most common
Common
Uncommon

- Nevi first appear as flat, round, uniformly colored papules.
- During this growth phase, nevi expand laterally while remaining flat and symmetric.
- Nevi may be slightly darker in color and slightly raised in the center and remain stable in size and appearance for several years.

- Then, over many years, nevi continue to become more elevated and uniformly lighter in color.
- Eventually, the nevus appears as a skin-colored papule or may completely disappear in later years.
- Residual nevi are uncommon after age 70.

Skin Findings

- Nevi are classified by the location and arrangement of nevus cells within the skin.

Junctional Nevi
- Junction nevi are flat or slightly raised, brown-tan papules.
- Skin markings are often preserved in the surface of the nevus.
- They are most commonly found in children.
- Nests of nevus cells cluster at the dermoepidermal junction.
- Nevi of the palms, soles, genitalia, and mucosa are usually junctional nevi.

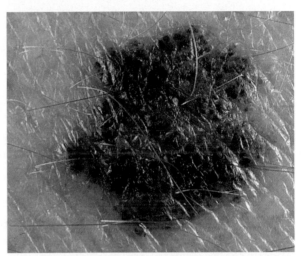

Compound Nevi
- Compound nevi are slightly to markedly raised, pigmented papules.
- Nests of nevus cells are found both at the dermoepidermal junction and within the dermis.
- Compound nevi can have an irregular border but are symmetric.
- The surface may be smooth or slightly papillomatous.
- The center tends to be more heavily pigmented than the periphery.
- These nevi tend to increase in thickness and pigmentation in late childhood and adolescence.

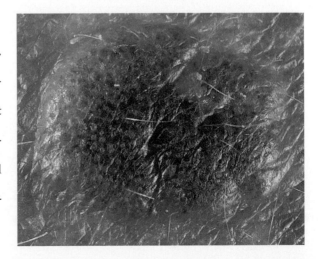

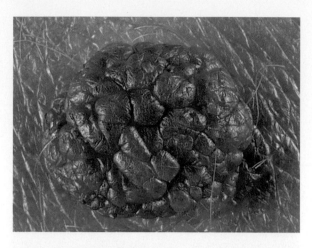

Intradermal Nevi

- Intradermal nevi are most commonly elevated, fleshy, slightly to moderately pigmented papules.
- The color varies from dark brown to normal skin color.
- Pigmentation may be arranged in flecks.
- Course, dark terminal hairs may grow from the nevus.
- Intradermal nevi are seen mainly after adolescence.
- Nests and cords of nevus cells are found within the dermis and may extend into the subcutaneous fat.
- Melanocytic cells are pale and fairly uniform in size and are found in cords or clusters surrounded by collagen bundles.

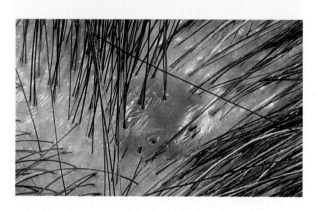

Blue Nevi

- Blue nevi are solitary, bluish macules or papules most commonly found on the head and neck or buttocks.
- Coloration is attributed to intensely pigmented melanocytes in the deep dermis.
- They commonly present in early childhood or at birth.
- They tend to slowly enlarge and persist for 10 to 15 years.
- Spindle-shaped, heavily pigmented nevus cells are located in the mid to lower dermis.

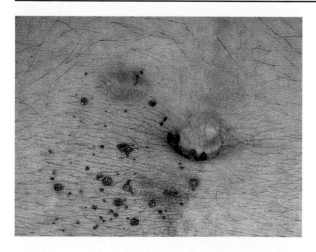

Nevus Spilus

- Nevus spilus is a sharply defined, tan to brown background macule similar to a café-au-lait spot, which also contains several small monomorphic, slightly raised, dark brown nevi.
- Nevus spilus does not have increased coarse hairs.
- Sun exposure does not seem to play a role in their development.
- Lesions usually develop before adulthood and follow a benign but persistent course.

Spitz Nevus

- Spitz nevus or spindle cell nevus is usually a red-pink, dome-shaped smooth papule.
- They most often occur on the face, scalp, or legs of preadolescent children.
- Skin biopsy reveals overall architectural order with nested spindle-shaped nevus cells and areas with large pleomorphic nevus cells.
- Such changes would be worrisome for melanoma in an adult.
- The lesion and its biologic course are benign.
- Most dermatologists favor complete excision of Spitz nevi to minimize the risk of recurrence and associated pleomorphism.

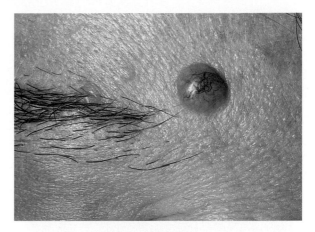

Halo Nevi

- Halo nevi occur primarily during adolescence.
- A preexisting nevus develops a surrounding rim of hypopigmentation that heralds the gradual disappearance of the nevus over several months.
- Skin biopsy shows a junction or compound nevus surrounded by a dense infiltrate of lymphocytes.
- This appears to be a host response directed against the nevus cells.
- Focal atypical nevus cells may be seen, although the majority of the preexisting nevi are benign.
- The halo usually eventually repigments.
- Halo nevi also occur in the setting of vitiligo and may develop in patients with melanoma.
- Patients with halo nevi should have a full skin examination to look for both vitiligo and melanoma.

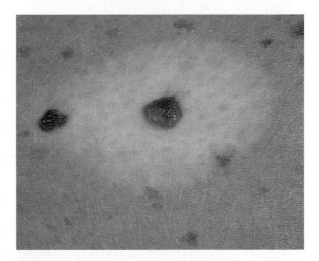

Recurrent Nevus Phenomenon

- Recurrent nevus phenomenon may occur at the site of a previously partially removed nevus.
- Randomly distributed pigmentation along with scar can be quite suspicious for melanoma.
- The biopsy may also be indistinguishable from that of melanoma.
- The history of previous biopsy and a review of the original specimen are critical to the correct diagnosis.

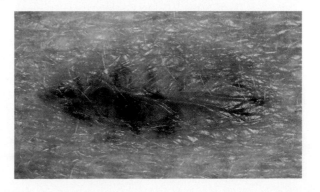

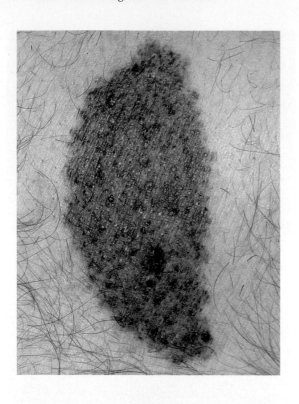

Congenital Melanocytic Nevi

- As previously discussed, any melanocytic nevus present at birth or appearing within infancy is considered to be a congenital melanocytic nevus.
- Congenital melanocytic nevi are usually dark brown and raised, with an irregular verrucous surface; most have increased terminal hairs.
- Congenital melanocytic nevi vary greatly in size.
- The risk of malignant degeneration occurring in congenital melanocytic nevi is controversial.
- There is general agreement that the risk of malignant change is increased in giant congenital melanocytic nevi (>20 cm); the lifetime risk is estimated at 10% to 20%.
- The lifetime risk of melanoma developing in smaller congenital nevi (<2 cm) is unclear but most likely falls in the 2% to 5% range, slightly higher than the background lifetime risk of melanoma.
- Because nevus cells in congenital nevi often extend into subcutaneous fat, such malignant change may not be easily detected.
- For this reason, many dermatologists favor elective excision of congenital nevi when feasible, usually around the time of puberty.

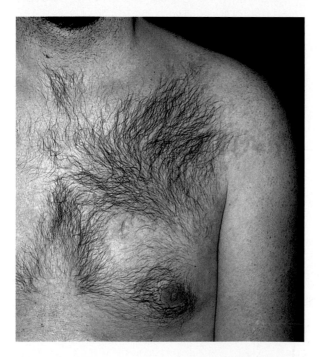

Becker's Nevus

- Becker's nevus is not a nevocellular nevus because it lacks nevus cells.
- The lesion is a developmental anomaly consisting of a brown macule, a patch of hair, or both. Nonhairy lesions may later develop hair.
- The lesions appear in adolescent men on the shoulder, submammary area, and upper and lower back.
- Becker's nevus varies in size and may enlarge to cover the entire upper arm or shoulder.
- The border is irregular and sharply demarcated.
- Malignancy has never been reported.
- Becker's nevus is usually too large to remove and is best left untouched. The hair may be shaved or permanently removed.

Dermal Melanocytosis (Mongolian Spot)

- Dermal melanocytoses are poorly defined, blue-black to gray patches.
- They are more commonly seen in newborns of darker skin types.
- They are most commonly found in the sacral region.
- They are equivalent to blue nevi histologically, with heavily pigmented, spindle-shaped nevus cells located deep in the dermis.
- They often fade in early childhood but may persist into adulthood.
- Such lesions are believed to represent incomplete migration of melanocytes to the epidermis.

NONSKIN FINDINGS

- Occasionally, benign nevus cells may be found within regional lymph nodes draining areas with congenital melanocytic nevi or dermal melanocytoses.
- Such findings are unusual but are not necessarily indicative of melanoma.

LABORATORY

- Nevus cells tend to cluster or nest in discrete areas of the skin.
- Junctional nevi have nested nevus cells at the dermoepidermal junction.
- Intradermal nevi have nests and cords of nevus cells within the dermis, sometimes extending into fat.
- Compound nevi have nested nevus cells at the junction and also in the dermis.
- The term *combined nevus* is used to designate a benign nevus with the typical features of a compound or junctional nevus but with a deeper blue nevus component.

COURSE AND PROGNOSIS

- The majority of melanocytic nevi are benign and follow the described course of maturation over years.
- Nevi that deviate from this pattern are suspicious, and biopsy is warranted.
- Junctional nevi are rare in adults.
- Unless known to be present since childhood, any biopsied junctional melanocytic lesion on an adult should be regarded as atypical if not melanoma in situ.

DIFFERENTIAL DIAGNOSIS

- Melanocytic nevi
  - Dysplastic nevi
  - Melanoma
- Junctional nevi in an adult: melanoma in situ
- Spitz nevi
  - Clinical: hemangioma, pyogenic granuloma, and juvenile xanthogranuloma
  - Histologic: melanoma

DISCUSSION

- The presence of halo nevi should initiate a screening examination for atypical melanocytic nevi and vitiligo.
- Great care must be taken to minimize the risk of misdiagnosis of melanocytic lesions.
- The clinician should provide the dermatopathologist with the age of the patient, location and clinical history of the lesion, any previous biopsy specimen, and the clinical differential diagnosis.
- An adequate biopsy specimen should be submitted.
- Similarly, it is the clinician's responsibility to correlate the pathologist's findings with the clinical diagnosis.

TREATMENT

- All of a patient's nevi should be assessed.
- With the exception of the dysplastic nevus syndrome, most nevi in most individuals have a fairly uniform pattern and appearance.
- There is little variability from one nevus to another on a given individual.
- The ABCDs of melanoma are a useful guide (see p. 408).
- Most benign nevi are symmetric, with a well-defined, regular border; they are uniform in color, with perhaps subtle variation in the hues of the dominant color, and are smaller than 6 mm in greatest diameter.
- Nevi that appear different from the remaining nevi should be regarded with suspicion.
- Suspicious nevi should be biopsied.
- Referral to a dermatologist should be considered.
- The current epidemic of skin cancers has prompted many patients to seek screening examination.
- Such an opportunity for early detection and treatment as well as patient education should not be missed.

- An examination of the entire cutaneous surface should be encouraged.
- Patients need to be educated on how to perform a self-skin examination and encouraged to do so on a regular basis.
  - Teaching about skin self-examination should be combined with the skin screening examination.
  - The patient should know the changes to watch for, including symptoms of itching and tenderness.
- The patient should feel comfortable in seeking care for any future changes or concerns.
- Sun awareness and regular use of sunscreens and sun-protective clothing should be also encouraged.

CAVEAT

- Benign nevi have a uniform appearance and a predictable life cycle. Nevi that deviate from this pattern are suspicious and should be biopsied.

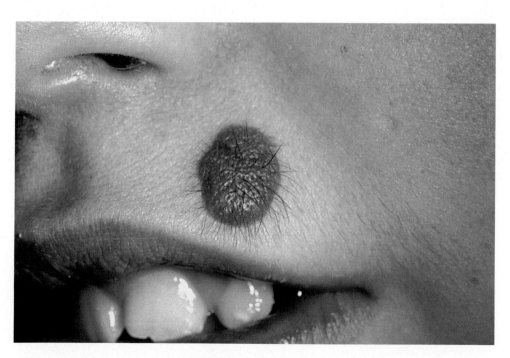

Dermal nevus with hair.

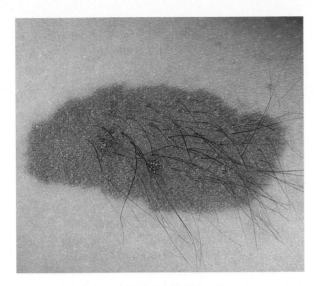

Congenital nevus. Uniform brown pigmentation with hair.

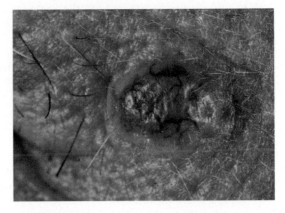

Dermal nevus. Flesh colored with surface vessels; resembles basal cell carcinoma.

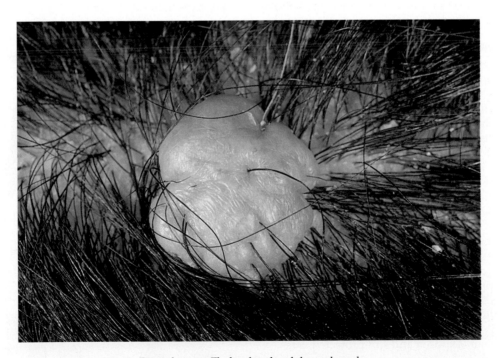

Dermal nevus. Flesh colored and dome shaped.

■ ATYPICAL MOLE SYNDROME

DESCRIPTION

- Atypical mole syndrome, consisting of multiple clinically atypical nevi along with an increased risk of melanoma, occurs as a familial syndrome and also occurs sporadically.

HISTORY

- Atypical mole syndrome was first described in 1978 by Clark and colleagues as *B-K mole syndrome.*
- Large, irregular nevi with variegated color and a palpable dermal component appear.
- Nevi were found in increased numbers in six families in which multiple members had a history of melanoma.
- The nevi were considered to be a phenotypic marker for family members at increased risk of developing melanoma.
- Inheritance is thought to be autosomal dominant with variable penetrance.
- These clinically and histologically distinctive melanocytic nevi occur as solitary lesions, as multiple lesions in sporadic cases, and as multiple lesions in the familial syndrome.
- In all three settings, atypical nevi are considered to be precursors for melanoma, most often the superficial spreading type.
- More than 90% of patients with familial melanoma have atypical nevi.
- Nomenclature and criteria have evolved over time and are confusing. Currently the term *atypical nevus* is favored.
- Depending on the criteria used, atypical nevi are common, with a prevalence estimated at 5% to 20%.
- Whereas solitary atypical nevi are common, the familial syndrome is uncommon.
- The incidence of sporadic (nonfamilial) occurrence of multiple atypical nevi is unknown.
- Male and female patients are equally affected.
- Atypical nevi are not present at birth and begin to appear during early childhood.
- The characteristic features of atypical moles are present at the time of puberty.
- Unlike common acquired melanocytic nevi that stop appearing after age 30, atypical nevi continue to appear well into adulthood.
- Although sun exposure does appear to influence the appearance of atypical nevi, lesions develop in both sun-exposed and sun-protected areas.

- Atypical nevi are best considered as part of a spectrum between benign nevi and melanoma.
- In patients with multiple atypical nevi, the number of nevi varies.
- Most affected individuals have more than 50 melanocytic nevi, some of which are atypical in appearance.
- There is striking heterogeneity from one nevus to another.
- Nevi are usually asymptomatic.

SKIN FINDINGS

- Atypical nevi differ from common acquired melanocytic nevi.
- Atypical nevi are usually larger, ranging from 6 to 15 mm in diameter.
- The border is irregularly outlined and indistinct, fading imperceptibly into the surrounding skin.
- The color is variegated with a haphazard mixture of pink, tan, brown, and black.
- The surface is irregular, often with a central or eccentric papule surrounded by a prominent macular component.
- Atypical nevi can appear anywhere in the skin, but occur most commonly on the trunk and upper extremities.

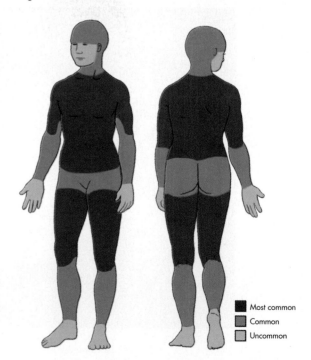

Most common
Common
Uncommon

- Affected persons often have nevi in sun-protected areas, such as the scalp, buttocks, female breasts, palms, and soles.
- The presence of nevi in these unusual locations in prepubertal children may be the first clinical sign of the syndrome.

NONSKIN FINDINGS
- Affected individuals may be a increased risk of ocular melanoma.

LABORATORY
- The nomenclature and histologic criteria for the diagnosis of atypical nevi remains controversial.
- There is general agreement on the following features:
  - Architectural disorder with asymmetry
  - Intraepidermal melanocytes extending beyond the main dermal component
  - Subepidermal fibroplasia
  - Lentiginous melanocytic hyperplasia with spindle or epithelioid melanocytes
  - Nevus cell nests that are of variable size and that form bridges between adjacent rete ridges
  - Variable degrees of melanocyte atypia

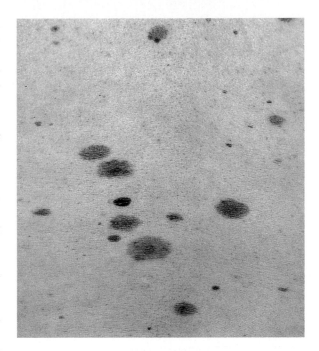

A cluster of atypical nevi.

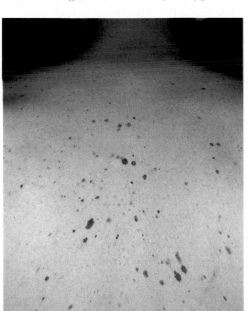

Common moles occur most often on sun-exposed areas. Atypical moles occur in those locations and at unusual sites such as the scalp, buttocks, and breast.

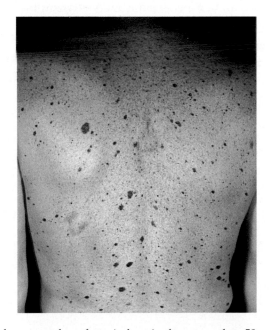

A larger number of atypical nevi, often more than 50, can occur.

COURSE AND PROGNOSIS

- The likelihood of an individual atypical nevus subsequently developing into melanoma cannot be estimated, although the risk of an individual with atypical nevi can be estimated.
- The lifetime risk of melanoma for the population born in the year 2000 is estimated at 1.3%.
- The lifetime risk of melanoma for people with atypical nevi but without family history of melanoma has been estimated at 6%.
- This risk increases to 15% in patients with atypical nevi and a family history of melanoma.
- The risk of a second melanoma is 10% in patients with atypical nevi and a personal history of melanoma.
- The lifetime risk approaches 100% in patients with multiple atypical nevi and two or more first-degree relatives with a history of melanoma.

DIFFERENTIAL DIAGNOSIS

- Benign nevi
- Melanoma

DISCUSSION

- Atypical nevi are best regarded as part of a continuum between benign and malignant melanocytic neoplasms.
- Biopsy may be required to establish the diagnosis.

TREATMENT

- Patients with atypical nevi should have routine skin examinations beginning around puberty.
- A referral to a dermatologist should be considered for regular monitoring of nevi.
- Referral to a tertiary center's pigmented lesion clinic should be considered for patients with numerous atypical nevi and a family history of melanoma.
- The frequency of follow-up examinations depends on a personal or family history of melanoma and the number of atypical nevi.
  - Follow-up examinations are usually performed every 3 to 12 months.

- Examination should not be limited to exposed areas and should include careful inspection of the scalp, genitalia, and acral regions.
- A baseline ophthalmologic examination should be obtained; patients may also be at increased risk for developing intraocular melanomas. Appropriate ophthalmologic follow-up should be done as warranted.
- Family members should also be examined.
- Photography can be extremely useful in identifying changes in nevi, with close-up views of the most clinically atypical moles taken during the initial examination.
- Any lesion with documented change should be removed in its entirety and sent for histopathologic examination.
- Nevi in which the patient has noted a change should also be removed.
- Patient education and awareness can not be overemphasized.
- Patients should start by becoming familiar with their own skin by performing monthly self-examinations.
- Sunlight has been implicated in the pathogenesis of malignant melanoma and the induction of melanocytic nevi in patients with atypical moles.
- Sun avoidance and sun-protective clothing are recommended to minimize ultraviolet exposure.
- Patients are also advised to use sunscreens with an SPF of 15 or greater each day, even on overcast or cloudy days.
- Reapplication of a sunscreen every 2 hours to 3 hours, particularly after swimming or exercising, should be strongly encouraged.

CAVEAT

- Atypical nevus syndrome represents a distinct, easily recognized clinical phenotype at increased risk of developing melanoma, particularly if there is a family history of melanoma.
- Management of such patients should focus on patient education, self-examination, and routine complete skin examinations.

ATYPICAL MOLES

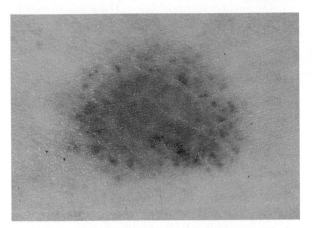

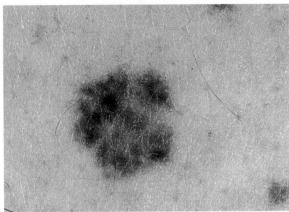

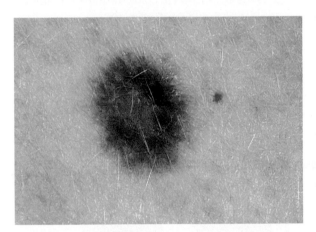

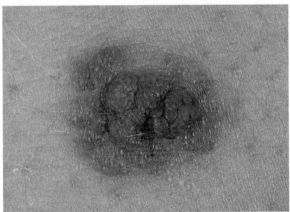

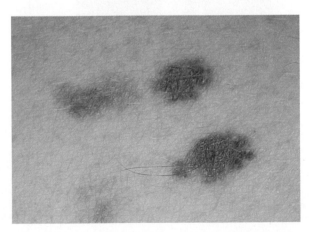

These moles are larger than common moles. They have a mixture of colors, including tan, brown, pink, and black. The border is irregular and indistinct and often fades into the surrounding skin. The surface is complex and variable, with both macular and papular components. A characteristic presentation is a pigmented papule surrounded by a macular collar of pigmentation ("fried-egg lesion").

■ MELANOMA

DESCRIPTION

- Melanoma is an increasingly common malignancy of melanocytes, most often arising in the skin; it is potentially curable with early detection and treatment.

HISTORY

- Melanoma is the eighth most common malignancy in the United States.
- It represents 4% of all cancers in men and 3% of all cancers in women.
- It is the most common malignancy in women age 25 to 29 years and second only to breast cancer in women age 30 to 35 years.
- The incidence of melanoma continues to rise at a rate faster than that of any other human cancer, and the increase in its mortality rate is second only to that of lung cancer.
- Between 1973 and 1994, the incidence of melanoma increased 120%, and the mortality rate attributed to melanoma rose 40%.
- The projected lifetime risk of melanoma for Americans born in the year 2000 is 1 in 75.
- Factors that increase the risk of developing melanoma include the following:
  - Fair skin (types I and II)
  - The presence of atypical nevi in both sun-exposed and sun-protected areas
  - A personal history of melanoma
  - A family history of atypical nevi or melanoma
  - A history of blistering sunburn or sunburn that was uncomfortable for more than 48 hours
  - Congenital nevi, in which the risk increases proportionally with increasing lesion size
- The most common early signs include an increase in nevus size and a change in its color or shape.
- The most common early symptom is itching.
- Later symptoms include tenderness, bleeding, and ulceration.
- Pigmented lesions may change slowly over months to years or may abruptly change.

SKIN FINDINGS

- It cannot be overemphasized that melanomas vary considerably in appearance; no one color or change is diagnostic.
- Some 30% of melanomas develop within a preexisting nevus, and the remaining 70% develop de novo.

- There are clinical clues that increase the index of suspicion and warrant biopsy. The following well-known guidelines are helpful in deciding which lesions are suspicious for malignant change:

ABCDs of melanoma

Asymmetry	Half of a lesion does not look like the remaining half.
Border irregularity	The border is scalloped or has focal "pseudopod" extension into the surrounding skin.
Color variegation	There are varying hues and varying colors.
Diameter >6 mm	The longest axis of the lesion is measured.

- When melanoma develops in a preexisting lesion, there is usually a focal area of color change.
  - It is the distinction in color from the remainder of the lesion, not necessarily the color itself, that is the clinical clue.
- No one specific color is by itself diagnostic, but the following should raise the index of suspicion:
  - Slate gray to black or deep blue may indicate melanin pigment deep within the dermis.
  - Pink or red may indicate localized inflammation.
  - White may indicate regression or scarring.

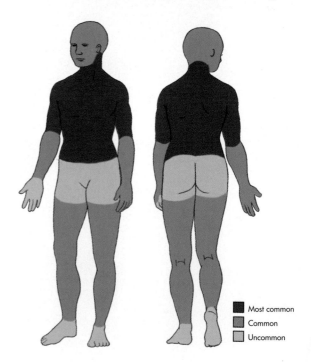

Most common
Common
Uncommon

- All pigmented lesions should be examined at regular intervals by both the patient and the provider. This is especially true of patients at increased risk of melanoma.
- The exact location, color, size, and pattern should be recorded.
- Photography can be extremely useful as a tool for recording such data, although it is only as useful as the photograph resolution allows.
- Although its value is operator dependent, epiluminescence microscopy allows examination of dermal pigmentation patterns within lesions.

NONSKIN FINDINGS

- The regional nodes should be palpated before biopsy, and the findings are documented.
- Postbiopsy inflammation may temporarily enlarge regional nodes.
- Any suspicious nodes should be evaluated by nodal biopsy.
- Such biopsy could be performed at the time of excision of the primary melanoma, with or without lymphatic mapping.

LABORATORY

- All suspect lesions warrant biopsy to confirm the presence of malignant melanocytes.
- The biopsy report should state the diagnosis, anatomic site, Breslow level, and presence or absence of biopsy margins.
- The Clark level, or anatomic level of invasion, is also helpful, especially for thin melanomas occurring on thin skin areas such as the eyelid, ear, and genitalia.
- The mitotic rate, degree of tumor lymphocyte infiltration, and presence or absence of histologic regression are often reported and may have prognostic significance.
- Ulceration or regression, if present, raises the possibility that the Breslow level may be underestimated.

COURSE AND PROGNOSIS

- In general, the thinner the melanoma, the better the prognosis.
- Localized disease has a far better prognosis than metastatic disease.
- Female patients and younger patients tend to have a more favorable prognosis.
- Melanoma on an extremity has a more favorable prognosis than melanoma on the trunk, head, or neck.
- Melanoma on the scalp has a worse prognosis than melanoma elsewhere on the head or neck.
- Some 85% of patients have stage I or II (local) disease.
- Some 13% of patients have stage III (regional) disease and an overall 5-year survival rate of 30%.
- Only 2% of patients have stage IV (distant) disease in which the 5-year survival rate is 6%.

DIFFERENTIAL DIAGNOSIS

- Superficial spreading melanoma
  - Benign nevi (moles)
  - Atypical (dysplastic) nevus
  - Seborrheic keratoses
  - Solar lentigo
- Nodular melanoma
  - Pigmented basal cell carcinoma
  - Angiokeratoma
  - Hemangioma
  - Traumatized nevus or acrochordon
  - Pyogenic granuloma
- Lentigo maligna
  - Spreading pigmented actinic keratosis
  - Bowen's disease
  - Solar lentigo

Melanoma staging

STAGE	DISEASE CATEGORY	BRESLOW LEVEL (THICKNESS)	RECOMMENDED SURGICAL MARGIN	5-YEAR SURVIVAL RATE
IA	Local	≤0.75 cm	1.0 cm	>95%
IB	Local	0.76-1.5 cm	1-2 cm	80%-95%
IIA	Local	1.50-4.0 cm	1-2 cm	60%-75%
IIB	Local	>4.0 cm	3.0 cm	<50%
III	Regional	Limited nodal metastasis	—	13%-45%
IV	Distant	Advanced regional metastasis or distant metastasis	—	<20%

MELANOMA SUBTYPES

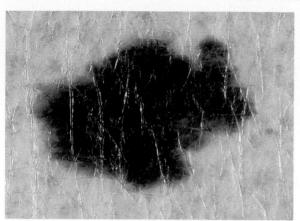

Superficial Spreading Melanoma

- Several clinical subtypes of melanoma are recognized; these types vary in clinical appearance, progression, anatomic site, and histologic appearance.
- Superficial spreading melanoma is the most common subtype, accounting for 70% to 80% of all melanomas arising in a preexisting lesion.
- They are usually seen on Caucasian skin.
- They may appear on any cutaneous site but most often are seen on the trunk and extremities.
- The lesions tend to be larger than 6 mm in diameter, flat, and asymmetric with varying coloration.
- Lesions appear and tend to spread laterally within the skin over a few years' time before nodules develop within the lesion.

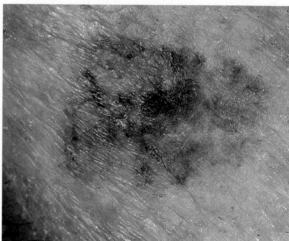

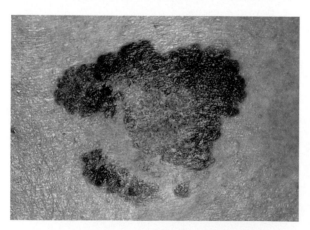

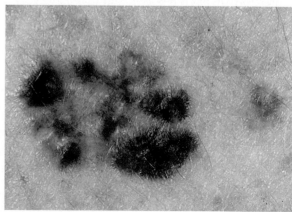

MELANOMA SUBTYPES

Nodular Melanoma

- Nodular melanoma accounts for 10% to 15% of all melanomas.
- They can occur on any cutaneous site but are found most often on the extremities.
- Lesions tend to be raised, brown to black, and rapidly appearing, growing papules; they may suggest a vascular lesion and may have focal hemorrhage.
- Lesions appear and evolve over months and tend to extend vertically in the skin.

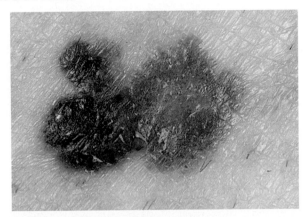

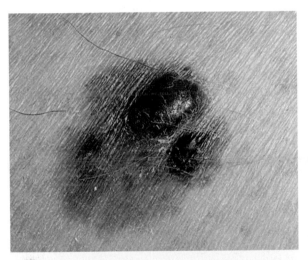

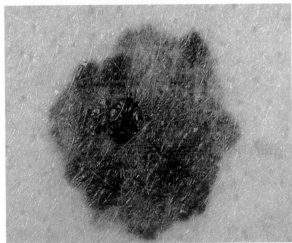

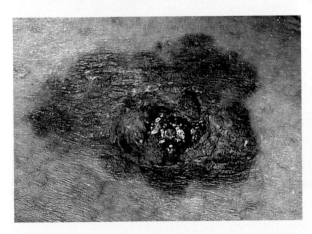

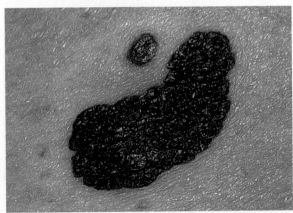

MELANOMA SUBTYPES

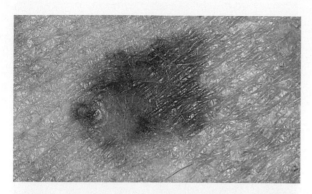

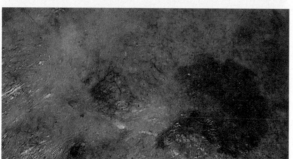

Lentigo Maligna and Lentigo Maligna Melanoma

- Lentigo maligna and lentigo maligna melanoma represent 5% to 10% of all cases of melanoma.
- Lentigo maligna represents in situ (intraepidermal) melanoma.
- Progression to invasive lentigo maligna melanoma occurs in roughly 5% of patients.
- It is usually seen in older individuals.
- It develops over years to decades on sun-exposed Caucasian skin, most often the face, neck, or dorsal arms.
- Lesions tend to be flat and irregularly outlined.
- The color is usually brown with some variation in epidermal pigment density.
- Lesions tend to look mottled or washed out and may contain areas of normal pigmentation.
- Examination under Wood's light often reveals irregular pigmentation extending well beyond the clinical lesion.
- Nodules and ulceration may indicate local invasion.

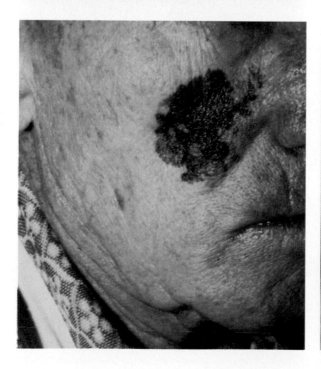

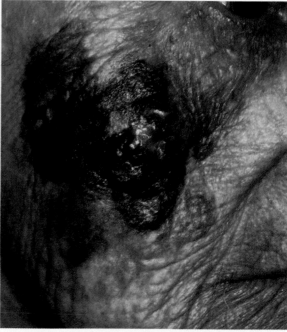

MELANOMA SUBTYPES

Acral Lentiginous Melanoma

- Acral lentiginous melanoma accounts for roughly 7% of all melanomas.
- It is more common in male than female patients and is usually found in older individuals.
- It occurs primarily on the hands and feet, including the nails of individuals with darker skin (types IV to VI).
- Similar lesions also occur on the modified skin around the mouth, anus, and genitalia.
- It is the most common form of melanoma in Asian-American and African-American skin, accounting for more than half of melanomas in these groups.
- It is the least common form of melanoma in Caucasian skin.
- Other than location, the lesion is similar in appearance to that of lentigo maligna and lentigo maligna melanoma: a flat, slowly expanding macule with a fairly uniform, mottled coloration.
- It appears and evolves over years.

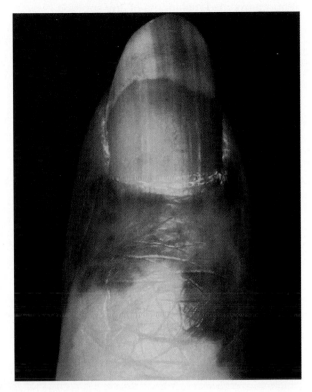

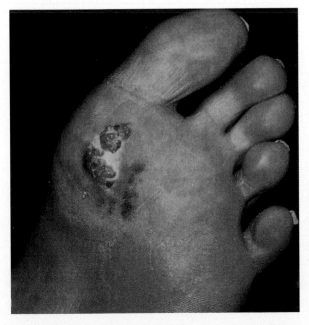

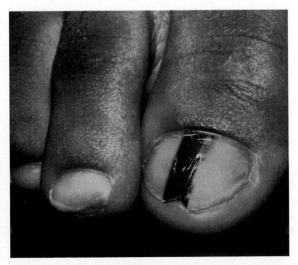

Amelanotic Melanoma

- *Amelanotic melanoma* is a descriptive term for a nonpigmented melanoma of any subtype.
- A total of 2% of all melanomas are amelanotic.
- Biopsy and diagnosis are often delayed.
- Malignant cells produce little if any melanin pigment.
- The lesion is an innocent-appearing, enlarging, pink to red papule.

DISCUSSION

- Biopsy discerns among the differential diagnoses.
- All nevi removed for diagnostic or cosmetic purposes should be submitted for histologic review.
- Incomplete excision or biopsy of nevi can lead to recurrence with epidermal hyperplasia of atypical-appearing melanocytes.
- This recurrent nevus phenomenon can be clinically and histologically indistinguishable from superficial spreading melanoma.
- The original excision or biopsy must be available for review to exclude a diagnosis of melanoma.

TREATMENT

- The risk of biopsy is far lower than the risk of missing a melanoma.
- Referral to a dermatologist should be considered.
- All suspect lesions warrant biopsy.
- The regional nodes should be palpated before biopsy, and the findings are documented.

- The only "perfect" biopsy technique is complete excision of the entire lesion into subcutaneous fat, which allows for accurate measurement of Breslow depth of invasion in a melanoma and avoids a sampling error (false-negative results).

- Shave biopsy is not recommended for suspect melanoma.
  - Shave biopsy specimen may not demonstrate the full Breslow depth of the lesion: the most important data for management and prognosis.
  - Shave biopsy is also subject to sampling error.

- An incisional or punch biopsy extending into subcutaneous fat may be considered when the clinical suspicion is low, when the lesions are large, or when lesions are in cosmetically important areas.
  - The most clinically suspicious areas should be included in the biopsy.
  - Incisional biopsy is still subject to sampling error, and false-negative results are possible.
  - Incisional biopsy does not appear to increase the risk of metastases.

- Reexcision of biopsy-confirmed melanoma with appropriate surgical margins determined by the Breslow depth is required.
- Melanoma in situ requires a 0.5-cm margin.
- Lentigo maligna tends to extend microscopically beyond the clinical lesion, even under Wood's light examination.

- For stage I and early stage II, surgical intervention might be the only necessary therapy.
- For advanced stage II to IV disease, adjuvant treatment may be considered.
- For advanced stage II and III disease, high-dose interferon-2α is the only systemic therapy shown to improve overall survival in clinical trials, although more recent studies have not confirmed this.

- Elective regional lymph node dissection improves the 5-year survival rate in some patients with stage II disease:
  - Those with thinner melanomas (Breslow level, 1.0 to 2.0 mm)
  - Patients younger than 60 years of age and with thinner melanomas
- Current research is focused on early detection of changes in cutaneous lesions with computer-enhanced imaging technologies.
- Methods of detecting early lymphatic spread, such as lymphatic mapping and sentinel node biopsy, are also being studied.
- Oncology referral and tumor board review should be considered.

- Follow-up examination should be performed at regular intervals and include the following:
  - Visual inspection and palpation of the excision site and surrounding skin
  - Visual examination of the entire cutaneous surface
  - Palpation of regional and distant nodes
  - Palpation of the liver
  - Baseline chest x-ray study
- Liver function tests are rarely revealing but are often obtained at baseline.
- First-degree relatives should be offered full skin examination for screening purposes.

Recommended interval between follow-up visits (months)

Year From Diagnosis	Primary Tumor Thickness			
	<0.76 mm	0.76-1.5 mm	1.5-4.0 mm	>4.0 mm
First	12	6	3	2
Second	12	6	3	2
Third	12	6	4	3
Fourth	12	12	4	3
Fifth	12	12	6	6
Subsequent	12	12	12	12

CAVEAT

- Full skin examination at regular intervals, especially of individuals at increased risk of melanoma, allows early detection and treatment of this serious health problem.

■ MELANOMA MIMICS

DESCRIPTION

- Melanoma mimics are a variety of melanocytic and nonmelanocytic skin lesions that may bear clinical and histologic resemblance to melanoma.

HISTORY

- Specific subtypes of benign melanocytic nevi may suggest melanoma.
- Benign melanocytic nevi, as discussed in detail on p. 397, are classified as junctional, compound, or intradermal based on the location of nevus cells within the skin.
- Most benign nevi have are symmetric, sharply defined, and less than 6 mm in greatest diameter; they usually have one dominant color and are usually asymptomatic.
- Roughly 30% of melanomas arise in preexisting melanocytic lesions.
- Nevi that develop symptoms such as itch or nevi that change in appearance are suspicious.
- Atypical nevi are often larger than 6 mm in greatest diameter and tend to have indistinct borders and variegated pigmentation.
- It may be impossible to distinguish visually atypical nevi from melanoma.
- This discussion focuses not on changing nevi or atypical nevi but rather on specific subtypes of benign nevi that may mimic melanoma.

SKIN FINDINGS

Blue Nevi

- Blue nevi are benign melanocytic nevi with nevus cells located deep within the dermis (see pp. 398 and 419).
- Their blue to black color may suggest melanoma.
- Blue nevi are sharply defined, are uniform in color, and remain stable in size or appearance over many years.

Combined Nevus

- *Combined nevus* refers to the combination of a blue nevus that is deep in the dermis and that is associated with an overlying benign junctional, compound, or intradermal nevus.
- Combined nevi are usually solitary and are often asymmetric with focal dark pigmentation.
- This presentation suggests melanoma, although the patient has not noted any change in the lesion's appearance.

Traumatized Nevi

- Traumatized nevi may be partially avulsed and have hemorrhagic crusting, suggesting ulceration.
- Patients are usually aware of the trauma.
- Nevi that have been partially removed either by trauma or biopsy can develop recurrent nevus phenomenon over several weeks to months (see p. 399).
- Melanocyte hyperplasia develops superficial to the scar, resulting in uneven pigmentation and irregular outlines as pigment extends into the surrounding skin; this is quite suggestive of melanoma.
- Recurrent nevus phenomenon can also resemble melanoma histologically.
- The history of trauma or biopsy along with review of the original biopsy helps exclude a diagnosis of melanoma.

Nonmelanocytic Lesions

- Nonmelanocytic lesions may also simulate melanoma.
- Pigmented basal cell carcinoma (see pp. 362 and 418-419) contains melanin pigment but is otherwise equivalent to nodular basal cell carcinoma.
- The amount of melanin and its distribution vary.
- Pigmented basal cell carcinoma can be mostly pink with focal blue-gray pigment, or it can be jet black.
- The surface has a pearl-like quality but may be ulcerated.
- The appearance may suggest nodular melanoma.

Seborrheic Keratoses

- Seborrheic keratoses (see p. 322) are benign keratinocyte tumors that also contain varying amounts melanin pigment.
- Pigmentation can be uneven and asymmetric within a single lesion.
- Seborrheic keratoses appear after age 30 and can grow quite rapidly.
- Lesions vary from flat to verrucous and from white to pink to jet black.
- Flat seborrheic keratoses may suggest lentigo maligna.
- Raised lesions may suggest superficial spreading melanoma.

MELANOMA MIMICS

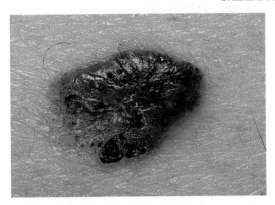

Darkly pigmented smooth surfaced seborrheic keratosis with horn pearls imbedded in the mass.

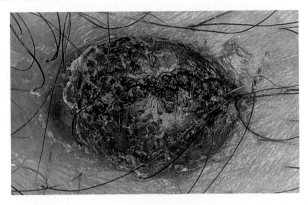

Inflamed seborrheic keratosis with a crusted surface and red border.

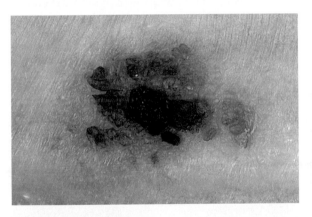

Rough-surfaced seborrheic keratosis with an irregular border.

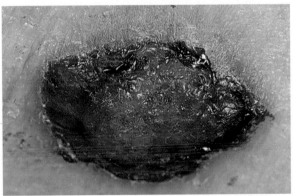

Inflamed seborrheic keratosis with a crusted surface and red border.

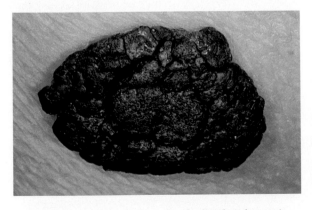

Darkly pigmented, rough-surfaced seborrheic keratosis.

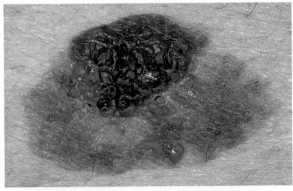

Rough-surfaced seborrheic keratosis with an asymmetric border.

Spreading Pigmented Actinic Keratosis

- Spreading pigmented actinic keratosis displays fine reticulated pigmentation and thin scale.
- Lesions appear on sun-damaged skin and simulate lentigo maligna melanoma.

Mature Hemangiomas

- Mature hemangiomas are often dark purple and can mimic nodular melanoma.
- Solitary angiokeratoma can be black and red.
- Trauma such as friction injury to the heel (talon noir) or injury to a nail may produce hemorrhage.
- Hemosiderin may be present in these lesions, suggesting melanin pigment.
- Dermatofibromas often contain hemosiderin, occasionally itch or are tender, and can suggest melanoma.
- Any questionable lesion should be biopsied to confirm the diagnosis.

LABORATORY

- Lesions that mimic melanoma clinically are usually discriminated from melanoma histologically.
- Histologic mimics of melanoma may require the use of special stains for accurate diagnosis.

- Melanoma, Bowen's disease, and Paget's disease may all show malignant cells within the epidermis. Special stain reveals the origin of the malignant cells in each disorder: melanocyte in melanoma, squamous cell in Bowen's disease, and adenocarcinoma in Paget's disease.
- Similarly, special stains are useful in spindle cell tumors to confirm the origin of the malignant cells.

- The nevus cells of Spitz nevus (see p. 399) may be pleomorphic and virtually indistinguishable from melanoma cells on histologic grounds.
  - The overall architecture of the lesion and age of the patient help discern Spitz nevus from melanoma.
  - Similarly, recurrent nevus phenomenon may show highly pleomorphic cells consistent with melanoma.
  - The history of previous biopsy and review of the original specimen establish the diagnosis.

- Lentigo maligna can be quite subtle and can resemble benign junctional nevi histologically.
  - As a rule, junctional nevi are lesions of childhood.

- Any melanocytic lesion from an adult diagnosed as junctional nevus should be considered suspicious.

DISCUSSION

- Questionable lesions should be biopsied.
- Histologic testing often discerns melanoma from lesions clinically suspicious for melanoma.
- Histologic mimics of melanoma include malignancies derived from nonmelanocytic cells.
- Special stains reveal the origin of the malignant cells.
- Melanocytic lesions that mimic melanoma histologically, such as Spitz nevus or recurrent nevus, require clinicopathologic correlation.

TREATMENT

- Treatment and follow-up are diagnosis dependent.

CAVEAT

- It is the responsibility of the clinician to correlate the histologic findings with the clinical impression.

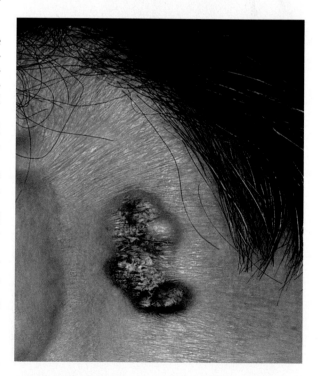

A pigmented basal cell carcinoma with a lobular surface and an irregular border.

MELANOMA MIMICS

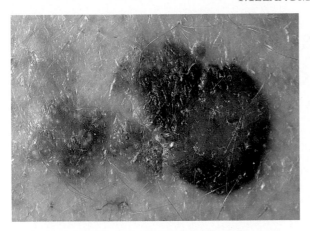

Smooth seborrheic keratosis with variation in pigmentation and an irregular border.

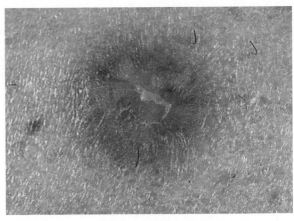

Dermatofibroma with a brown, irregular border and central clearing.

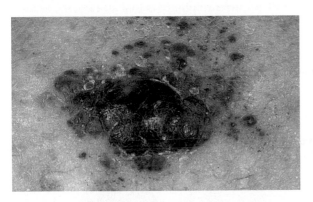

Hemangiomas vary in size and color. This complex lesion resembles a nodular melanoma.

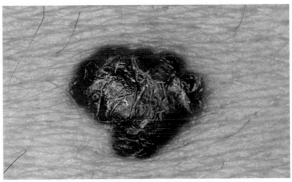

Traumatized hemangioma.

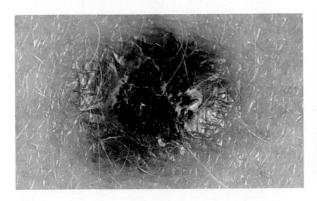

Blue nevus.

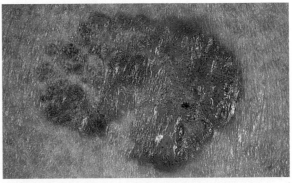

A pigmented basal cell carcinoma with areas of regression.

19

Vascular Tumors and Malformations

■ HEMANGIOMAS

DESCRIPTION

- Hemangiomas are benign, red to purple to blue vascular neoplasms occurring within the first year of life.
- Most lesions follow a predictable clinical course, with early rapid growth over weeks, stabilization over months, and ultimately involution over years.

HISTORY

- Hemangiomas are the most common vascular tumor of infancy, accounting for 32% to 42% of all vascular tumors in this age group.
- The incidence is slightly higher in female patients and in premature infants.
- The prevalence is estimated at 1% to 3% of neonates, perhaps as high as 10% by age 1.
- Traditionally, two lesions were described under the term *hemangioma:* strawberry hemangioma and the less common "cavernous" hemangioma.
  - Both occur in infancy, more often in girls, and with a predilection for the head and neck.
  - Cavernous hemangioma has been considered to be a deeper variant of the strawberry hemangioma.
  - Cavernous hemangiomas are more often multiple, involve deeper tissue levels possessing a bluish color with overlying skin possessing a normal color, and tend to persist rather than involute.

- The current opinion is that strawberry lesions are benign neoplasms of endothelial cells and thus are true hemangiomas.
- Cavernous hemangioma is now considered to be a venous malformation rather than a benign neoplasm.
- *Capillary hemangioma* and *strawberry hemangioma* are considered synonyms.

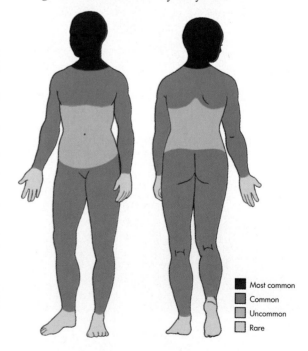

Most common

Common

Uncommon

Rare

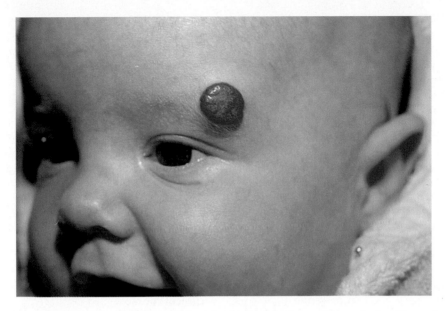

Strawberry hemangiomas. Most are small, harmless birthmarks that proliferate for 8 to 18 months and then slowly regress over the next 5 to 8.

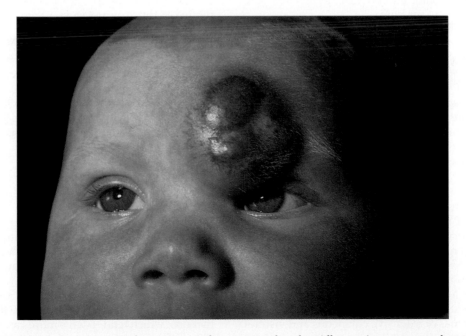

Strawberry hemangioma. Vital structures can be compressed, and rapidly growing areas may ulcerate.

SKIN FINDINGS

- Strawberry hemangiomas may be present at birth but more commonly appear within the first month of life.
- They occur most often on the head and neck.
- They may appear at any anatomic site, including the oral and genital mucosa.
- Usually, there is a single lesion; 15% to 20% of infants with capillary hemangiomas have more than one lesion.
- Multiple cutaneous hemangiomas may be associated with visceral hemangiomas (diffuse neonatal hemangiomatosis).
- The lesion initially appears as a poorly defined, pink, mottled vascular macule.
- Over a few weeks to several months, the lesion organizes into a sharply demarcated, strawberry to crimson red lobular plaque or nodule.
- During this time, the hemangioma grows rapidly and is firm, rubbery, and compressible.
- Capillary hemangiomas may be located in the papillary dermis, reticular dermis, or subcutaneous fat or may involve more than one tissue level. The color of the lesion suggests the level of tissue involvement.
  - Lesions in the papillary dermis are bright red.
  - Those involving the reticular dermis and subcutaneous fat are blue.

A violaceous color suggests both deep and superficial involvement or a superficial hemangioma with an underlying venous malformation.

NONSKIN FINDINGS

- Hemangiomas can extend quite deeply and compress underlying structures.
- The possibility of visceral hemangiomas in the setting of multiple cutaneous hemangiomas (diffuse neonatal hemangiomatosis) must also be considered.
- Any organ system may be involved and its function compromised.
- The risk of mortality is high in neonates with extensive visceral involvement.
- In addition to compression of vital structures, there is a risk of high-output congestive heart failure and consumptive coagulopathy.
- Kasabach-Merritt syndrome, a rare complication, occurs most often in neonates with large capillary hemangiomas or extensive cutaneous and visceral hemangiomas.
  - This syndrome is a consumptive coagulopathy related to platelet sequestration and consumption of clotting factors within the hemangiomas.
- Rapid change in the size or appearance of a large hemangioma, pallor, or ecchymoses in a neonate suggest this diagnosis.

LABORATORY

- In early lesions, there are solid masses of endothelial cells with few vascular cells.
- As lesions mature, they become less cellular, and vascular spaces are more organized.
- Involuting lesions have progressive fibrosis with loss of vascular spaces.
- Imaging studies are indicated for patients with multiple cutaneous hemangiomas to look for visceral involvement.

COURSE AND PROGNOSIS

- Most hemangiomas follow a benign, predictable clinical course.
- Initial growth is rapid over weeks, which is followed by a stable phase lasting months and then slow involution with residual fibrosis and lightening in color over years.
- Roughly 50% of lesions involute by the time the patient is 5 years old, and 70% do so by age 7.
- Neither the initial size nor the lesion site is predictive of future regression.
- A lesion that does not show signs of regression by age 6 is unlikely to resolve completely.
- Depending on location, vital structures may be compressed during the rapid-growth phase; intervention is required in such cases.
- Surface epithelium may ulcerate with recurrent bleeding.
- Superficial infection can occur but is rarely a serious problem.

DISCUSSION

- Capillary hemangiomas are distinguished from vascular malformations.
- Hemangiomas are often not apparent at birth, whereas vascular malformations usually are.
- Hemangiomas have a rapid growth phase, during which malformations grow in proportion with the child.
- Early hemangiomas are usually more cellular in composition and are firmer in texture than malformations, which tend to have more vascular spaces.
- This difference in composition may be confirmed by ultrasound.

TREATMENT

- Hemangiomas, which follow a benign course and pose no risk to vital structures, are best left to mature and involute without intervention.
  - After involution, the overlying skin may appear normal but more often has some degree of atrophy.
  - The ultimate cosmetic appearance is usually acceptable.
  - Intervention is required for hemangiomas that because of location, interfere with normal development and function.
  - Lesions that threaten the airway or interfere with feeding require immediate attention.
  - Periorbital hemangiomas may block the visual field at a critical age of visual development.
    - Amblyopia and strabismus are frequent complications.
    - Lesions on the ear may obstruct the auditory canal and impair hearing as well as language development.
- Systemic corticosteroids and interferon-alpha may be indicated for rapidly growing lesions.
- Laser surgery may be help as well, although it is less effective for deeper lesions.
- Referral to a tertiary care center that offers laser surgery should be considered.

CAVEAT

- Parents need to know what the clinical course is likely to be.
- Usually, periodic follow-up, reassurance, and time are all that are needed.

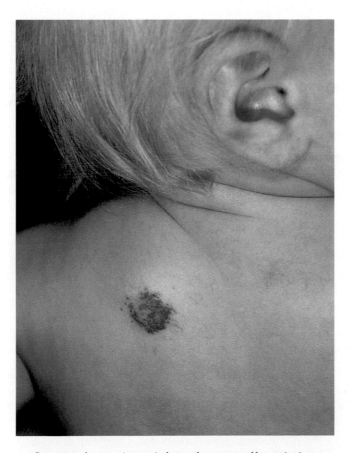

Cavernous hemangiomas (a form of venous malformation) are skin-colored, red or blue masses that are ill defined.

■ VASCULAR MALFORMATIONS

DESCRIPTION

- Vascular malformations are a clinically heterogeneous group of vascular lesions with a common etiology.
- Lesions represent abnormally arranged or abnormally functioning normal tissue.

HISTORY

- Malformations represent an abnormal arrangement or function of normal tissue as a result of an error in embryonic development.
- Vascular malformations may be classified by the vessels affected: capillary, venous, arterial, lymphatic, or a combination thereof.
- Lesions are usually present at birth.

Nevus Flammeus or Salmon Patch

- Nevus flammeus is a pink-red, midline macular lesion commonly known as an *angel kiss* on the glabella and as *stork bites* in the nuchal region.
- Sacral lesions are also common.
- Some 25% to 40% of newborns of both genders and of all races have small midline nevus flammeus lesions.
- Larger, less common, usually unilateral nevus flammeus lesions known as *port-wine stains* affect perhaps 0.3% of all newborns. They are bilateral in 40% of patients.

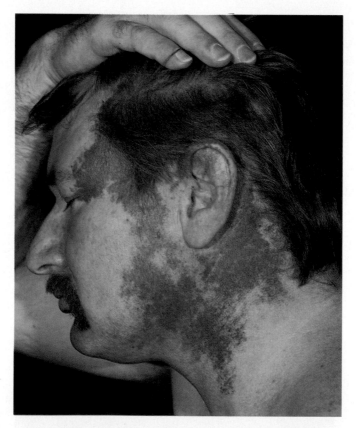

Nevus flammeus appears at birth as flat, irregular, red to purple patches. Later, they may become papular, simulating a cobblestone surface.

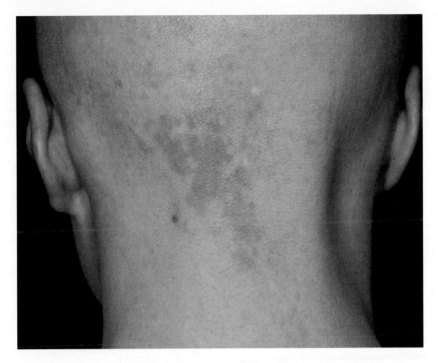

Salmon patches (stork bite) are variants of nevus flammeus. They are red, irregular patches resulting from dilation of dermal capillaries.

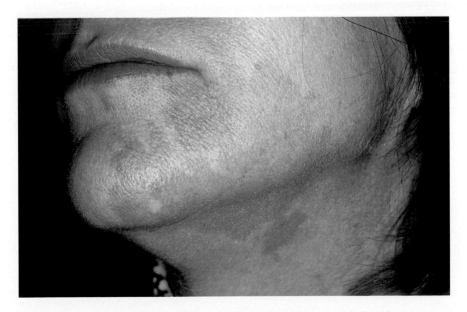

Port-wine stains are a significant cosmetic problem that do not fade with age.

Nevus Anemicus

- Nevus anemicus is a pale, irregular macule. The lesional vessels are abnormally reactive to catecholamines.
- It is more common in female than male patients.
- The most common location is the upper chest, although any skin site can be affected.
- Cutaneous vessels within the lesion are morphologically normal but functionally abnormal.
- Because of localized vasoconstriction, lesion skin appears blanched compared with the normal surrounding skin in the presence of normal physiologic levels of circulating catecholamines.
- The lesion is obscured by diascopic examination when the surrounding skin blanches under applied pressure.
- Wood's light (365 nm) does not accentuate the lesion.
- Applied heat or cold does not induce erythema within the lesion as it does in normal skin.

Cavernous Hemangioma

- The current opinion is that the lesions represent venous malformations rather than benign neoplasms.
- Bluish nodules, which are usually noted in infancy, occur more often in female patients and with a predilection for the head and neck.
- Unlike the strawberry hemangioma, venous malformations tend to persist.

Lymphangioma

- Lymphangioma is an uncommon, distinctive lesion consisting of dilated cutaneous lymph vessels.
- Surface papules communicate with lymphatic vessels deeper in the skin.

SKIN FINDINGS

Nevus Flammeus

- Nevus flammeus is a well-defined but irregularly outlined, deep red to salmon pink vascular macule or patch.
- Most are isolated small lesions favoring the midline on the glabella, nuchae, or sacrum.
- The color intensifies with emotion and crying.
- Port-wine stains tend to be deeper in color and are unilateral.
- Underlying soft tissue hypertrophy may be palpable as a plaque on the face or as diffuse hypertrophy of an entire involved limb.

Nevus Anemicus

- Nevus anemicus is an irregularly outlined, pale macule or patch.
- It is most commonly found on the upper chest.

Venous Malformations

- Venous malformations are blue to purple, soft to rubbery, compressible, roughly 1.0-cm nodules.
- They are usually solitary and tend to occur on the head and neck.
- Multiple cutaneous venous malformations may suggest the rare blue rubber bleb nevus syndrome, an autosomal dominant inherited condition.

Lymphangioma Circumscriptum

- Lymphangioma is a discrete group of 1- to 5-mm, clear to blood-tinged papules that appear at first glance to be vesicles.
- The appearance has been likened to that of frog eggs.

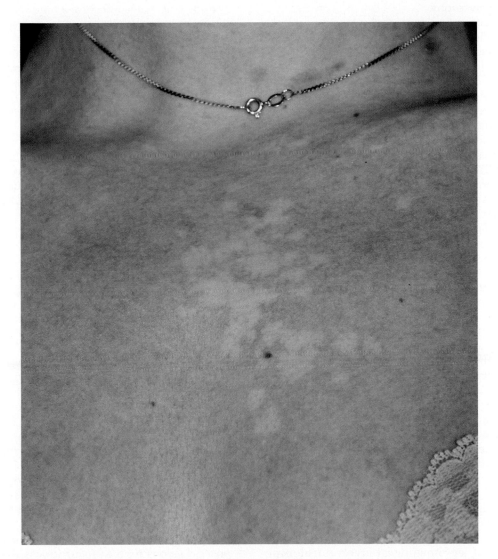

Nevus anemicus is a rare congenital lesion most frequently observed on the chest or back of females. The lesion usually consists of a well-defined, white macule with an irregular border, often surrounded by smaller white macules beyond the border of the major lesion.

Nonskin Findings

- Port-wine stains involving at least the ophthalmic division of the trigeminal nerve may be associated with underlying angiomatosis and soft tissue and bony hypertrophy.
- Potential complications include glaucoma, seizures, and intellectual impairment with leptomeningeal involvement.

Laboratory

- Nevus anemicus is indistinguishable from nonlesional normal skin on biopsy.
- Nevus flammeus, both isolated lesions and port-wine stains, have an increased number of dilated capillaries and venules within the dermis.
- Skull radiographs reveal "tram track" calcifications along the cerebral cortex in patients with the Sturge-Weber syndrome.
  - Computed tomography and magnetic resonance imaging confirm leptomeningeal angiomatosis.
  - The electroencephalogram may reveal associated seizure activity.
- Multiple cutaneous and gastrointestinal venous malformations occur in the rare blue rubber bleb nevus syndrome.

Course and Prognosis

- Nevus anemicus tends to persist indefinitely.
- Nevus flammeus on the glabella tends to fade during childhood but often becomes visible when the face becomes flushed (e.g., when the child cries).
- Nuchal and sacral nevus flammeus lesions tend to persist throughout life, as do port-wine stains.
- Port-wine stains persist into adulthood, with progressive dermal fibrosis giving a cobblestone appearance to the overlying skin.
  - Early intervention with pulsed dye laser treatment appears to limit future fibrosis.
  - Roughly 10% of patients with facial port-wine stains develop ipsilateral glaucoma in the absence of leptomeningeal involvement, especially if the port-wine stain simultaneously involves both the ophthalmic and maxillary distributions of the trigeminal nerve.
- Sturge-Weber syndrome is the association of nevus flammeus involving at least the ophthalmic and maxillary divisions of the trigeminal nerve with underlying leptomeningeal involvement.

- The incidence is estimated to be between 0.3% and 0.6% of patients with facial port-wine stains.
- Epilepsy and mental retardation are the most common sequelae.
- Port-wine stains affecting a limb may be associated with soft tissue and bony hypertrophy (Klippel-Trenaunay syndrome).
- Lymphangiomas persist indefinitely and may be subject to repeated trauma or infection.

Differential Diagnosis

- Nevus achromicus
- Vitiligo

Discussion

- Both nevus achromicus and vitiligo have decreased melanin pigment and are thus accentuated by Wood's lamp examination, whereas nevus anemicus is not.
- Vitiligo is not present at birth.

Treatment

- No treatment is required for nevus anemicus.
- Reassurance is often all that is required for small nevus flammeus lesions.
- Patients with suspected Sturge-Weber syndrome should have neurologic and ophthalmologic evaluations.
  - Some 30% to 60% of patients have eye involvement and are at risk for glaucoma.
  - Imaging of the central nervous system should be performed to look for leptomeningeal angiomatosis.
  - There is no correlation between the extent of cutaneous involvement and leptomeningeal involvement.
  - Pulsed dye laser is quite effective for cosmetic improvement of port-wine stains and is best performed early, before the lesions mature with fibrosis.
- Lymphangiomas may be treated for cosmetic purposes. Lesions tend to recur unless the deeper lymphatic channels are destroyed, either by excision or electrosurgery.

Caveat

- Pediatric neurology consultation and imaging studies should be obtained for patients suspected of having the Sturge-Weber syndrome.

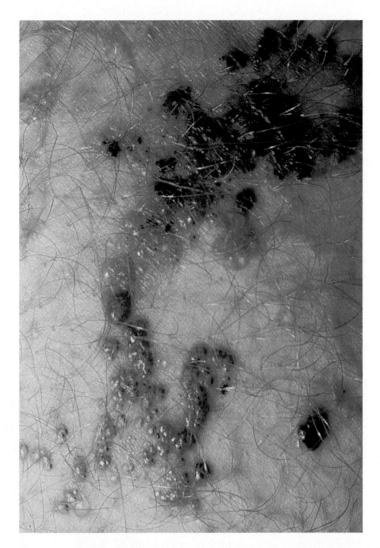

Lymphangioma circumscriptum. These hamartomatous malformations consist of grouped, translucent or hemorrhagic vesicles on a dull red or brown base. The appearance has been compared to a mass of frog's eggs ("frog spawn").

■ CHERRY ANGIOMA

DESCRIPTION

- Cherry angioma is a clinically distinct, benign vascular neoplasm found on nearly all people older than 30 years of age.

HISTORY

- Lesions appear in early adulthood and increase in number and size with age.
- Individual lesions are asymptomatic, slowly increase in size, and persist indefinitely.

SKIN FINDINGS

- A discrete, 0.5- to 5.0-mm, smooth, dome-shaped to polypoid vascular papule appears.
- Its color varies from a cherry red to a deeper maroon as the lesion increases in size.
- Angiomas are less easily blanched under diascopy than telangiectases.
- They are scattered randomly on the body surface and are found in greatest density on the trunk and less densely on the head, neck, and extremities.
- The number of lesions may range from a few to hundreds.

LABORATORY

- Skin biopsy is rarely needed but demonstrates a sharply defined, benign proliferation of dilated capillaries and postcapillary venules within the papillary dermis.
- Larger lesions show flattening of the overlying epidermis and a collarette of epithelium at the periphery.

COURSE AND PROGNOSIS

- Isolated reports of patients with hundreds of cherry angiomas arising in association with pregnancy and also in patients with elevated prolactin levels suggest that hormonal factors may play a role.
- The sign of Leser-Trélat is the eruptive onset of innumerable cutaneous lesions in association with occult internal malignancies. Both cherry angiomas and seborrheic keratoses have been reported as the cutaneous lesions in this rare condition.
- The sudden appearance of such lesions may warrant a search for occult malignancy, especially for small tumors capable of hormone production (those in the pancreas, small bowel, and respiratory system).

- Undisturbed angiomas typically persist indefinitely.
- Superficial trauma may produce bleeding, which is best managed with direct pressure.

DISCUSSION

- Telangiectases, dilatations of previously existing vessels, are less papular in appearance and are more easily blanched.
- Pyogenic granulomas are often confused with larger cherry angiomas.
- Typically, pyogenic granuloma presents as a solitary lesion arising in an area of prior trauma or during pregnancy, although multiple clustered lesions can occur.
- Pyogenic granulomas are more friable, are more often tender, and bleed more easily.
- Bacillary angiomatosis is an infectious disease caused by *Bartonella* species.
- Bacillary angiomatosis occurs in the setting of advanced acquired immunodeficiency syndrome when the CD4$^+$ count is below 200 cells/mm^3. Early lesions may resemble a cherry angioma or pyogenic granuloma and often involve mucosal surfaces.

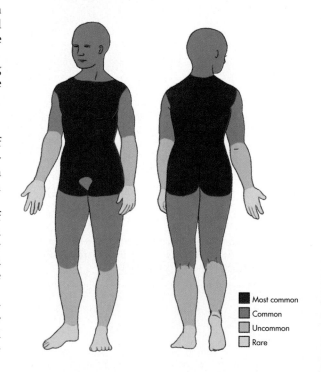

- Most common
- Common
- Uncommon
- Rare

TREATMENT

- Reassurance usually suffices, although individual lesions may be ablated by electrocautery, laser surgery, or cryosurgery.
- There is a slight risk of scarring and dyspigmentation with treatment.

CAVEAT

- Although the sign of Leser-Trélat is extremely rare, cherry angiomas are extremely common.
- The *presence* of numerous lesions should not prompt a search for malignancy, although the *explosive appearance* of such lesions should raise concern.

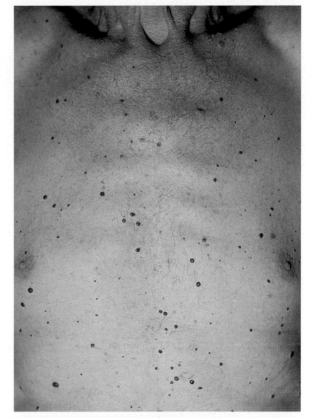

Cherry angioma are most commonly seen on the trunk and vary in number from a few to hundreds.

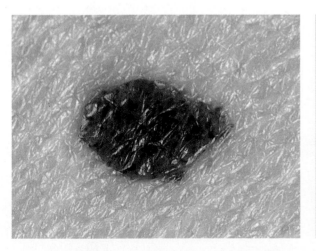 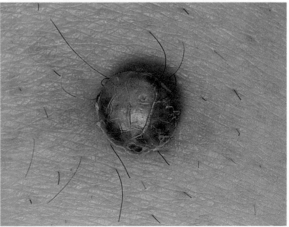

Cherry angioma. These 0.5- to 5-mm, smooth, firm, deep red papules occur in virtually everyone after age 30 and numerically increase with age.

■ ANGIOKERATOMA

DESCRIPTION

- Angiokeratomas are common, usually asymptomatic, vascular papules with overlying hyperkeratosis.
- They are most often seen as multiple lesions restricted to specific body sites.

HISTORY

- Four clinical variants of acquired angiokeratomas are recognized.
- Variants are distinguished by the distribution of lesions on the body and the age of onset.

Angiokeratoma of Fordyce

- Angiokeratoma of Fordyce is the most common form.
- Asymptomatic multiple angiokeratomas occur symmetrically on the scrotum and vulva.
- Lesions begin to appear in middle to later life and persist indefinitely.
- The onset may relate to increased venous pressure.
- Scrotal angiokeratomas may be associated with inguinal hernia, varicosities of the leg, or varicocele.
- Vulvar angiokeratomas may develop in younger woman during pregnancy or oral contraceptive use, possibly from increased venous pressure.

Solitary or Papular Angiokeratomas

- Solitary or papular angiokeratomas are equally common among men and women.
- They arise in younger adults and may occur at any cutaneous site, although the legs are most common.
- Usually, one angiokeratoma is present, and rarely, several appear.
- Lesions tend to be larger than other variants of angiokeratoma and are more likely to be traumatized.

Angiokeratoma of Mibelli

- Angiokeratomas of Mibelli are symmetric, grouped multiple angiokeratomas occurring on the dorsal aspect of the fingers and toes.
- Lesions first appear during childhood and adolescence and increase in number into adulthood.
- Because of their location, lesions may be frequently traumatized and painful.
- Lesions may be associated with acrocyanosis and pernio.

- Lesions seem to occur more commonly in female than male patients, although autosomal dominant inheritance of angiokeratomas on the hands and feet is described in one family.

Angiokeratoma Corporis Diffusum

- Angiokeratoma corporis diffusum is the rarest variant; it is quite striking clinically.
- Lesions begin to appear around the time of puberty; they appear symmetrically in the bathing trunk area and become nearly confluent.
- Generally, they are asymptomatic unless they are traumatized.
- They are associated with several metabolic enzyme deficiency syndromes, classically X-linked inherited alpha-galactosidase A deficiency or Fabry's disease.

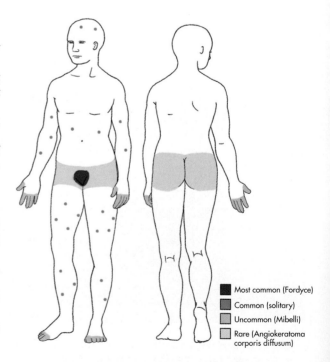

Most common (Fordyce)
Common (solitary)
Uncommon (Mibelli)
Rare (Angiokeratoma corporis diffusum)

Skin Findings

- Angiokeratoma is a deep red to maroon, or blue to black, sharply defined, 0.5- to 1.0-cm papule.
  - Early lesions are lighter in color, are soft, and are more easily compressed.
  - Older lesions tend to be firmer, more raised, and darker and have more surface keratin.
- Angiokeratomas of Fordyce are monomorphic in appearance, range in size from 0.1 and 0.4 cm, and have a shiny surface.
  - Early lesions are soft and compressible with a red to maroon color, whereas older lesions are darker and firmer but less keratotic than other mature angiokeratomas.
- Solitary angiokeratomas tend to be blue to black with increased surface keratin.
  - On close inspection, thrombosed vessels, surface crust, and hemosiderin can often be seen at the edge of lesions.
- Solitary angiokeratomas can easily be confused with melanoma.
- Angiokeratomas of Mibelli are monomorphic, 0.3 to 0.5 cm in size, deep red to purple with thickened surface keratin in an acral distribution.
  - Lesions extend from the dorsal aspect of the fingers and toes into the web spaces.
- The lesions in angiokeratoma corporis diffusum tend to be monomorphic, 0.5 to 5.0 cm in size, and burgundy to deep purple.
  - Lesions approach confluence on the genitalia, buttocks, lower abdomen, and upper thighs.
  - Older lesions are firm in contrast to the surrounding supple genital skin.
  - Other cutaneous findings include generalized xerosis and anhidrosis.
  - Hyperthermic crises can occur in such patients.

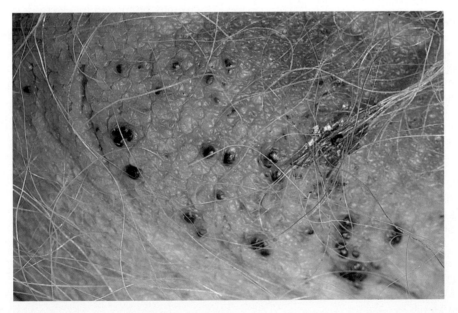

Angiokeratomas are lesions characterized by dilation of the superficial dermal blood vessels and hyperkeratosis of the overlying epidermis.

Nonskin Findings

- Angiokeratoma corporis diffusum is seen with several enzyme-deficiency states.
- Fabry's disease is caused by a deficiency in alpha-galactosidase A, resulting in the accumulation of neutral glycosphingolipids within the lysosomes of endothelial cells, fibroblasts, neurons, and myocytes.
  - Painful paresthesia of the hands and feet after a temperature change occurs early and may precede the skin findings.
  - Death usually occurs by age 50 from chronic renal failure or acutely from myocardial infarction or cerebrovascular accident.
  - Cornea verticillata is a distinctive, superficial corneal dystrophy found on slit-lamp examination in patients with Fabry's disease. This diagnostic finding is often present in mild cases of Fabry's disease as well as in carrier females.
- Other, rarer inherited disorders that may present with clinically identical lesions include deficiencies in galactosidase B 1-fucosidase, beta-mannosidase, and neuraminidase.
- There are rare reports of patients with angiokeratoma corporis diffusum in whom an enzyme defect could not be found.

Laboratory

- Angiokeratomas are not proliferations of endothelial cells and thus are not true hemangiomas.
- All variants of angiokeratomas are indistinguishable histologically with hematoxylin and eosin.
- Dilated, thin-walled capillaries are seen in the superficial papillary region.
- The degree of hyperkeratosis and benign epidermal hyperplasia may vary from pronounced in solitary angiokeratomas to nearly absent in angiokeratoma of Fordyce.
- Vacuolization of endothelial cells and smooth muscle cells in angiokeratoma corporis diffusum lesions is difficult to detect by routine microscopy and is best demonstrated by special stains and with electron microscopy.

Course and Prognosis

- Undisturbed angiokeratomas tend to persist indefinitely.
- Surface trauma often results in bleeding but not resolution of the lesions.

Discussion

- When multiple angiokeratomas are present in specific body surface areas as in angiokeratoma corporis diffusum and the Fordyce and Mibelli variants, the diagnosis is obvious.
- The differential diagnosis for a solitary angiokeratoma may be more difficult, and skin biopsy should be considered.
- A black, thrombosed angiokeratoma might easily be confused with melanoma.
- Hemosiderin from prior hemorrhage can mimic melanin pigment in the surrounding skin.
- Other lesions that may resemble a solitary angiokeratoma include thrombosed common wart, Kaposi's sarcoma, pyogenic granuloma, pigmented basal cell carcinoma, and squamous cell carcinoma.

Treatment

- Treatment is indicated for repeatedly traumatized lesions or for cosmetic purposes. Individual lesions may be treated by electrodesiccation or ablated with carbon dioxide laser.
- Extensively involved areas of the scrotum may do well with excision.
- Ophthalmologic and neurologic consultation should be considered in cases of angiokeratoma corporis diffusum.
- Genetic counseling and screening of family members are appropriate.

Caveat

- Patients with angiokeratomas of Fordyce should be reassured that the lesions are not sexually transmitted.

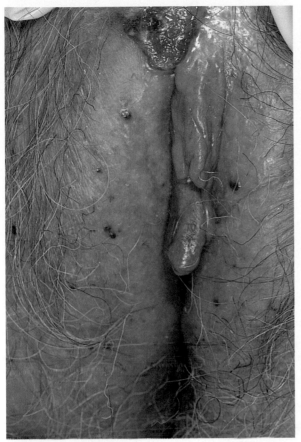

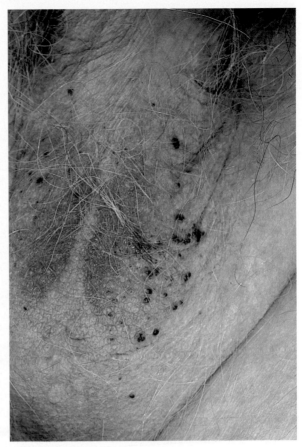

Angiokeratomas of the scrotum (Fordyce) or vulva. Increased venous pressure, such as occurs with pregnancy and hemorrhoids, may be implicated.

Angiokeratomas are characterized by multiple 2- to 3-mm, red to purple papules that occasionally bleed with trauma.

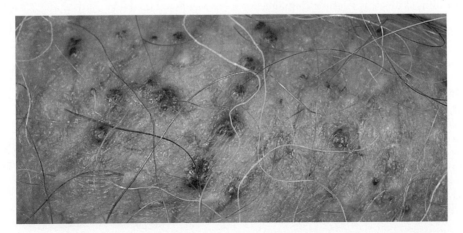

Angiokeratomas (Fordyce). Multiple red to purple papules consisting of many small blood vessels.

■ VENOUS LAKE
DESCRIPTION
- A venous lake is a common, soft, compressible, dark blue to purple papule found on sun-exposed skin or the mucosal lip in older patients.

HISTORY
- Venous lakes are often multiple and small; they are of long duration.
- Flatter lesions are usually asymptomatic.
- Raised lesions, depending on location, can become intermittently pruritic or tender.
- Lesions on the mucosal lip are subject to repeated trauma while the patient eats or speaks.
- Lesions may present acutely and with tenderness suggestive of an acute change in a chronic lesion.
- Lesions are more easily seen and are perhaps more commonly found in older Caucasian men.
- No racial or gender predilection has been described.
- Acquired sun damage and loss of dermal elasticity may play a causal role in the development of venous lakes.

SKIN FINDINGS
- A venous lake is a dark blue to purplish, 2- to 10-mm, well-defined papule with the look and feel of a varicose vein.
- The papule feels soft and cystic.
- Sustained pressure usually forces blood from the lesion, although it quickly refills on release.
- Several lesions may be present on sun-exposed skin and oral mucosae, especially the lower lateral vermilion lip and the ears.
- The surrounding skin shows actinic damage.
- Tenderness on palpation suggests thrombosis, usually with a history of trauma.
- Traumatized lesions often have hemorrhagic crust and bleed easily.

LABORATORY
- Any removed tissue should be submitted for histologic review.
- The histologic characteristics are those of a dilated, thin-walled venule located high in the dermis or submucosa.
- Thrombus is often seen in the vessel lumen.
- Associated actinic damage is present in the surrounding dermis.

COURSE AND PROGNOSIS
- Some consider "capillary aneurysm" and venous lake to be different stages of the same process: dilatation of a preexistent vessel with associated thrombus.
- Left undisturbed, venous lakes persist indefinitely.
- Further dilatation may occur over years.
- Thrombosis and surface trauma usually heal with persistence of the venous lake.

DISCUSSION
- It is important to recognize a venous lake because of its resemblance to melanoma.
- Diascopic examination of the lesion helps discern between these two entities.
- Biopsy is rarely necessary but should be considered if doubt exists.
- Some vascular neoplasms may appear similar to a venous lake when present on the lip or on sun-exposed areas.
  - Kaposi's sarcoma arising in the setting of advanced acquired immunodeficiency syndrome often affects mucosal surfaces.
- Angiosarcoma also occurs on the face in older patients and can be quite subtle. Angiosarcoma does not typically blanch with pressure.

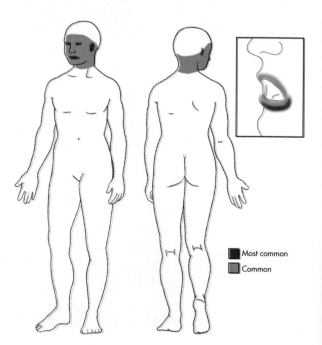

Most common

Common

- Biopsy is diagnostic and should be performed if doubt exists.
- Cavernous hemangiomas can resemble a venous lake.
  - This vascular malformation lies deeper in the skin, arises in infancy, and is not related to sun exposure.
  - Numerous cavernous hemangiomas occur in two rare disorders: Maffucci's syndrome and the blue rubber bleb nevus syndrome.
- Traumatized venous lakes might be confused with herpes labialis when they are tender and crusted and when they involve the mucosal lip.

TREATMENT

- Reassurance of the patient is often all that is needed for venous lakes.
- Treatment is indicated if the lesion is frequently traumatized, interferes with eating or speaking, or is of cosmetic concern.
- Treatment involves unroofing the vascular space with iris scissors and electrocautery under local anesthesia or regional nerve block.
- Recurrences are common and are similarly treated.

CAVEAT

- Venous lakes may be perceived as arising acutely and may be quite tender with acute thrombosis.
- Lesions should resemble a varicosity occurring in sun-damaged skin.

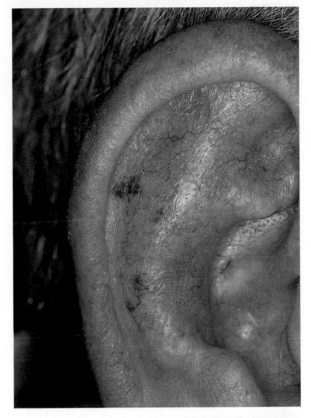

Venous lakes are common on sun-exposed surfaces of the ears.

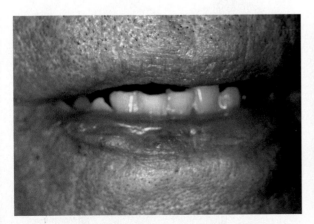

Venous lakes are dark, and patients are concerned about malignancy. The lesion should be firmly depressed to force the blood out and blanch the lesion.

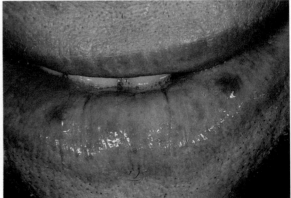

Venous lakes are common on sun-exposed surfaces of the vermilion border of the lip. Venous lakes are dark blue, slightly elevated, 0.2- to 1-cm, dome-shaped lesions composed of a dilated, blood-filled vascular channel.

■ PYOGENIC GRANULOMA

DESCRIPTION

- Pyogenic granuloma is a common, friable vascular papule arising at sites of previous trauma on the skin or mucosa.

HISTORY

- Pyogenic granulomas occur more frequently in children and young adults and are less common with increasing age.
- Both genders are affected equally.
- Pyogenic granulomas occurring on the gingiva in pregnant women are referred to as *epulis gravidarum*.
- The term *pyogenic granuloma* is misleading. It was once assumed that these lesions were caused by pyogenic infection.
- Controversy exists as to whether this lesion represents neoplasia or hyperplasia.
- Most authors consider pyogenic granuloma to be a reactive response to injury.
- Hormonal factors almost certainly play a modulatory role.

SKIN FINDINGS

- Pyogenic granuloma is a yellow to deep red, glistening, dome-shaped to polypoid, 3- to 10-mm papule.
- The base of the papule is often surrounded by a collarette of scale as though the rapidly growing papule has pushed aside the surrounding skin.
- Thin, moist, yellow crusting develops on the surface but is easily removed, often producing oozing hemorrhage.
- Pyogenic granuloma appears suddenly, often at a site of minimal trauma.
- The lesion grows rapidly to a stable size within a few weeks and then persists as an elevated, friable papule that bleeds easily.
- The lesion itself may be quite tender.
- With time, a pyogenic granuloma becomes more fibrous but retains its tendency to bleed easily with surface trauma.
- Lesions may occur anywhere but are most commonly found on the head and neck.
- Lesions of the oral mucosa, especially the lips and gingiva, are very common, as are lesions on the fingers.

LABORATORY

- The histologic characteristics are similar to those of granulation tissue.
- A superficial, somewhat lobular mass of proliferating endothelial cells and fibroblasts expand the papillary dermis.
- This vascular mass protrudes above the surrounding surface epithelium, creating a surrounding collarette of thickened epidermis.
- The overlying epidermis is flattened and often eroded, exposing the underlying capillary spaces.
- A mixed inflammatory infiltrate is often present in the dermis beneath eroded lesions.
- Recurrent lesions often extend deeper into the dermis.

COURSE AND PROGNOSIS

- Pyogenic granulomas arise suddenly, attain stable size, and tend to persist without treatment.
- With aggressive treatment, most resolve with a single crateriform scar.
- Recurrences are common and imply incomplete destruction of the initial lesion.

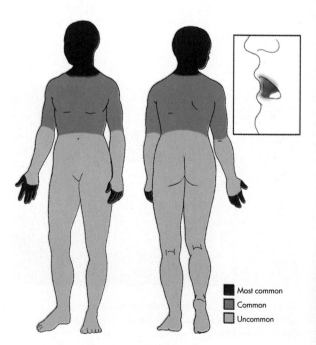

■ Most common
■ Common
□ Uncommon

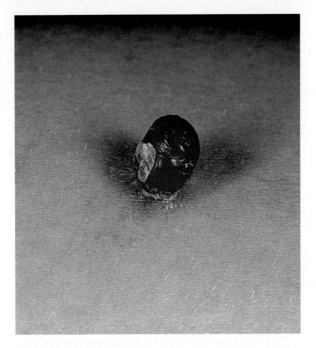

Pyogenic granuloma is a small, rapidly growing, yellow to bright red, dome-shaped, fragile protrusion that has a glistening, moist to scaly surface.

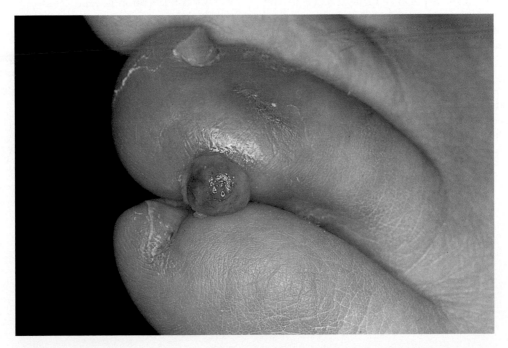

Pyogenic granulomas may protrude and bleed profusely if traumatized.

DISCUSSION

- When a single lesion is present, the diagnosis is usually straightforward.
- Pyogenic granuloma has a unique appearance and clinical course.
- Biopsy obtained at the time of treatment is sufficient to confirm the diagnosis.
- When multiple lesions are present, especially in a patient with disease caused by the human immunodeficiency virus (HIV), the possibilities of bacillary angiomatosis and Kaposi's sarcoma must be considered.
- Bacillary angiomatosis is an infectious disease caused by organisms of the genus *Bartonella* seen in the setting of advanced acquired immunodeficiency syndrome.
  - Lesions in this disease are clinically and histologically similar to those of pyogenic granuloma.
  - Special stains demonstrate the causative bacilli within biopsy material.
- Kaposi's sarcoma also occurs in the setting of advanced HIV disease.
  - The lesions are rarely as raised as those of pyogenic granuloma.
  - Skin biopsy discerns between the two entities.
- Angiosarcoma should be considered in the differential diagnosis, especially for lesions occurring in older patients.
  - This uncommon malignancy occurs most frequently in older Caucasians and usually on the head and neck.
  - Angiosarcoma also occurs in the setting of long-standing lymphedema (Stewart-Treves syndrome) and after radiation therapy.
- Biopsy is mandatory when pyogenic granuloma is considered in these clinical settings.

TREATMENT

- Pyogenic granulomas are best treated by aggressive electrodesiccation and curettage of the base and border of the lesion.
  - This is necessary to control bleeding and to ensure complete tissue destruction.
  - Inadequate treatment results in recurrences that require repeated electrodesiccation and curettage.
- Treatment leaves a crateriform scar.
- Recurrences do occur, most often in adolescents, even after seemingly adequate treatment.
- Patients and parents should be advised of this possibility, and a follow-up appointment is recommended.
- Occasionally multiple satellite lesions develop at and around the site of a previously treated pyogenic granuloma.
- This occurs most often on the shoulder and trunk in younger patients.
- Referral to a dermatologist should be considered.
- During a course of isotretinoin (Accutane), patients with severe acne may develop numerous lesions of pyogenic granuloma within previous acne lesions.
  - This occurs rarely.
  - This complication is best referred to a dermatologist for management.

CAVEAT

- Patients and parents should be advised of the possibility of recurrence after treatment.
- A follow-up appointment is recommended.

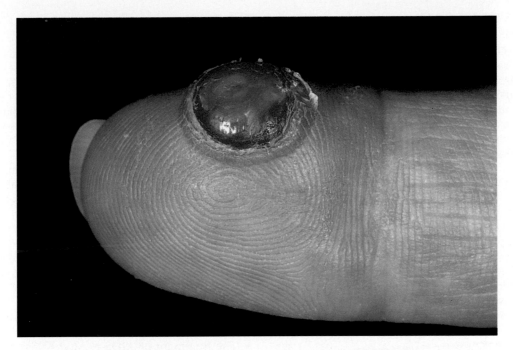

Pyogenic granulomas grow rapidly and look like nodular melanoma.

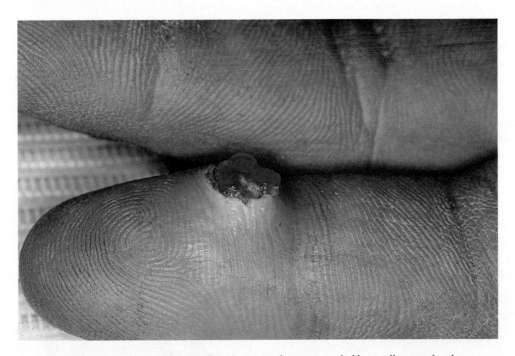

Pyogenic granuloma. The base of the lesion is often surrounded by a collarette of scale.

■ KAPOSI'S SARCOMA

DESCRIPTION

- Kaposi's sarcoma (KS) is a malignant tumor of lymphatic endothelial cells recently linked to herpesvirus type 8.
- KS can be divided into five subsets based on clinical and epidemiologic criteria: classic, African cutaneous, African lymphadenopathic, acquired immunodeficiency syndrome (AIDS) related, and immunosuppressive.

HISTORY

- Classic KS is sporadic and slowly progressive and occurs predominantly in 50- to 70-year-old men of Jewish, Greek, or Italian descent. Lesions typically appear on the feet or lower legs.
- African KS involves the lymph nodes or localized nodular lesions, most commonly in men.
- Azathioprine, cyclophosphamide, cyclosporine, and prednisone, singly or in combination, have been implicated in sporadic cases of KS, particularly in patients who have undergone renal transplant.
- Homosexual men are at greatest risk of AIDS-related KS. Lesions are often multifocal and widespread, occurring commonly on the trunk, head and neck, and oral mucosa.

SKIN FINDINGS

- Lesions are slightly raised, oval or elongated, poorly demarcated, rust or purple-red macules, patches, plaques, and nodules.
- The distribution is often multifocal at the time of the diagnosis.
- Lesions may resemble granulation tissue, ulceration, stasis dermatitis, pyogenic granuloma, or capillary hemangiomas.

NONSKIN FINDINGS

- Patients with AIDS-related KS often have systemic involvement, particularly of the gastrointestinal tract.
- Fever, night sweats, and weight loss may be present.

LABORATORY

- Skin biopsy is indicated to confirm the diagnosis.
- The CD4 count in AIDS-related cases is often less then 200 cells/mm^3.

TREATMENT

- In endemic KS, local radiation therapy or chemotherapy is suggested. Radiation is the treatment of choice.
- In KS related to immunosuppression and renal transplantation, some tumors regress after therapy is withdrawn, and others respond to radiation.
- In AIDS-related KS, radiation therapy is very effective; it is often the treatment of choice for larger, localized, or ulcerative lesions.
- Liquid nitrogen cryotherapy is another choice. Treatment is repeated at 3-week intervals. Cryotherapy yields excellent cosmetic results, but deeper lesions often remain.
- Other options include intralesional injection of vincristine; systemic, palliative single or multiagent chemotherapy for rapidly progressive and visceral disease; and the administration of interferon-alpha.

DISCUSSION

- Some 95% of epidemic, AIDS-related KS occurs in homosexual men.
- The treatment of AIDS-related KS is often performed for cosmesis because often the cutaneous lesions are otherwise asymptomatic.
- Newer antiretroviral treatment regimens are associated with the regression of KS in some cases.

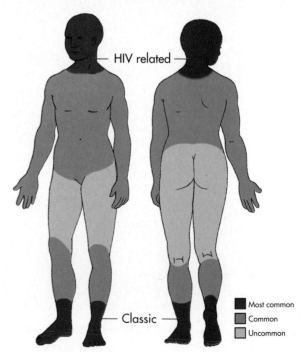

HIV related

Classic

Most common

Common

Uncommon

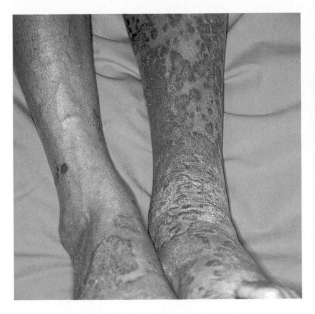

Kaposi's sarcoma related to acquired immunodeficiency syndrome occurs as a multifocal and widespread disease. It begins as violaceous macules and papules and progresses to plaques with multiple red-purple nodules.

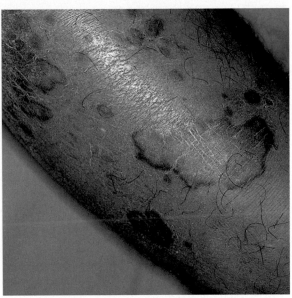

Classic Kaposi's sarcoma.

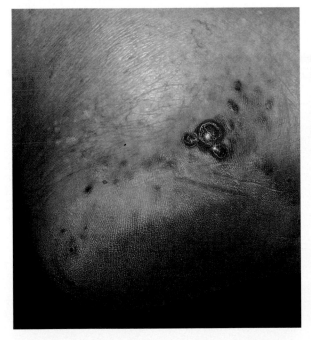

Classic Kaposi's sarcoma typically appears as nodules on the lower legs.

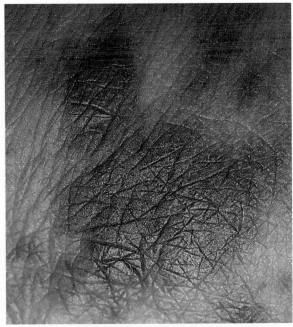

AIDS-related Kaposi's sarcoma.

■ TELANGIECTASIAS

DESCRIPTION

- Telangiectasias are common, asymptomatic, permanent abnormal dilatations of vessels within the subpapillary plexus.

HISTORY

- Telangiectasias occur in a variety of clinical settings.
- Although there is little variation in the appearance of individual telangiectasias from one disorder to another, the age of onset, distribution, and progression vary among disorders.
- Recognition of this along with other associated clinical findings helps discern between the various disorders associated with telangiectasias.
- It is useful to distinguish between disorders in which telangiectasias are a primary pathologic feature and disorders in which telangiectasias arise secondarily.

Primary Telangiectasias

Hereditary hemorrhagic telangiectasia (Osler-Rendu-Weber syndrome)

- Hereditary hemorrhagic telangiectasia is an autosomal dominant condition in which telangiectasias are found on the mucosae, skin, and internal organs.
- The earliest sign of the disorder is recurrent epistaxis in childhood.
- Characteristic telangiectasias do not appear until early adulthood.
- Telangiectasias are prominent on the tongue, palate, nasal mucosa, palms, soles, and nailbeds.
- Telangiectasias and arteriovenous fistulas may involve the gastrointestinal tract, liver, brain, and lungs.
- Bleeding from the gastrointestinal tract may present as melena or more insidiously as anemia.
- Abnormal perivascular connective tissue has been implicated as the cause of the abnormal bleeding.
- Most affected individuals have a normal life span but are at risk of life-threatening hemorrhage.

Hereditary benign telangiectasia

- Hereditary benign telangiectasia is an autosomal dominant condition.
- Widespread telangiectasias are found on the skin but not on the mucosa and internal organs.
- There is no associated bleeding diathesis.

Ataxia-telangiectasia (Louis-Bar syndrome)

- Ataxia-telangiectasia is an autosomal recessive condition with progressive cerebellar ataxia, telangiectasias, and immune dysfunction.
- The earliest sign, ataxia, is evident when the child begins to walk and usually by age 3.
- Telangiectasias appear on the conjunctivae, face, neck, and upper trunk by age 5.
- Café au lait macules may also be present.
- Affected individuals have defective DNA repair of chromosomal breaks and an increased sensitivity to ionizing radiation.
- Most patients die before age 20 from lymphoreticular malignancy or infection.

Generalized essential telangiectasia

- Women are affected by generalized essential telangiectasia more often than men.
- Telangiectasias first appear on the legs and then gradually, progressively, and symmetrically extend to involve the trunk and arms.
- The pathogenesis is unknown.
- Neither extracutaneous lesions nor increased bleeding has been reported.

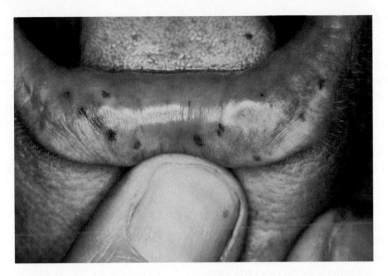

Hereditary hemorrhagic telangiectasia is an autosomal dominant, inherited malformation of blood vessels. Few to numerous lesions occur primarily on the lips, tongue, nasal mucosa, forearms, hands, and fingers and throughout the gastrointestinal tract.

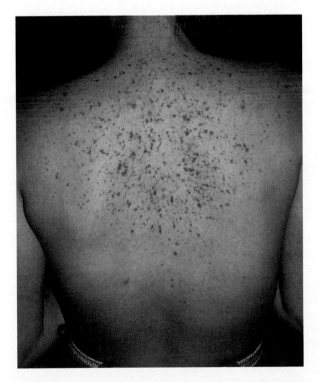

Generalized essential telangiectasia is seen primarily in women. The telangiectasias slowly progress over years and are not accompanied by associated systemic problems.

Unilateral nevoid telangiectasia

- There is a unilateral dermatomal distribution of fine telangiectasias.
- The most commonly affected dermatomes are the trigeminal and the third and fourth cervical.
- This condition may be congenital or acquired.
  - The congenital form affects male patients more often, whereas the acquired form is seen more often in female patients.
  - Estrogen may play a role in the acquired form. In some patients, lesions appear at times of increased estrogen levels, such as puberty and pregnancy, and subsequently resolve when estrogen levels decrease.

Secondary Telangiectasias

- Secondary disorders include basal cell carcinoma, rosacea, collagen vascular disease, steroid atrophy, and chronic graft-versus-host disease.
- Though perhaps an oversimplification, secondary telangiectasias occur in the setting of altered dermal connective tissue as a result of injury or chronic inflammation.
- Damage may be from ultraviolet radiation (actinic damage), ionizing radiation given therapeutically for cancer, or overtreatment with topical or intralesional corticosteroids.
- Telangiectasias also occur secondarily in scleroderma and the CREST syndrome.
  - Telangiectasias in scleroderma and the CREST syndrome appear as discrete, 5-mm macular clusters referred to as *telangiectatic mats* on the face, lips, neck, upper trunk, and dorsal and palmar aspects of the hands.
  - The skin of the fingers feels waxy, and Raynaud's phenomenon, cutaneous calcinosis, and ulceration may also be present.

SKIN FINDINGS

- The lesion is a dilated dermal vessel with a diameter of 1 mm or less, is not palpable, and is easily blanched with diascopy.
- Lesions may appear as discrete vessels or clustered as telangiectatic mats.
- The distribution of lesions varies among disorders, as previously discussed.

LABORATORY

- Skin biopsy reveals a thin-walled vessel in close approximation to the overlying epidermis.
- A sparse infiltrate of lymphocytes is often seen surrounding the vessels in hereditary hemorrhagic telangiectasia.
- The telangiectatic vessel is usually a postcapillary venule but may also be a capillary or arteriole.
- Depending on the clinical setting and suspicion, diagnosis-specific testing may be indicated.
  - Imaging studies of the brain and internal organs should be considered for hereditary hemorrhagic telangiectasia.
  - Specific serologic testing is indicated for suspected forms of scleroderma.
  - Autoantibodies directed against centromere proteins and DNA topoisomerase type I are found in a high number of patients with the CREST syndrome and in patients with diffuse scleroderma, respectively.

DISCUSSION

- Telangiectasias are easily overlooked; lesions occur in a wide range of disorders.
- Distinguishing between primary and secondary disorders narrows the differential diagnosis.

TREATMENT

- Cosmetically objectionable telangiectasias may be ablated with laser surgery or pinpoint electrocautery.
- Multiple treatments may be required.

CAVEAT

- Careful attention to the distribution, age of onset, and clinical progression of telangiectasias may provide useful diagnostic clues to underlying disease.

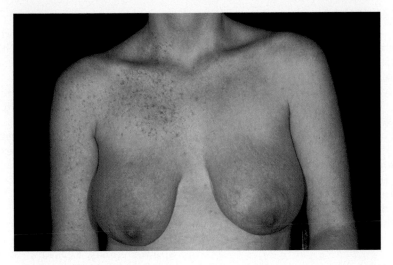

Unilateral nevoid telangiectasia syndrome. Telangiectasias appear in a segmental distribution. The acquired form begins with states of increasing estrogen blood levels: (1) at puberty in females, (2) during pregnancy, or (3) with alcoholic cirrhosis.

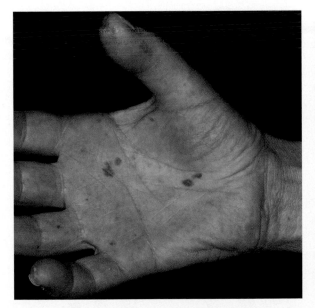

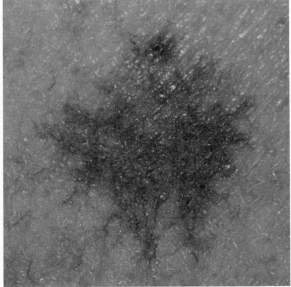

The telangiectasias of CREST syndrome and scleroderma occur as flat (macular), 0.5-cm, rectangular collections of uniform tiny vessels; these are the so-called telangiectatic mats.

■ SPIDER ANGIOMA

DESCRIPTION

- Spider angioma is a common, asymptomatic vascular papule with a distinct clinical appearance and distribution.

HISTORY

- Spider angiomas are found in 10% to 15% of normal adults and are also quite common in young children.
- Because the lesions are asymptomatic, the patient or parent often perceives the lesion to have suddenly appeared.
- Lesions represent dilatations of a previously existing vessel rather than a neoplasm.

SKIN FINDINGS

- Spider angiomas bear a vague resemblance to a spider.
- There is a central, slightly raised, bright red vascular papule from which fine blood vessels radiate.
- The application of gentle pressure with a glass slide (diascopy) tends to blanch the radiating vessels, whereas the central papule is less easily blanched. Pulsation of the central papule with this technique confirms the arteriolar nature of the papule.
- Spider angiomas are most commonly found on the face and also on the neck, upper trunk, and upper arms in adults.
- In children, lesions are also frequently present on the hands and fingers.

NONSKIN FINDINGS

- Spider angiomas occur with increased frequency in pregnancy and in the setting of chronic liver disease.
- It has been suggested that spider angiomas occur in a state of relative estrogen excess.
- Lesions arising during pregnancy tend to resolve after the birth.
- Those found in patients with liver disease tend to persist. Other stigmata of chronic liver disease such as gynecomastia, testicular atrophy, palmar erythema, ascites, and perhaps icterus should also be present.

LABORATORY

- Skin biopsy is rarely indicated but demonstrates a central arteriole ascending high into the papillary dermis, there giving rise to a subepidermal ampulla.
- Thin-walled arterioles radiate outward into the surrounding papillary dermis and branch into delicate capillaries.
- If chronic liver disease is suggested by clinical examination, laboratory studies to assess hepatic function and hepatitis serologic testing may be warranted.

COURSE AND PROGNOSIS

- Spider angiomas arising during pregnancy and those occurring in children tend to disappear spontaneously. Reassurance is often all that is needed.
- If cosmetic treatment is desired, efforts should be focused on the central papule.
- Ablation of the ampulla with either a pulsed dye laser or electrocautery usually results in resolution of the entire lesion.
- Treatment carries a risk of scarring and dyspigmentation.
- Recurrences are frequent.

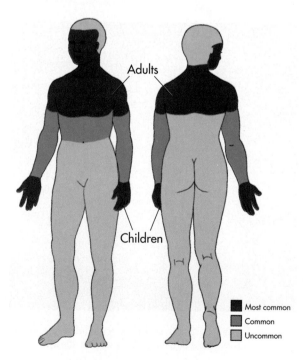

Adults

Children

■ Most common
■ Common
□ Uncommon

DISCUSSION

- Telangiectasias are persistent dilatations of venules and occasionally arterioles.
- Although similar in color and size to spider angiomas, telangiectasias lack the central papule and radiating vessels.

TREATMENT

- The patient should be reassured that spider angiomas are common, benign lesions that usually resolve without treatment.
- If the lesion is persistent and cosmetically bothersome, it may be treated with either pulsed dye laser or electrocautery.

- The patient should know that treatment is a cosmetic procedure, that there is a slight risk of dyspigmentation and scarring, and that lesions may recur.
- Consultation with a specialist in laser treatment should be considered.

CAVEAT

- The association between spider angiomas and chronic liver disease is overstated.
- Spider angiomas occurring in an otherwise healthy person without other signs of hepatic dysfunction are far more likely to be a normal finding than a sign of occult liver disease.

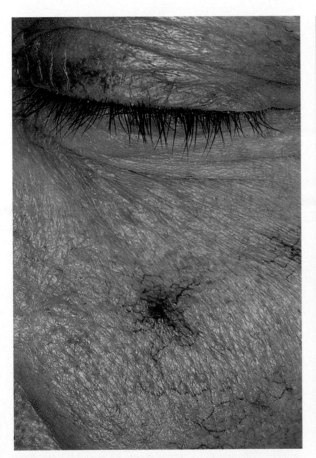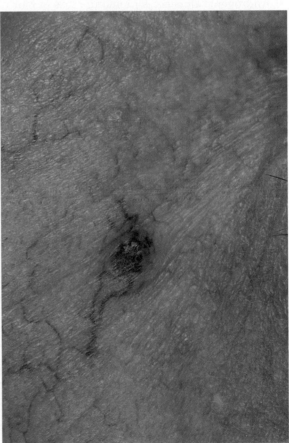

Spider angiomas form as arterioles (spider bodies), become more prominent near the surface of the skin, and radiate capillaries (spider legs). They blanch with firm pressure. They are most common on the exposed surfaces of the face and arms. They increase in number with liver disease and during pregnancy and are probably stimulated by higher-than-normal estrogen concentrations.

■ ANDROGENIC ALOPECIA (MALE PATTERN BALDNESS)

DESCRIPTION

- Androgenic alopecia is premature loss of hair of the central scalp.

HISTORY

- Alopecia is a physiologic reaction induced by androgens in genetically predisposed men.
- The pattern of inheritance is probably polygenic.
- It begins with bitemporal thinning that then progresses to an M-shaped recession. Then there is a loss of hair focally in the crown of the scalp, which extends to total hair loss in the central scalp.
- It can begin any time after puberty and usually is fully expressed by the time the patient is in his forties.

SKIN FINDINGS

- Terminal hair follicles are transformed into velluslike follicles.
- Terminal hair is replaced by fine, light vellus hair, which is shorter and has a reduced diameter.
- With time, further atrophy occurs, leaving the scalp shiny and smooth. The follicles disappear.
- There is increased growth of secondary sexual hair (e.g., that on the chest, in the axillae, and in pubic and beard areas).

TREATMENT

Minoxidil (Rogaine), a topical 2% or 5% solution, is available over the counter.

- It is applied to a dry scalp twice a day.
- Ideal candidates are men under 30.
- Regrowth takes 8 to 12 months.
- It may help stop further loss but must be used continually to preserve growth.

Propecia is a 1-mg formulation of finasteride.

- The drug works by blocking 5α-reductase in the scalp.
- It must be used daily and chronically to stabilize or reverse balding.
- Decreased libido and erectile dysfunction occur in less than 2% of men taking the drug.
- It is contraindicated for women.
- Hair transplants have been used successfully for years to permanently restore hair.
- Hair weaves have been refined in a process whereby strands of human hair are applied to a thin nylon filament anchored to the scalp with the individual's own hair.
- An anteroposterior elliptic excision of bald vertex scalp with primary closure can provide an instant hair effect.

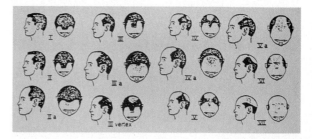

The progression and various patterns of hair loss have been classified by Hamilton. Triangular frontotemporal recession occurs normally in most young men (type I) and women after puberty. The first signs of balding are increased frontotemporal recession accompanied by midfrontal recession (type II). Hair loss in a round area on the vertex follows, and the density of hair decreases, sometimes rapidly, over the top of the scalp (types III through VII).

ANDROGENETIC ALOPECIA IN WOMEN (FEMALE PATTERN HAIR LOSS)

DESCRIPTION

- Androgenetic alopecia in women is a common hereditary, central, diffuse hair thinning that begins at a relatively early age. This is in contrast to hair loss that occurs as part of the aging process that begins in the patient's fifties, sixties, or seventies.

HISTORY

- Alopecia can be inherited from either side of the family.
- Women rarely become bald like men.
- Hereditary hair thinning begins in the patient's teens, twenties, or thirties, and is usually fully expressed by the forties.
- Hair loss is gradual, not abrupt or massive.
- Menses is normal and regular. Heavy menses causes iron deficiency and increased hair shedding. Pregnancies are normal, and there is no infertility or galactorrhea.
- Certain drugs cause hair thinning. Hair regrows when the drug is stopped.

SKIN FINDINGS

- Most women experience a gradual loss of hair on the central scalp, with retention of the normal hairline without frontotemporal recession, and the scalp becomes more visible.
- There is increased spacing between hairs.
- There are a variety of hair diameters in the central scalp. Many of the hairs are miniaturized (thin and short). Hairs along the frontal hairline are normal.
- Hair diameter becomes thinner over time. This is noticed when the hair is gathered into a ponytail.

LABORATORY

- Most patients do not require hormonal evaluation.
- Dehydroepiandrosterone sulfate (DHEAS), serum free or total testosterone, and prolactin levels should be determined if one or more of the following is present: irregular menses, hirsutism, virilization, cystic acne, galactorrhea, and infertility.
- The thyroid-stimulating hormone level should be determined to rule out a treatable thyroid disease.
- Patients with heavy menses should have the following tests: serum iron determination, total iron-binding capacity, and ferritin level.
- Scalp biopsy is performed in patients suspected of having a scarring alopecia.

TREATMENT

- The term *female pattern baldness* should be avoided. Instead, the terms *hereditary hair thinning* or *female pattern hair loss* should be used when talking to patients.
- A 2% topical minoxidil solution (Rogaine) may be effective in some women. It is applied twice a day. The 5% solution is approved for use on men. Women who use this stronger concentration may experience increased hair on the forehead and face.
- Patients with abnormal laboratory studies can be referred to an endocrinologist or gynecologist.
- There are no restrictions on frequency of washing, combing, hair coloring, or permanents.
- Estrogen is not usually prescribed to treat women for androgenetic alopecia.
- Women with androgenetic alopecia who desire an oral contraceptive should use a progestin with little androgenic activity, such as norgestimate or ethynodiol diacetate.

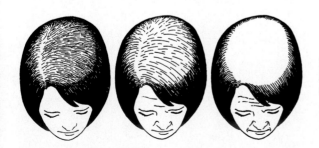

Evolution of the female type of androgenetic alopecia. (*From Montagna W, Parakkal PF: The structure and function of skin, ed 3, New York, 1974, Academic Press.*)

■ ALOPECIA AREATA

DESCRIPTION

- Alopecia areata is rapid-onset total hair loss in a sharply defined, usually round area.

HISTORY

- Alopecia areata is most common in children and young adults.
- There is a sudden occurrence of one or several, 1- to 4-cm areas of hair loss.
- The eyelashes, beard, and rarely, other parts of the body may be involved.
- Total hair loss of the scalp (alopecia totalis) is seen most frequently in young people; it may be accompanied by cycles of growth and loss.
- Total hair loss of the body (alopecia universalis) is very rare.
- Stress is frequently cited as the cause, but there is little evidence that it plays a role.
- Regrowth begins in 1 to 3 months and may be followed by loss in other areas.
- The prognosis for total permanent regrowth in cases with limited involvement is good, but it is poorer for patients with more involvement.

SKIN FINDINGS

- A wide spectrum of involvement is seen.
- The skin is smooth or may have short stubs of hair.
- The hair shaft is poorly formed and breaks on reaching the surface.
- New hair is usually the same color and texture but may be fine and white.

NONSKIN FINDINGS

- Thyroid structural and functional abnormalities may occur.
- Diffuse fine nail pitting occurs in 3% to 30% of cases.

LABORATORY

- Alopecia areata may be associated with thyroid disease, pernicious anemia, Addison's disease, vitiligo, lupus erythematosus, ulcerative colitis, diabetes mellitus, and Down syndrome.
- Triiodothyronine, thyroxine, thyroid-stimulating hormone, antithyroglobulin, and antimicrosomal antibody testing should be considered, especially for children.
- The presence of eosinophils in a biopsy is a helpful diagnostic sign in difficult-to-diagnose cases.

DIFFERENTIAL DIAGNOSIS

- "Moth-eaten" or diffuse alopecia of secondary syphilis

TREATMENT

- In most areas, hair regrows, and no treatment is needed.
- Group I topical steroids applied twice a day are minimally effective. They should be used in cycles (e.g., 2 weeks of treatment and 1 week of no treatment).
- Intradermal injection of triamcinolone acetonide (Kenalog), 2.5 to 10 mg/ml, is effective.
  - Injections may be repeated at 4-week intervals.
  - Atrophy is the major side effect.
  - This treatment should be reserved for patients with a few small areas of hair loss.
- Anthralin (Drithocreme 1%, 0.5%, 0.25%, or 0.1%), applied once a day in concentrations high enough to induce a visible dermatitis, is occasionally effective.

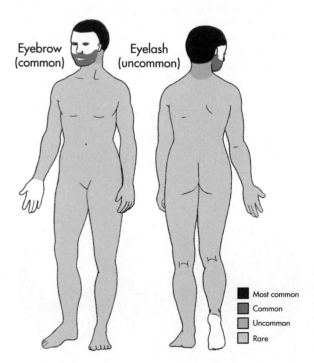

Eyebrow (common)   Eyelash (uncommon)

■ Most common
■ Common
□ Uncommon
□ Rare

- An intravenous pulse of methylprednisolone may be effective in patients with rapidly progressing extensive multifocal alopecia areata.
- Oral corticosteroid therapy does not prevent the spread or relapse of severe alopecia areata, and when regrowth is obtained, it is rarely maintained off therapy.
- A wig might be considered.
- A network of support groups across the country is available to help patients cope: Alopecia Areata Foundation, 710 C Street, Suite 11, San Rafael, CA 94901, (415) 456-4644, www.alopeciaareata.com.

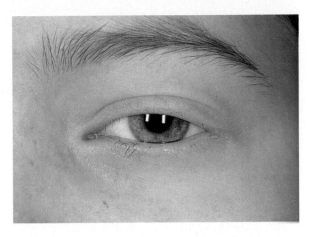

Alopecia areata. The eyelashes, beard, and rarely, other parts of the body may be involved.

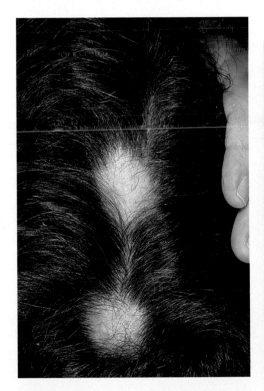

Alopecia areata is characterized by the rapid onset of total hair loss in a sharply defined, usually round area.

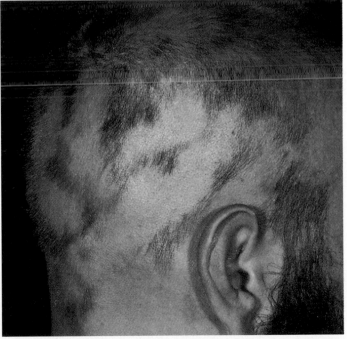

Alopecia areata. A wide spectrum of involvement is seen. The majority of patients report the sudden occurrence of one or several, 1- to 4-cm areas of hair loss on the scalp.

■ TRICHOTILLOMANIA

DESCRIPTION

- Trichotillomania is recurrent pulling of one's hair, resulting in significant hair loss.
- It may involve many hours each day of pulling the hair or thinking about pulling it.

HISTORY

- Trichotillomania is a habit tic commonly performed by young children.
- It is also seen in adolescents and adults.
- The female/male ratio is 2.5:1.
- Hair is twisted around finger, pulled, and rubbed until it is extracted or broken.
- Favorite sites are the easily reached frontoparietal scalp, eyebrows, and eyelashes.
- It first manifests during inactive periods (e.g., while watching television, before falling asleep).
- Parents seldom notice the behavior.
- It is triggered by stress and may be an obsessive-compulsive disorder.
- It can be a chronic problem and often resolves spontaneously.

SKIN FINDINGS

- There is a patch of hair loss with an irregular, angulated border.
- The hair density is greatly reduced; the involved area is not bald and smooth like in alopecia area.
- Short, broken hairs of varying lengths are randomly distributed in the involved site.

LABORATORY

- A potassium hydroxide test rules out noninflammatory tinea capitis.
- A plucked hair shows no telogen hair roots (100% in active-growing, anagen phase).
- Gentle hair traction produces no hair.
- Skin biopsy reveals normal hairs, absence of hairs in follicles, and no inflammation.

DIFFERENTIAL DIAGNOSIS

- Alopecia areata
- Tinea capitis
- Syphilis

TREATMENT

- Discussion with an understanding physician or parent is helpful for the child.
- The child's attention should be diverted when hair is being pulled.
- The parents and physician should be accepting and supportive rather than judgmental and punitive.
- Extensive involvement or persistence requires psychiatric evaluation.
- Clomipramine (Anafranil), fluoxetine (Prozac), and pimozide (Orap) are effective, and other drugs have been reported to be effective as well.

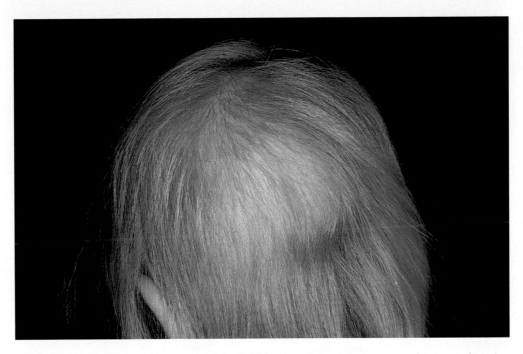

The favorite site is the easily reached frontoparietal region of the scalp, but any scalp area or the eyebrows and eyelashes may be attacked.

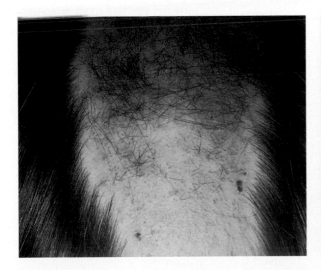

The affected area has an irregular angulated border, and the density of hair is greatly reduced, but the site is never bald, as in alopecia areata.

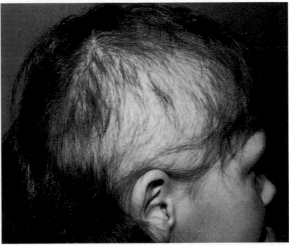

Several short, broken hairs of varying lengths are randomly distributed in the involved site. Hair that grows beyond 0.5 to 1 cm can be grasped by small fingers and extracted.

21 Cutaneous Manifestations of Internal Disease

■ ACQUIRED CUTANEOUS PARANEOPLASTIC SYNDROME

DESCRIPTION

- Acquired cutaneous paraneoplastic syndrome involves cutaneous findings attributed to internal malignancy.

HISTORY

- Internal malignancy may manifest though a variety of cutaneous signs and symptoms.
- Some cutaneous signs are specific enough to warrant a search for occult internal malignancy.
- *Carcinoid syndrome* refers to episodic intense flushing of the face, neck, and upper chest.
  - The syndrome is caused by a release of vasoactive mediators from carcinoid tumors into the systemic circulation.
  - Most carcinoid tumors arise in the small bowel, usually the appendix.
  - Vasoactive mediators released from the tumor are inactivated in the liver before reaching the systemic circulation.
  - When carcinoid tumors metastasize to the liver, mediators have access to the systemic circulation.
  - Carcinoid tumors also arise in the lung and as such, release mediators into the systemic circulation.

- Adults with dermatomyositis are more likely to have an internal malignancy than age-matched controls.
  - The prevalence has been estimated at 6% to 50%, with the greatest prevalence among older patients.
  - The prevalence of malignancy does not appear to be increased in children with dermatomyositis.
  - Most malignancies are diagnosed when the dermatomyositis is diagnosed.
  - The most common associated malignancies are in the breast, lung, ovary, and gastrointestinal system.
- Glucagonoma syndrome is a rare, clinically distinctive syndrome consisting of a dynamic generalized cutaneous eruption associated with a glucagon-secreting alpha-cell tumor.
- Paraneoplastic pemphigus presents as a sign of internal malignancy, most often hematologic and chronic lymphocytic leukemia.
  - Most patients die from complications of paraneoplastic pemphigus or the malignancy.
- The sudden, eruptive appearance of numerous seborrheic keratoses may indicate internal malignancy.
  - This exceedingly rare and ominous entity is known as the *sign of Leser-Trélat*.
  - Adenocarcinoma is the most common associated type of malignancy.
- Pruritus is a symptom of many dermatoses.
  - In the absence of skin findings, pruritus may indicate occult malignancy.

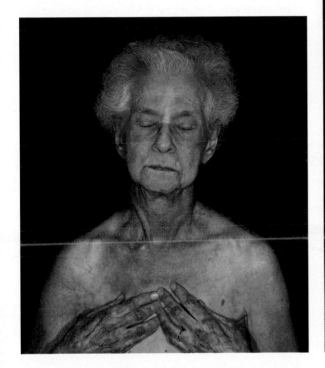

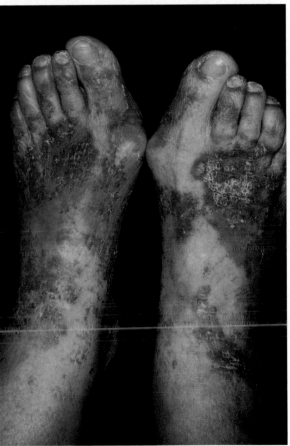

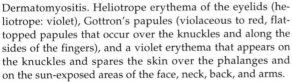

Dermatomyositis. Heliotrope erythema of the eyelids (heliotrope: violet), Gottron's papules (violaceous to red, flat-topped papules that occur over the knuckles and along the sides of the fingers), and a violet erythema that appears on the knuckles and spares the skin over the phalanges and on the sun-exposed areas of the face, neck, back, and arms.

Glucagonoma syndrome (necrolytic migratory erythema). The dermatitis begins as an erythematous area, progresses to superficial blisters, and gradually spreads ("migrates"), with central crusting and then healing, followed by hyperpigmentation 7 to 14 days after the initial erythema.

- Pruritus is a common symptom of lymphoreticular malignancies, especially Hodgkin's disease.
- The term *Sweet's syndrome,* or *acute febrile neutrophilic dermatosis,* describes recurrent, painful papules in association with fever, elevated white blood cell count, and arthralgias.
  - Female patients are affected more often than male patients.
  - Sweet's syndrome may be associated with acute infection or with hematologic malignancy, most often acute myelogenous leukemia.

Skin Findings

- Carcinoid syndrome presents as an acute flushing of the face, neck, and chest, lasting usually less than 30 minutes. Flushing episodes are often associated with dyspnea, abdominal cramping, and diarrhea.
- The findings of dermatomyositis include Gottron's papules, periorbital heliotrope coloration, photosensitive violaceous eruption, poikiloderma, and periungual telangiectasia.
- *Necrolytic migratory erythema* describes the eruption of the glucagonoma syndrome.
  - The eruption is generalized but favors the groin, buttocks, and thighs.
  - Bright dermal erythema is soon followed by flaccid bullae that desquamate, leaving denuded areas and advancing polycyclic collarette scales.
  - The process is dynamic, changing and extending each day.
- Paraneoplastic pemphigus presents as ocular inflammation, oral erosions, generalized erythema multiforme–like bullous lesions, and denuded areas with crusting.
- Widespread seborrheic keratoses are seen in the sign of Leser-Trélat. Lesions are small, monomorphic, and widespread.
- The lesion of Sweet's syndrome is a red edematous, succulent plaque. Lesions vary from 0.5 to 5.0 cm and are tender to palpation.

Nonskin Findings

- Carcinoid syndrome is associated with an internal bronchial carcinoid tumor or a small bowel carcinoid tumor with hepatic metastases.
- Dermatomyositis may be associated with muscle weakness and internal malignancies.
- Glucagonoma syndrome is often associated with an alpha-cell tumor of the pancreas.
- Paraneoplastic pemphigus is often associated with a hematologic malignancy.
- Sweet's syndrome may be associated with an acute infection, in which case there is usually a prodrome of fever and myalgias. The most common associated malignancy is acute myelogenous leukemia.

Laboratory

- Dermatomyositis shows an interface dermatitis with increased dermal mucin.
- In necrolytic migratory erythema, characteristic hydropic degeneration of the superficial epidermis is seen along with intracellular edema.
- The seborrheic keratoses in the sign of Leser-Trélat are not unique.
- In paraneoplastic pemphigus, there is suprabasilar acantholysis, as in pemphigus vulgaris.
  - Unlike pemphigus vulgaris, there is also an interface dermatitis.
  - Direct immunofluorescence confirms immunoglobulin G within the epidermis and at the dermoepidermal junction.
  - Indirect immunofluorescence using rat bladder substrate confirms the diagnosis.

Course and Prognosis

- The clinical course and prognosis usually depend on the internal malignancy.

Differential Diagnosis

- Necrolytic migratory erythema: acrodermatitis enteropathica
- Paraneoplastic pemphigus: other blistering disorders

Discussion

- The clinical and histologic features of necrolytic migratory erythema and acrodermatitis enteropathica are similar, although necrolytic migratory erythema does not respond to zinc supplementation.
- When paraneoplastic pemphigus is suspected, immunofluorescence testing is used to discern among the differential diagnoses.

TREATMENT

- Patients with cutaneous findings suggestive of internal malignancy without known malignancy should be carefully evaluated.
- With the exception of dermatomyositis, the search is directed by the most likely tumor to be found based on the presentation.
- Patients with dermatomyositis should be evaluated first by age-appropriate screening for malignancy; they should be followed closely.

CAVEAT

- The importance of recognizing the cutaneous findings associated with internal malignancy lies in the fact that the earliest possible detection of tumor usually may offer the best prognosis.

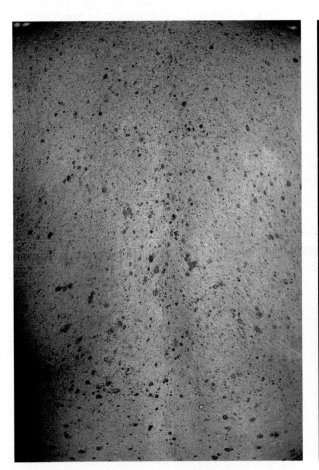

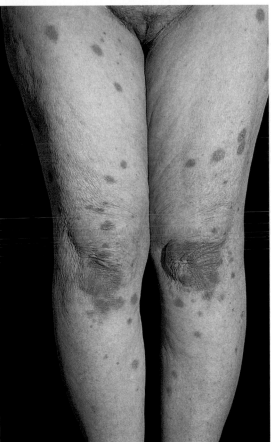

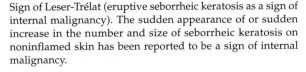

Sign of Leser-Trélat (eruptive seborrheic keratosis as a sign of internal malignancy). The sudden appearance of or sudden increase in the number and size of seborrheic keratosis on noninflamed skin has been reported to be a sign of internal malignancy.

Sweet's syndrome. Acute, tender, erythematous plaques, pseudovesicles, and occasionally, blisters with an annular or arciform pattern occur on the head, neck, legs, arms, and particularly the back of the hands and fingers. Careful systemic evaluation is indicated, especially when cutaneous lesions are severe or hematologic values are abnormal. Approximately 20% of cases are associated with malignancy.

■ INHERITED CUTANEOUS PARANEOPLASTIC SYNDROME

DESCRIPTION

- Inherited cutaneous paraneoplastic syndrome involves cutaneous findings associated with heritable conditions that carry an increased risk of internal malignancy (Box 21-1).

HISTORY

- A variety of cutaneous lesions may be associated with internal malignancy.
- Recognition of such signs is only of value if it leads to the prevention, early detection, or treatment of internal malignancy.
- Several genodermatoses carry an increased risk of malignancy.
- Patients with such an inherited disorder may benefit from increased surveillance for likely tumors.
- Similarly, genetic testing and counseling may be important to patients and their families.
- Cowden's syndrome, or multiple hamartoma syndrome, is a rare, often undiagnosed disorder affecting multiple systems.
  - Inheritance is autosomal dominant with incomplete penetrance and variable expression.
  - Affected individuals develop hamartomatous growths of various tissues.
  - Thyroid adenoma is the most common neoplasm with occasional malignant degeneration.
  - Ductal carcinoma of the breast occurs in more than 30% of female patients with Cowden's syndrome.
- Gardner's syndrome consists of multiple epidermal cysts, fibrous tumors of the skin and subcutaneous tissue, and intestinal polyposis.
  - Inheritance is autosomal dominant.
  - Intestinal polyps are usually limited to the colon.
  - Malignant degeneration of polyps occurs in 50% of patients.
  - There is usually a family history of colon cancer.
- Muir-Torre syndrome consists of multiple benign sebaceous tumors and colonic polyps with increased risk of malignant degeneration. Inheritance is autosomal dominant.

SKIN FINDINGS

- In Cowden's syndrome, characteristic facial and oral papules develop during early adulthood.
  - The facial papules are 1- to 3-mm, smooth, and skin-colored and are concentrated on the pinnae and around the eyes, nose, and mouth.
  - Biopsy usually confirms the papule as a trichilemmoma, a benign adnexal tumor.
  - The oral papules are 1- to 3-mm, smooth, and white, coalescing into a cobblestone pattern on the tongue and gingiva.
  - Two thirds of patients also develop flat-topped, 1- to 4-mm, skin-colored, wartlike keratoses on the dorsal hands.
  - Punctate keratoses of the palms and soles occur in roughly half of patients.
- Individuals with Gardner's syndrome develop multiple epidermal cysts, most commonly on the face and scalp.
  - Multiple pilar cysts of the scalp are not associated with Gardner's syndrome.
  - Discrete fibrous tumors of the skin are rarely symptomatic.
- Muir-Torre syndrome is suggested by the presence of multiple benign tumors of the sebaceous glands, including sebaceoma, sebaceous adenoma, and basal cell carcinoma with sebaceous differentiation.
  - Of these, the most specific for Muir-Torre is the sebaceous adenoma.
  - Patients with Muir-Torre syndrome also develop keratoacanthomas with distinctive sebaceous differentiation.
- Sebaceous hyperplasia is a common condition in otherwise healthy people and is not considered part of the Muir-Torre syndrome.

Box 21-1   Familial Multiple Cancer Syndromes and Autosomal Dominant "Cancer Family Syndromes"

Cowden's disease
(multiple hamartoma syndrome)

Muir-Torre syndrome

Gardner's syndrome
(familial adenomatous polyposis
with extraintestinal manifestations)

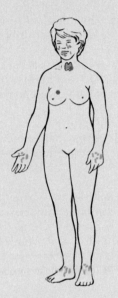

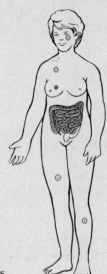

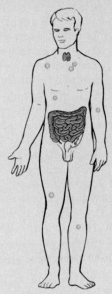

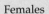 • Solid tumors

Females

Mucocutaneous
  lesions
  Facial papules
  Oral papules
  Hand keratosis

Breast lesions
  Cancer
  Fibrocystic

Thyroid
  Goiter
  Carcinoma

Males = females

Skin tumors
  Sebaceous gland
  (at least 1)

Keratoacanthomas

Internal tumors
  Colorectal
  Genitourinary
  Breast

Males = females

Skin signs
  Epidermal cysts

Osteomas
  (palpable)
  Skull
  Jaw

Pigmented ocular
  fundus lesions

Colon
  Polyps >100
  Adenocarcinoma

Thyroid carcinoma

NONSKIN FINDINGS

- A variety of benign and malignant neoplasms have been reported in individuals with Cowden's syndrome.
  - The most common neoplasm is thyroid adenoma.
  - Female patients have a significantly increased risk of ductal carcinoma of the breast.
- Patients with Gardner's syndrome develop osteomas of the membranous bones of the head, which are visible on x-ray films.
  - Pigmented lesions of the retinal fundus are found in 90% of patients.
  - Fundal lesions are usually present in infancy and are useful as a screening finding.
- A variety of genitourinary malignancies have been described in the Muir-Torre syndrome, all with low incidence.
  - The most common malignancy is colon carcinoma, usually proximal to the splenic flexure.
  - Individuals suspected of having the Muir-Torre syndrome should be screened by colonoscopy.

LABORATORY

- Skin biopsy of the facial papules seen in Cowden's syndrome most often confirms the lesion as a trichilemmoma, a benign tumor of hair differentiation.
- Epidermal rather than trichilemmal keratinization is seen.
- In Gardner's syndrome, histologic testing confirms the scalp cysts as epidermal rather than pilar cysts.
- Sebaceous adenoma is the most characteristic lesion of Muir-Torre syndrome. Such lesions may have an architecture reminiscent of keratoacanthoma.

COURSE AND PROGNOSIS

- The prognosis depends on the malignancy, stage at the time of diagnosis, and treatment.

DISCUSSION

- Patients with genodermatoses may benefit from increased surveillance for likely tumors.
- Families of affected individuals may benefit from screening examination and from genetic counseling.

TREATMENT

- Screening of family members and genetic counseling are indicated for genodermatoses with an increased risk of malignancy.
- Female patients suspected of having Cowden's syndrome should have regular breast examinations, mammograms, and close follow-up.
- Prophylactic bilateral mastectomy has been suggested by some authors.
- Patients suspected of having Gardner's syndrome or Muir-Torre syndrome should undergo colonoscopy.
- Prophylactic colectomy is recommended for patients with Gardner's syndrome.

CAVEAT

- A skin biopsy showing trichilemmoma should raise the possibility of Cowden's syndrome.
- A patient with multiple epidermal cysts of the face and scalp should raise suspicion of Gardner's syndrome.
- A skin biopsy showing sebaceous adenoma or keratoacanthoma with sebaceous differentiation should suggest Muir-Torre syndrome.

■ ACANTHOSIS NIGRICANS

DESCRIPTION

- Acanthosis nigricans is thickened, velvety, hyperpigmented skin.
- It is most commonly associated with obesity and diabetes.
- Other, less common associations are other endocrine disorders, pineal tumors, occult malignancy, and the use of drugs such as nicotinic acid, estrogens, and corticosteroids.
- Rarely, it is an autosomal dominant trait.

HISTORY

- Usually, there is a gradual onset when it is associated with diabetes and obesity.
- Malignancy-associated acanthosis nigricans develops more rapidly and suddenly.

SKIN FINDINGS

- There is a symmetric, velvety brown thickening of the skin.
- The surface is leathery, warty, or papillomatous.
- The axillae are most commonly involved; other favored areas are the flexural areas of the neck and groin, the belt line, the dorsal fingers, the mouth, the umbilicus, and the breast areolae.
- The severity is variable: from mild to extensive.
- Acanthosis nigricans is asymptomatic or pruritic.

NONSKIN FINDINGS

- Acanthosis nigricans is a cutaneous marker of tissue insulin resistance.
- Patients without diabetes have high levels of circulating insulin or an impaired response to exogenous insulin.
- The vulva is commonly affected in obese, hirsute, hyperandrogenic, insulin-resistant women.
- HAIR–AN syndrome is *h*yper*a*ndrogenism, *i*nsulin *r*esistance, and *a*canthosis *n*igricans.

LABORATORY

- Glucose levels may be elevated. Other studies are not routinely done.
- There are high levels of circulating insulin.
- There is an impaired response to exogenous insulin.

DISCUSSION AND TREATMENT

- Lesions are usually asymptomatic and do not require treatment.
- Reducing thick lesions in areas of maceration may decrease the odor and promote comfort.
- Lac-Hydrin, a 12% lactic acid cream, is applied twice a day.
- Retinoic acid (Retin-A cream or gel) applied each day, or less often if irritation occurs, can be helpful.

CAVEAT

- A sudden onset and extensive acanthosis nigricans should prompt an evaluation for internal malignancy. Stomach adenocarcinoma is the most common finding.

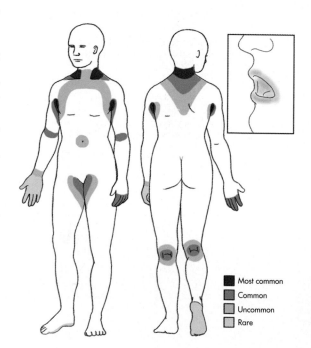

Most common
Common
Uncommon
Rare

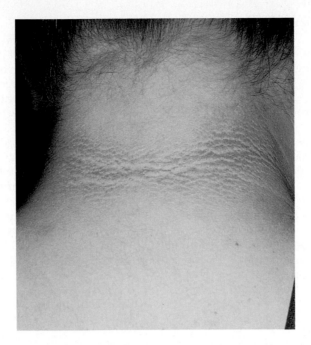

The most common site of involvement is the axilla, but the changes may be observed in the flexural areas of the neck and groin, at the belt line, over the dorsal surfaces of the fingers, in the mouth, and around the areolae of the breasts and umbilicus.

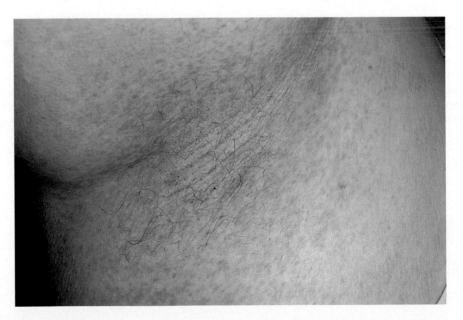

There is a symmetric, brown thickening of the skin. In time the skin may becomes thickened as the lesion develops a leathery, warty, or papillomatous surface.

■ NEUROFIBROMATOSIS

DESCRIPTION

- Neurofibromatosis is an autosomal dominant inherited disorder affecting the ectodermal tissues.

HISTORY

- The inheritance is autosomal dominant; the gene locus is 17q11.2.
- Neurofibromatosis is the most common form of neurofibromatosis, with 50% of cases arising from spontaneous mutation. (That is, there is no family history.)
- The incidence is estimated at 1 in 3000 live births.
- It affects male and female patients equally; there is no racial predilection.
- The pathogenesis is believed to be a defect in the neurofibromin gene.
- Neurofibromin is a suppressor of products of ras protooncogenes, and its loss leads to tumor progression.

SKIN FINDINGS

- Neurofibromatosis presents from birth to early childhood.
- Café au lait macules increase in number and size in the first 5 years of life; more than six suggests the presence of neurofibromatosis-1.
- Axillary or inguinal freckling (Crowe's sign) occurs.
- Dermal and subcutaneous neurofibromas start appearing around puberty and increase in number with age and with pregnancy.
- Plexiform neuromas occur along the course of peripheral nerves, often with overlying hyperpigmentation and hypertrichosis.
- Malignant degeneration of cutaneous neural tumors occurs in 2% of patients but is rare before age 40.

NONSKIN FINDINGS

- Lisch nodules, or asymptomatic iris hamartomas, occur in more than 90% patients over age 6.
- Optic gliomas occur in two thirds of patients; they are asymptomatic but may lead to blindness.
- Other tumors of the central nervous system (CNS) seen with increased frequency include astrocytomas, meningioma, vestibular schwannoma (acoustic neuroma), and ependymoma.
- Patient may have seizures, learning disabilities, incoordination, and hydrocephalus.
- Non-CNS tumors occurring in neurofibromatosis-1 include neurofibrosarcoma, rhabdomyosarcoma, pheochromocytoma, and Wilms' tumor.
- Renovascular abnormalities may include renal artery stenosis.
- Skeletal abnormalities may include short stature, scoliosis, sphenoid wing dysplasia, and macrocephaly.
- Peer relationships and psychosocial adjustment are often major issues during adolescence.

LABORATORY

- Magnetic resonance imaging of the brain and spinal cord is recommended.

COURSE AND PROGNOSIS

- There is great variation in the severity of the disorder.
- Vision and cognitive function may be impaired by CNS tumors.
- Life-threatening complications may include seizures, increased intracranial pressure, vascular complications from hypertension, and malignancy.

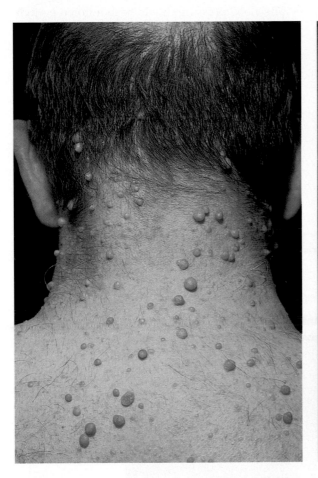

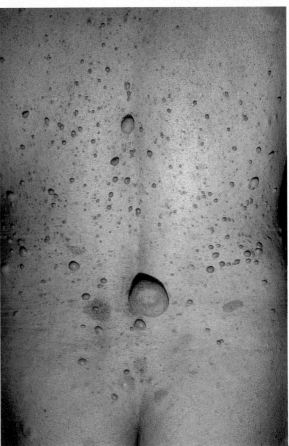

Tumors are usually not present in childhood, but they begin to appear at puberty. Tumors increase in both number and size as the patient ages.

Tumors. The most common is sessile or pedunculated. Early tumors are soft, dome-shaped papules or nodules that have a distinctive violaceous hue. Most are benign.

DISCUSSION

- The differential diagnosis includes other, less common forms of neurofibromatosis, including the McCune-Albright, Noonan, and Proteus syndromes.
- Consensus criteria for diagnosis were adopted in 1987 by the National Institutes of Health. These criteria require two or more of the following features:
  - Six or more café au lait macules over 5 mm in greatest diameter in prepubertal individuals and over 15 mm in greatest diameter in postpubertal individuals
  - Two or more neurofibromas of any type or one plexiform neurofibroma
  - Freckling in the axillary or inguinal regions
  - Optic glioma
  - Two or more Lisch nodules
  - A distinctive osseous lesion such as sphenoid dysplasia or thinning of long bone cortex with or without pseudoarthrosis
  - A first-degree relative with neurofibromatosis-1

TREATMENT

- Care is best performed via a multidisciplinary approach with regular follow-up by the primary care physician, ophthalmologist, neurologist, and dermatologist.
- The head circumference should be monitored closely in children.
- The blood pressure should be monitored periodically.
- Hypertension in a child may indicate renal artery stenosis. In an adult, it may suggest pheochromocytoma.
- The patient should be referred to an orthopedist, a psychiatrist, and a neurosurgeon as indicated.
- First-degree relatives should be screened for cutaneous and ophthalmologic signs of neurofibromatosis.
- Genetic counseling of patients and their families is recommended.
- There is a 50% chance of inheritance with nearly 100% penetrance.

CAVEAT

- Patients and their families should be encouraged to contact local neurofibromatosis support groups.

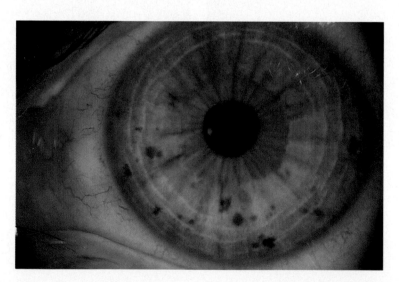

Lisch nodules are pigmented, melanocytic, iris hamartomas. They increase in number with age and are asymptomatic. All adults with neurofibromatosis who are 21 years of age or older have Lisch nodules. Slit-lamp examination is essential for differentiation from iris freckles or nevi.

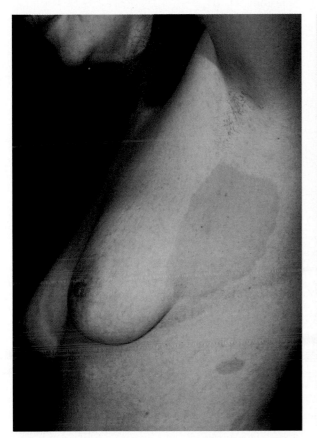

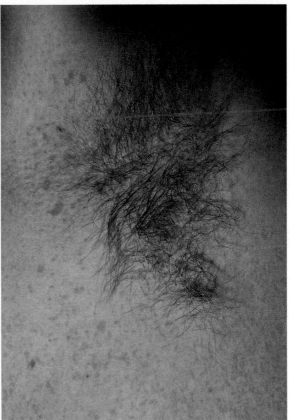

Café au lait spots are light-colored to brown macules. The spots are present, usually at birth, but they may not appear for months. Their size and number increases with age. Presumptive evidence of neurofibromatosis: six or more café au lait macules over 5 mm in greatest diameter if the patient is prepubertal or six or more café au lait macules over 15 mm in greatest diameter if the patient is postpubertal.

Intertriginous freckling, a pathognomonic sign, may occur in the axillae, inframammary region, and groin.

■ TUBEROUS SCLEROSIS

DESCRIPTION

- Tuberous sclerosis is an autosomal dominant inherited disorder with characteristic signs of skin and central nervous system (CNS) problems.

HISTORY

- The incidence is estimated at 1:10,000.
- Male and female patients are affected with equal frequency.
- There is no racial predilection.
- Spontaneous mutations account for 75% of cases.
- Inheritance is autosomal dominant in 25% of cases.
- Two separate genes have been implicated; the locus is 9q34,16p13.
- The pathogenesis is as yet incompletely understood.

SKIN FINDINGS

- The disorder typically presents at birth.
- The earliest sign is the ash-leaf macule: hypopigmented macules on the trunk and extremities.
- Hypopigmented macules are also found in 0.2% to 0.3% of normal neonates but are present in at least half of individuals with tuberous sclerosis.
- Polygonal, hypopigmented "confetti" macules are also common, especially in the pretibial area.
- Facial angiofibromas, so-called adenoma sebaceum, appear in early childhood and increase in number throughout adolescence.
- These benign hamartomas are smooth, firm, pink, 1- to 5-mm papules appearing on the nasolabial folds, cheeks, and chin.
- The shagreen patch is a connective tissue nevus seen in roughly 80% of patients with tuberous sclerosis. Typically located in the lumbosacral area, the shagreen patch is a 1- to 5-cm, white to yellow plaque with a pebbled surface similar to that of tanned pigskin.
- Periungual fibromas are conical, pink, firm projections from the posterior nailfolds of the fingers and toes. They appear around the time of puberty and persist indefinitely.
- Fibrous, flesh-colored, discrete plaques on the forehead are sometimes seen and, if present, are considered to be pathognomonic of tuberous sclerosis.

NONSKIN FINDINGS

- Cortical tubers consisting of astrocytes and giant cells, paraventricular calcification, subependymal hamartomas, and astrocytomas may be seen via imaging studies of the head.
- Seizures occur in 75% of patients with CNS lesions.
- Infantile spasms and mental retardation are also reported.
- Retinal hamartomas (phakomas) may be seen on funduscopic examination.
- Angiomyolipoma and cysts may be seen on renal ultrasound.
- Cardiac rhabdomyoma may be seen by echocardiogram.
- Careful examination of the oral cavity may reveal enamel pits and gingival fibromas.
- Phalangeal cysts and periosteal thickening may be seen on plain films of the hands.
- Pulmonary cysts may be seen on chest film and may occasionally result in spontaneous pneumothorax.

LABORATORY

- Wood's light examination accentuates the appearance of the ash-leaf macules.
- Skin biopsy of ash-leaf macules confirms the presence of melanocytes, thus excluding a diagnosis of vitiligo.
- Skin biopsy of shagreen patches shows an increased number of collagen bundles, which is consistent with connective tissue nevus.
- Transfontanelle ultrasound, computed tomography, and magnetic resonance imaging may demonstrate CNS lesions.
- An electrocardiogram may reveal areas of seizure activity.
- Funduscopic examination confirms the presence of retinal hamartomas.
- Renal ultrasound and echocardiogram should be performed in neonates when the diagnosis of tuberous sclerosis is suspected.

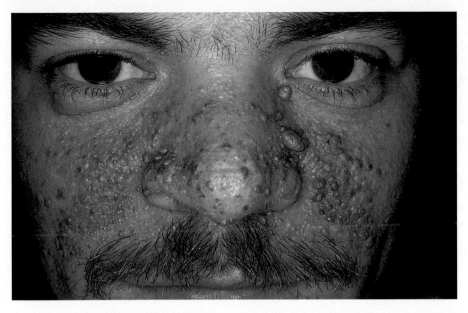

Adenoma sebaceum is the most common cutaneous manifestation of tuberous sclerosis. The lesions consist of smooth, firm, 1- to 5-mm, yellow-pink papules with fine telangiectasia.

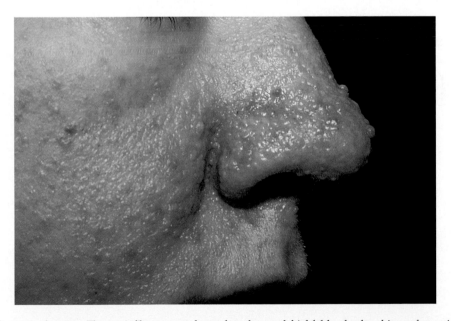

Adenoma sebaceum. The angiofibromas are located on the nasolabial folds, cheeks, chin, and occasionally, forehead, scalp, and ears. The number varies from a few inconspicuous lesions to dense clusters of papules. They are rare at birth but may begin to appear by ages 2 to 3 and proliferate during puberty.

COURSE AND PROGNOSIS

- Some 40% of affected individuals have normal intelligence; the remainder have mild to moderate mental retardation.
- Cutaneous manifestations may not correlate with mental ability.
- Premature death occurs rarely, most often from status epilepticus or malignant brain tumor.

DIFFERENTIAL DIAGNOSIS

- Hypopigmented macules
  - Nevus anemicus
  - Vitiligo
  - Idiopathic guttate hypomelanosis
  - Hypomelanosis of Ito

DISCUSSION

- Nevus anemicus is a functional lesion of normal vasculature, which is abnormally sensitive to circulating catecholamines.
- The other disorders reveal decreased melanocytes and melanosomes.

TREATMENT

- Complete physical examination with routine follow-up by the primary care physician is recommended.
- Imaging studies should be performed to look for visceral and CNS tumors.
- Referral to a pediatric neurologist, including long-term follow-up, should be considered for seizure management.
- Baseline ophthalmologic evaluation should be performed.
- Neurosurgery referral is made for the removal of CNS tumors if indicated.
- Carbon dioxide laser ablation of facial angiofibromas can significantly improve an individual's quality of life and peer interactions.
- If needed, special educational planning should help an individual reach maximal potential.
- Careful cutaneous and general examination of first-degree relatives, as well as genetic counseling, is recommended.

CAVEAT

- Local and national support groups can be valuable sources of information and comfort to affected families.

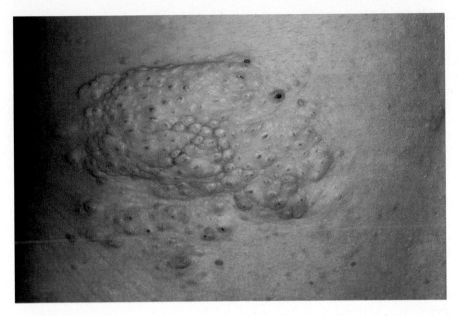

The shagreen patch. There is usually one lesion, but several may be present. They are soft, flesh-colored to yellow plaques with an irregular surface that has been likened to pigskin. The lesion consists of dermal connective tissue and appears most commonly in the lumbosacral region.

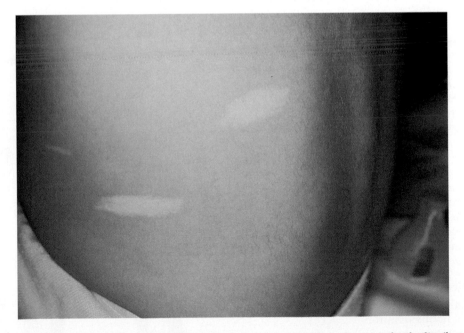

Hypomelanotic macules (oval, ash-leaf shaped, stippled, or confetti shaped) are randomly distributed with a concentration on the arms, legs, and trunk. They are the earliest sign of tuberous sclerosis.

■ GRANULOMA ANNULARE

DESCRIPTION

- Granuloma annulare is a benign, uncommon, slowly progressive, but self-limited disease of unknown etiology.
- It begins with a small, flesh-colored papule or papules and slowly progresses to an irregular ring of firm papules that may spontaneously disappear after a number of years.
- There is a localized and a rare disseminated form.

HISTORY

- Some 70% of patients are younger that 30 years of age, and 40% are younger than 15 years.
- The male/female ratio is 2:1.
- The duration is highly variable; 50% of patients are "clear" in 2 years, but 40% experience recurrence in the same site.

SKIN FINDINGS

- A ring of small, firm, flesh-colored or violaceous papules appears.
- The localized form, most common in young women, is most frequently found on the lateral or dorsal surfaces of the hands and feet.
- The disease begins with an asymptomatic, flesh-colored papule that undergoes central involution. Over months, a ring of papules slowly increases in diameter to 0.5 to 5 cm.
- Disseminated granuloma annulare occurs in adults and appears with numerous flesh-colored or violaceous papules, some of which form annular rings. The papules may be accentuated in sun-exposed areas. The course is variable; many lesions persist for years.

NONSKIN FINDINGS

- There are conflicting reports about the association of granuloma annulare with diabetes mellitus.
- Most patients with the localized form do not have clinical or laboratory evidence of diabetes.
- The association between disseminated granuloma annulare and diabetes has been established, but the frequency is unknown.

LABORATORY

- The clinical presentation is characteristic, and biopsy may not be required.
- Histologic testing shows collagen degeneration, chronic inflammation, and fibrosis.

DIFFERENTIAL DIAGNOSIS

- Necrobiosis lipoidica
- Ring worm pattern of fungal infection (There is no scaling on the border, as is seen in tinea.)

TREATMENT

- Localized lesions are asymptomatic and are best left untreated.
- Group I topical steroids used in 2- to 3-week intervals are sometimes effective. Group II topical steroids with plastic-wrap occlusion for 2 to 8 hours each day for 10 to 14 days is more effective.
- Intralesional triamcinolone acetonide (2.5 to 5 mg/ml) should be injected only into the elevated border. This is predictably effective and induces long periods of remission. Local atrophy is the potential side effect.
- Disseminated granuloma annulare has been reported to respond to dapsone, isotretinoin, etretinate, hydroxychloroquine, and niacinamide.

CAVEAT

- Granuloma annulare is often diagnosed as tinea because of the round pattern. The border of granuloma annulare does not scale, whereas the border of tinea usually does.

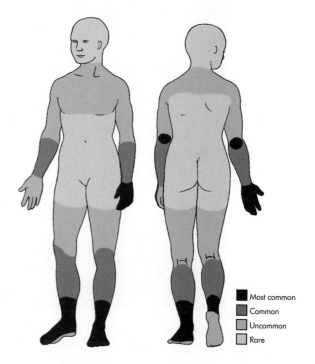

Most common
Common
Uncommon
Rare

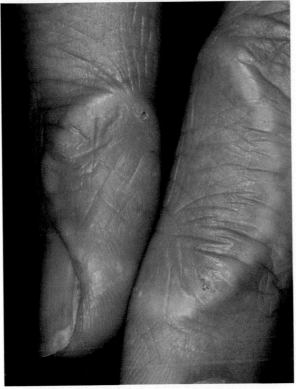

Granuloma annulare. The localized form, most common in young women, is most frequently found on the lateral or dorsal surfaces of the hands and feet.

Granuloma annulare. The disease begins with an asymptomatic, flesh colored papule that undergoes central involution.

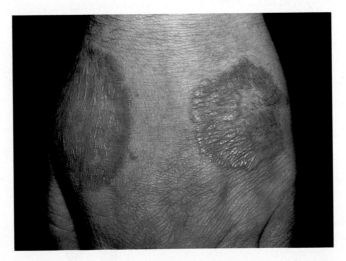

Granuloma annulare. Granuloma annulare is characterized by a ring of small, firm, flesh-colored or red papules.

■ NECROBIOSIS LIPOIDICA

DESCRIPTION

- Necrobiosis lipoidica is an idiopathic inflammatory condition characterized by collagen degeneration (necrobiosis).
- Because of its association with diabetes, necrobiosis lipoidica is often called *necrobiosis lipoidica diabeticorum (NLD);* more than 50% of individuals with necrobiosis lipoidica also have insulin-dependent diabetes.
- Less than 1% of diabetic patients develop necrobiosis lipoidica.

HISTORY

- Lesions usually develop slowly and are often asymptomatic.
- They may appear years before the onset of diabetes.
- The onset may occur at any age but the disease most commonly starts in the third and fourth decades.
- About 75% of those affected are women.

SKIN FINDINGS

- Lesions are often limited to the anterior surfaces of the shins but may be seen on the calves, thighs, arms, hands, feet, and scalp.
- They begin as round, violaceous patches and slowly expand.
- The advancing border is red, and the central area turns a characteristic yellow-brown.
- The central area atrophies and has a shiny, waxy surface with prominent telangiectasias.
- Ulceration may occur, particularly after trauma, in 13% of cases. Ulcerations are usually exquisitely tender.

NONSKIN FINDINGS

- The term *necrobiosis lipoidica diabeticorum* has fallen out of favor because a significant minority of affected individuals do not have diabetes.

LABORATORY

- Clinical features are often so characteristic that biopsy is not required, although in some cases it can be helpful.
- Since NLD may be the presenting sign of diabetes, a glucose tolerance test may be considered.

COURSE AND PROGNOSIS

- The number or severity of lesions or ulcerations has not been correlated with the degree of diabetic control.
- The course is unpredictable; lesions are often chronic.

TREATMENT

- Topical and intralesional steroids arrest inflammation but promote further atrophy.
- Middle-to-high potency corticosteroids are used under occlusion.
- Intralesional injections can be helpful; the concentration of triamcinolone acetonide [Kenalog], 10 mg/ml, should be diluted with saline or xylocaine, up to 2.5 mg/ml, to avoid atrophy.
- A short course (5 to 6 weeks) of oral corticosteroids can be considered if disease activity and symptoms are severe.
- Pentoxifylline (Trental), 400 mg three times a day, is helpful in some and has been used in combination with low-dose aspirin for ulcerating NLD.
- Skin grafting is effective for extensive disease.

CAVEAT

- Patients with NLD without overt diabetes should be evaluated periodically for the development of diabetes.

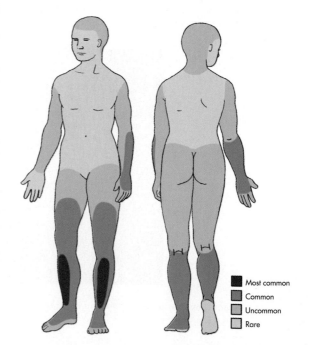

Most common
Common
Uncommon
Rare

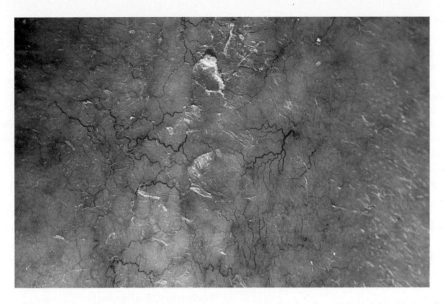

The eruption begins as an oval, violaceous patch and expands slowly. The advancing border is red, and the central area turns yellow-brown. The central area atrophies and has a waxy surface; telangiectasias become prominent.

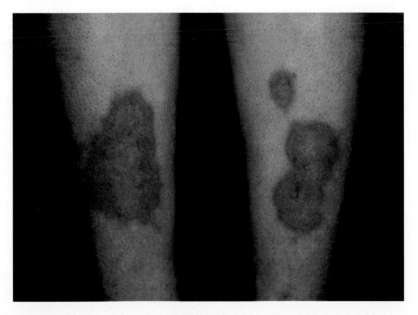

More than 50% of patients with this condition are generally insulin dependent. Most are females, and in most cases the lesions are confined to the anterior surfaces of the lower legs.

LABORATORY

- The diagnosis is based on clinical features, since the pathologic characteristics are nonspecific. Infection should be excluded by appropriate cultures.
- Serum protein electrophoresis may show a monoclonal gammopathy in 10% of patients.
- The sedimentation rate is often elevated.
- Pathologic testing is not specific but can exclude other entities. The ulcer base shows neutrophilic infiltrate with abscess formation; peripherally, infiltrate is mixed and then lymphocytic. Fibrin may be present in vessel walls.

DIFFERENTIAL DIAGNOSIS

- Infection
  - Atypical mycobacteria
  - Gummatous syphilis
  - Amebiasis
  - Deep fungal infection
  - Viral infection
  - Synergistic gangrene
  - Clostridial infection
- Spider bite ischemic ulceration
- Chloroma
- Halogenoderma
- Systemic vasculitis
- Antiphospholipid antibody syndrome
- Neoplasm
- Stasis ulceration

TREATMENT

General Measures

- Any associated conditions should be sought and any infection excluded.
- The patient is taught to protect the lesion, avoid trauma, and get plenty of bed rest.
- Analgesia is often required.
- The ulcer can be treated locally with compresses with silver nitrate (1/8%) or Burow's solution (wet) applied two or three times a day, followed by topical antibacterial creams.
- Hydrocolloid dressings can relieve pain but may result in excess granulation tissue.
- Small lesions may be aborted with intralesional injection of triamcinolone acetonide (Kenalog), 10 or 40 mg/ml.
- Group II to V topical steroids with or without occlusion may be effective.

Systemic Medication

- For larger and rapidly expanding lesions, systemic corticosteroids are usually first-line treatment. Prednisone, 1 mg/kg/day with slow tapering, is required to gain control and effect healing.
- Treatment alternatives include the following:
  - Dapsone, 100 to 400 mg/day, with or without prednisone is effective; it may be steroid sparing.
  - Pulse methylprednisolone, 1000 mg/day for 1 to 5 days, may decrease the side effects of prolonged high-dose oral therapy.
  - Other effective drugs include cyclosporine (5 to 8 mg/kg/day), clofazimine, chlorambucil, minocycline (100 mg twice a day), potassium iodide, topical cromolyn sodium 2% aqueous solution, and thalidomide.

COURSE AND PROGNOSIS

- Pyoderma gangrenosum tends to recur and persist; without treatment, lesions may last from months to years.
- It recurs in approximately 30% of patients.
- Ulcers can expand rapidly, and in such instances, treatment should begin as soon as possible.

DISCUSSION

- Although 50% of cases are idiopathic, patients with pyoderma gangrenosum should be evaluated for associated diseases.

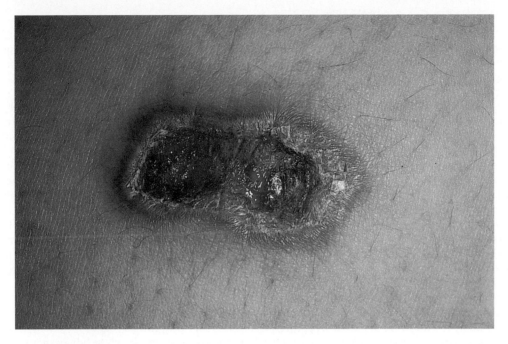

The initiating lesion consists of discrete pustules surrounded by an inflammatory areola. The lesion then degenerates into an ulcer.

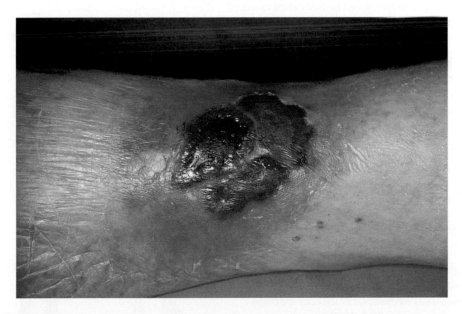

Differentiation from other diseases causing ulcers is sometimes very difficult. Malignancies may present as ulcers with exactly the same appearance. A biopsy is therefore justified.

■ PYODERMA GANGRENOSUM
DESCRIPTION
- Pyoderma gangrenosum is a poorly understood ulcerating skin disease characterized by a rapidly enlarging, exudative ulcer with undermined borders.
- Pathergy (enlargement of the lesion) with trauma is typical.

HISTORY
- Lesions may begin spontaneously or at the site of trauma.
- The majority of cases occur in patients between the ages of 25 and 54. Pyoderma gangrenosum is rare in children.
- The male/female ratio is 1:1.
- A total of 15 cases occur for every ½ million people every 10 years.
- The disease is associated with inflammatory bowel disease, rheumatoid arthritis, chronic active hepatitis, immunoglobulin G monoclonal gammopathy, myelodysplasia, polycythemia rubra vera, paraproteinemia, acute or chronic myeloid leukemia, myeloma (usually, the immunoglobulin A type), Waldenström's macroglobulinemia, and myelofibrosis. Lymphoma and solid tumors (colon, bladder, prostate, breast, bronchus, ovary) are less common but have been described.
- Postsurgical pyoderma gangrenosum may masquerade as wound dehiscence or infection.

SKIN FINDINGS
- The most common sites are the lower legs, buttocks, and abdomen; it is rare to see pyoderma gangrenosum on the face.
- The lesion begins as a very tender, red or dusky macule, papule, pustule, nodule, or bulla.
- The initial lesion is often described as a pustule or inflamed nodule that then ulcerates, forming an extremely painful, sharply marginated, violaceous bordered ulcer with a purulent base.
- The edge of the ulcer is elevated (undermined) and violaceous and may have tiny pustules along the border.
- Ulceration and expansion can occur rapidly.
- The fully evolved, classic ulcerated lesion is generally smaller than 10 cm.
- Lesions heal with irregular, cribriform scarring.

- There are four clinical variants:
  - In the ulcerative form, there is skin ulceration with a purulent base and an undermined, violaceous border. Arthritis, monoclonal gammopathy, and inflammatory bowel disease may be associated with this variant.
  - In the pustular form, discrete tender pustules with inflammatory borders appear. This variant may be associated with inflammatory bowel disease.
  - The bullous form is characterized by tender bullae that erode and lead to superficial ulceration. Often, myeloproliferative disorder is present.
  - The vegetative form extends peripherally from the primary lesion, resulting in a necrotic ulcer or ulcers with purulent bases; undetermined, purple to red margins; and erythematous halos.

NONSKIN FINDINGS
- Findings not involving the skin are uncommon; occasionally, fatigue occurs.
- See sections on associated diseases.

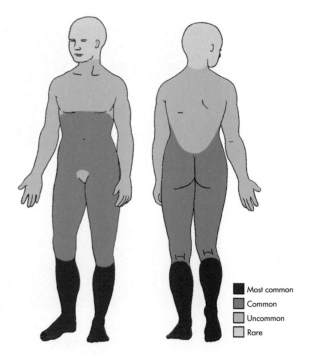

Most common
Common
Uncommon
Rare

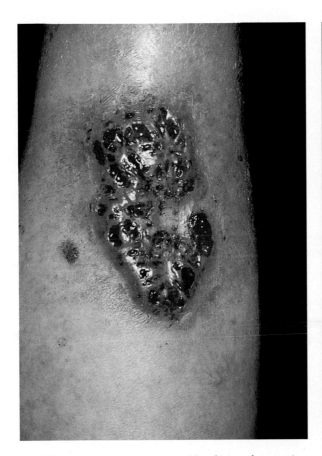

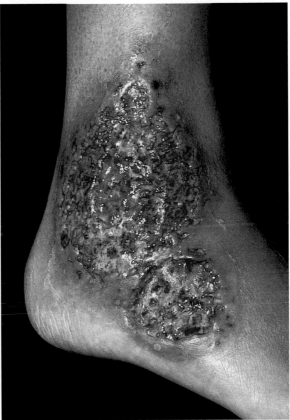

The legs are the most common site. New lesions form at sites of injury a phenomenon called *pathergy*. The new lesions become much large than the lesion created by the initial injury.

Eventually a lesion with multiple ulcers with craterlike holes form. This is a highly characteristic feature. The lesions consist of small fistula tracks from which pus can be obtained with pressure.

Appendixes

A

Primary, Secondary, and Special Lesions *

■ PRIMARY LESIONS

Most skin diseases begin with a basic lesion that is referred to as a *primary lesion*. Identification of the primary lesion is the key to accurate interpretation and description of cutaneous disease. Its presence provides the initial orientation and allows the formulation of a differential diagnosis. Definitions of the primary lesions and their differential diagnoses follow.

■ SECONDARY LESIONS

Secondary lesions develop during the evolutionary process of skin disease or are created by scratching or infection. They may be the only type of lesion present, in which case the primary disease process must be inferred. The differential diagnoses of secondary lesions follow.

■ SPECIAL LESIONS

A certain number of unique structures and changes called *special lesions* occur. The lesions and their definitions follow.

■ PRIMARY SKIN LESIONS
MACULE AND PATCH

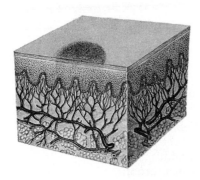

A circumscribed, flat discoloration. A macule is smaller than 0.5 cm, and a patch is larger than 0.5 cm. They that may be brown, blue, red, or hypopigmented

Brown
Becker's nevus
Café au lait spot
Erythrasma
Fixed drug eruption
Freckle
Junction nevus
Lentigo
Lentigo maligna
Melasma
Photoallergic drug eruption
Phototoxic drug eruption
Stasis dermatitis
Tinea nigra palmaris

Blue
Ink (tattoo)
Maculae ceruleae (lice)

Mongolian spot

Red
Drug eruptions
Juvenile rheumatoid arthritis
Rheumatic fever
Secondary syphilis
Viral exanthems

Hypopigmented
Idiopathic guttate hypomelanosis
Nevus anemicus
Piebaldism
Postinflammatory psoriasis
Radiation dermatitis
Tinea versicolor
Tuberous sclerosis
Vitiligo

*Art from Seidel HM et al: *Mosby's guide to physical examination*, ed 4, St Louis, 1999, Mosby.

PAPULE

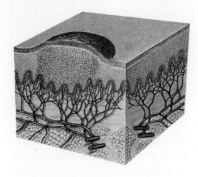

A palpable lesion up to 0.5 cm in diameter; color varies; papules may become confluent and form plaques

Flesh Colored, Yellow, or White

Achrochordon (skin tag)
Adenoma sebaceum
Basal cell epithelioma
Closed comedo (acne)
Flat warts
Granuloma annulare
Lichen nitidus
Lichen sclerosis et atrophicus
Milium
Molluscum contagiosum
Neurofibroma
Nevi (dermal)
Pearly penile papules
Pseudoxanthoma elasticum
Sebaceous hyperplasia
Skin tags
Syringoma

Brown

Dermatofibroma
Keratosis follicularis
Melanoma
Nevi
Seborrheic keratosis
Urticaria pigmentosa
Warts

Red

Acne
Atopic dermatitis
Cat-scratch disease
Cherry angioma
Cholinergic urticaria
Chondrodermatitis helicis
Eczema
Folliculitis
Insect bites
Keratosis pilaris
Leukocytoclastic vasculitis
Miliaria
Polymorphous light eruption
Psoriasis
Pyogenic granuloma
Scabies
Urticaria

Blue or Violaceous

Angiokeratoma
Blue nevus
Lichen planus
Lymphoma
Kaposi's sarcoma
Melanoma
Mycosis fungoides
Venous lake

PLAQUE

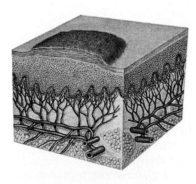

A circumscribed, palpable, solid lesion more than 0.5 cm in diameter, often formed by the confluence of papules

Eczema
Cutaneous T-cell lymphoma
Discoid lupus erythematosus
Lichen planus
Paget's disease
Papulosquamous (papular and scaling lesions)
Pityriasis rosea
Psoriasis
Seborrheic dermatitis
Sweet's syndrome
Syphilis (secondary)
Tinea corporis
Tinea versicolor

NODULE

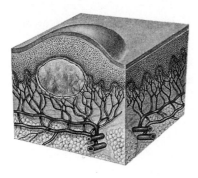

A circumscribed, often round, solid lesion more than 0.5 cm in diameter; a large nodule is referred to as a *tumor*

Basal cell carcinoma
Cutaneous T-cell lymphoma
Erythema nodosum
Furuncle
Hemangioma
Kaposi's sarcoma
Keratoacanthoma
Lipoma
Lymphoma
Melanoma
Metastatic carcinoma
Neurofibromatosis
Prurigo nodularis
Sporotrichosis
Squamous cell carcinoma
Warts
Xanthoma

PUSTULE

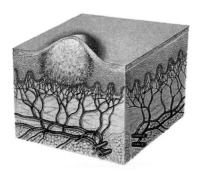

A circumscribed collection of leukocytes and free fluid that varies in size

Acne
Candidiasis
Chicken pox
Dermatophyte infection
Dyshidrosis
Folliculitis
Gonococcemia
Hidradenitis suppurativa
Herpes simplex
Herpes zoster
Impetigo
Keratosis pilaris
Pseudomonas folliculitis
Psoriasis
Pyoderma gangrenosum
Rosacea
Scabies
Varicella

VESICLE

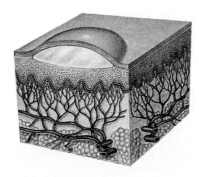

A circumscribed collection of free fluid up to 0.5 cm in diameter

Benign familial chronic pemphigus
Cat-scratch disease
Chicken pox
Dermatitis herpetiformis
Eczema (acute)
Erythema multiforme
Herpes simplex
Herpes zoster
Impetigo
Lichen planus
Pemphigus foliaceus
Porphyria cutanea tarda
Scabies

Bulla

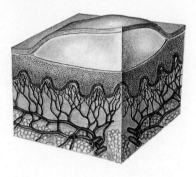

A circumscribed collection of free fluid more than 0.5 cm in diameter

Bullae in diabetics
Bullous pemphigoid
Cicatricial pemphigoid

Epidermolysis bullosa acquisita
Fixed drug eruption
Herpes gestationis
Lupus erythematosus
Pemphigus

Wheal (Hive)

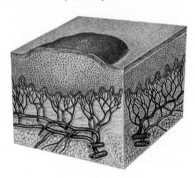

A firm edematous papule or plaque resulting from infiltration of the dermis with fluid; wheals are transient and may last only a few hours

Angioedema
Cholinergic urticaria
Dermographism
Hives
Urticaria pigmentosa (mastocytosis)

■ SECONDARY SKIN LESIONS
Scales

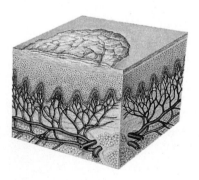

Fine to Stratified
Erythema craquelé
Ichthyosis: dominant (quadrangular)
Ichthyosis: sex-linked (quadrangular)
Lupus erythematosus (carpet tack)
Pityriasis rosea (collarette)
Psoriasis (silvery)
Scarlet fever (fine, on trunk)
Seborrheic dermatitis

Syphilis (secondary)
Tinea (dermatophytes)
Tinea versicolor
Xerosis (dry skin)

Scaling in Sheets (Desquamation)
Kawasaki syndrome
Scarlet fever (hands and feet)
Staphylococcal scalded skin syndrome
Toxic shock syndrome

CRUST

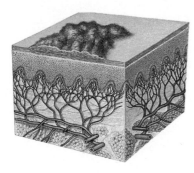

A collection of dried serum and cellular debris; a scab

Acute eczematous inflammation
Atopic (face)

Impetigo (honey colored)
Pemphigus foliaceus
Tinea capitis

EROSION

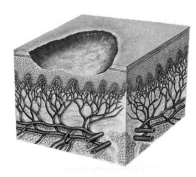

A focal loss of epidermis; erosions do not penetrate below the dermoepidermal junction and therefore heal without scarring

Candidiasis
Dermatophyte infection
Eczematous diseases
Herpes simplex

Intertrigo
Neurotic excoriations
Perlèche
Senile skin
Toxic epidermal necrolysis
Vesiculobullous diseases

ULCER

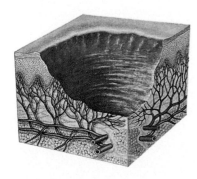

A focal loss of epidermis and dermis; ulcers heal with scarring

Aphthae
Chancroid
Decubitus
Factitial

Ischemic
Necrobiosis lipoidica
Neoplasms
Pyoderma gangrenosum
Radiation dermatitis
Stasis ulcers
Syphilis (chancre)

FISSURE

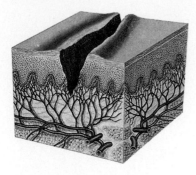

A linear loss of epidermis and dermis with sharply defined, nearly vertical walls

Chapping (hands, feet)
Eczema (fingertip)
Intertrigo
Perlèche

ATROPHY

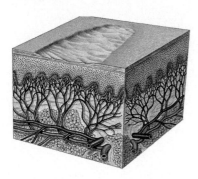

A depression in the skin resulting from thinning of the epidermis or dermis

Aging
Dermatomyositis
Discoid lupus erythematosus
Lichen sclerosis et atrophicus

Morphea
Necrobiosis lipoidica diabeticorum
Radiation dermatitis
Striae
Topical and intralesional steroids

SCAR

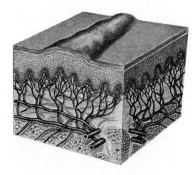

An abnormal formation of connective tissue implying dermal damage; after injury or surgery, scars are initially thick and pink but with time become white and atrophic

Acne
Burns
Herpes zoster
Hidradenitis suppurativa
Keloid
Porphyria
Varicella

■ SPECIAL SKIN LESIONS

DESCRIPTION	DIFFERENTIAL DIAGNOSIS

EXCORIATION
An erosion caused by scratching; excoriations are often linear

Scabies
Atopic dermatitis
Primary pruritus
Dermatitis herpetiformis
Prurigo
Acne excor
Dry skin

COMEDO
A plug of sebaceous and keratinous material lodged in the opening of a hair follicle; the follicular orifice may be dilated (blackhead) or narrowed (whitehead or closed comedo)

Acne
Epidermal cyst
Discoid lupus erythematosus
Solar comedones

MILIA
A small, superficial keratin cyst with no visible opening

Chronic solar damage
Porphyria cutanea tarda
Inherited blistering disorders

CYST
A circumscribed lesion with a wall and a lumen; the lumen may contain fluid or solid matter

Epidermal
Pilar

BURROW
A narrow, elevated, tortuous channel produced by a parasite

Scabies
Creeping eruption

LICHENIFICATION
An area of thickened epidermis induced by scratching; the skin lines are accentuated so that the surface looks like a washboard

Atopic dermatitis
Lichen simplex chronicus
Chronic eczematous dermatitis

TELANGIECTASIA
Dilated superficial blood vessels

Actinically damaged skin
Adenoma sebaceum
Ataxia-telangiectasia
Basal cell carcinoma
Bloom's syndrome
CREST syndrome
Hereditary hemorrhagic
  telangiectasia
Keloid
Lupus erythematosus
Necrobiosis lipoidica diabeticorum

Continued

■ SPECIAL SKIN LESIONS—cont'd

DESCRIPTION	DIFFERENTIAL DIAGNOSIS

TELANGIECTASIA—CONT'D
Dilated superficial blood vessels—cont'd

Of the proximal nailfold
    Dermatomyositis
    Lupus erythematosus
    Scleroderma
Poikiloderma
Radiation dermatitis
Rosacea
Scleroderma
Vascular spiders
    Pregnancy
    Cirrhosis
Xeroderma pigmentosum

PETECHIAE
A circumscribed deposit of blood less than 0.5 cm in diameter

Gonococcemia
    Leukocytoclastic vasculitis
    Meningococcemia

PURPURA
A circumscribed deposit of blood greater than 0.5 cm in diameter

Platelet abnormalities
    Progressive pigmentary
      purpura
    Rocky Mountain spotted fever
    Scurvy
    Senile traumatic purpura
    Vascular spider

Differential Diagnoses
by Body Region

Common and important diseases are included. Body regions and then diseases are listed alphabetically. Some common diseases that are obvious to most practitioners are not included.

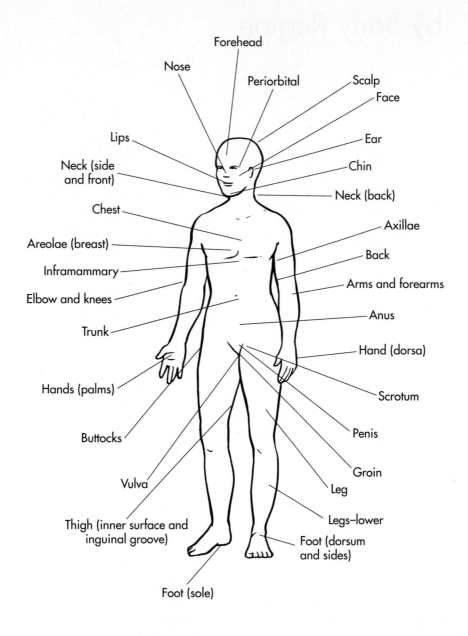

Anus

Hidradenitis suppurativa
Lichen sclerosis et atrophicus
Lichen simplex chronicus
Psoriasis (gluteal pinking)
Streptococcal cellulitis
Vitiligo
Warts

Areolae (Breast)

Eczema
Paget's disease
Seborrheic keratosis

Arms and Forearms

Acne
Atopic dermatitis
Dermatitis herpetiformis (elbows)
Dermatomyositis
Erythema multiforme
Granuloma annulare
Insect bite
Keratoacanthoma
Keratosis pilaris
Lichen planus
Neurotic excoriations
Nummular eczema
Pityriasis alba (white spots)
Polymorphic light eruption
Prurigo nodularis
Purpura (in sun damaged skin)
Scabies
Seborrheic keratosis (flat)
Squamous cell carcinoma
Stellate pseudo scars
Sweet's syndrome
Tinea

Axillae

Acanthosis nigricans
Acrochordons
Candidiasis
Contact dermatitis
Erythrasma
Freckling: Crowe's sign (von Recklinghausen's disease)
Furunculosis
Hailey-Hailey disease

Hidradenitis suppurativa
Impetigo
Lice
Trichomycosis axillaris

Back

Acne
Becker's nevus
Cutaneous T-cell lymphoma
Dermatographism
Keloids (acne scars)
Melanoma
Nevus anemicus
Seborrheic keratosis
Tinea versicolor

Buttocks

Cutaneous T-cell lymphoma
Furunculosis
Herpes simplex (females)
Hidradenitis suppurativa
Psoriasis
Tinea

Chest

Acne
Actinic keratosis
Darier's disease
Eruptive syringoma
Keloids
Seborrheic dermatitis
Steatocystoma multiplex
Tinea versicolor
Transient acantholytic dermatitis (Grover's disease)

Chin

Acne
Atopic dermatitis
Impetigo
Perioral dermatitis
Warts (flat)

Ear

Actinic keratosis
Basal cell carcinoma
Cellulitis
Chondrodermatitis nodularis chronica helicis

Eczema (infected)
Epidermal cyst
Keloid (lobe)
Lupus erythematosus (discoid)
Psoriasis
Ramsey-Hunt syndrome (herpes zoster)
Seborrheic dermatitis
Squamous cell carcinoma
Venous lake

Elbows and Knees

Dermatitis herpetiformis
Lichen simplex chronicus
Psoriasis

Face

Actinic keratosis
Adenoma sebaceum
Angioedema
Atopic dermatitis
Basal cell carcinoma
Cowden's disease
Eczema
Erysipelas
Favre-Racouchot (solar comedones)
Herpes zoster
Impetigo
Lentigo maligna
Lupus erythematosus (discoid)
Lupus erythematosus (systemic)
Melasma
Molluscum contagiosum
Nevus sebaceus
Perioral dermatitis
Pityriasis alba (white spots)
Psoriasis
Sebaceous hyperplasia
Seborrheic dermatitis
Seborrheic keratosis
Spitz nevus
Squamous cell carcinoma
Steroid rosacea
Sycosis barbae (folliculitis [beard])
Tinea
Warts (flat)

Foot (Dorsum and Sides)

Contact dermatitis
Cutaneus larva migrans
Erythema multiforme
Granuloma annulare
Hand, foot, and mouth disease
Lichen simplex chronicus
Stucco keratosis
Tinea

Foot (Sole)

Cutaneus larva migrans
Dyshidrotic eczema
Erythema multiforme
Hand, foot, and mouth disease
Hyperkeratosis
Juvenile plantar dermatosis
Melanoma
Nevi
Pitted keratolysis
Psoriasis (pustular)
Scabies (infants)
Syphilis (secondary)
Tinea
Wart

Forehead

Actinic keratosis
Basal cell carcinoma
Flat warts
Herpes zoster
Psoriasis
Sebaceous hyperplasia
Seborrheic dermatitis
Seborrheic keratosis

Groin

Acrochordons (skin tags)
Candidiasis
Condyloma
Erythrasma
Extramammary Paget's disease
Hidradenitis suppurativa
Intertrigo
Lichen simplex chronicus
Molluscum contagiosum
Psoriasis (without scale)
Seborrheic keratosis
Striae (topical steroids)
Tinea

Hand (Dorsa)

Actinic keratosis
Atopic dermatitis
Contact dermatitis
Cowden's disease
Erythema multiforme
Granuloma annulare
Keratoacanthoma
Lentigo
Paronychia (acute, chronic)
Polymorphous light eruption
Porphyria cutanea tarda
Psoriasis
Scabies
Seborrheic keratosis
Squamous cell carcinoma
Stucco keratosis
Tinea
Vesicular "id reaction"

Hands (Palms)

Basal cell nevus syndrome (pits)
Calluses/corns
Contact dermatitis
Cowden's disease
Dyshidrotic eczema
Eczema
Erythema multiforme
Hand, foot, and mouth disease
Keratolysis exfoliativa
Pompholyx
Psoriasis
Pyogenic granuloma
Rocky Mountain spotted fever
Scabies (infants)
Syphilis (secondary)
Tinea
Vesicular "id reaction"
Wart

Inframammary

Acrochordon (skin tags)
Candidiasis
Contact dermatitis
Intertrigo
Psoriasis (without scale)
Seborrheic keratoses
Tinea versicolor

Leg

Basal cell carcinoma
Bowen's disease
Eruptive xanthomas
Kaposi's sarcoma
Livedo reticularis
Melanoma
Nummular eczema
Panniculitis
Prurigo nodularis
Pyoderma gangrenosum
Squamous cell carcinoma

Leg (Lower)

Bites
Cellulitis
Dermatofibroma
Diabetic bullae
Diabetic dermopathy (shin spots)
Erysipelas
Erythema nodosum
Flat warts
Folliculitis
Granuloma annulare
Henoch-Schönlein purpura
Ichthyosis vulgaris
Idiopathic guttate hypomel-anosis
Leukocytoclastic vasculitis
Lichen planus
Lichen simplex chronicus
Majocchi's granuloma (tinea)
Necrobiosis lipoidica
Schamberg's purpura
Stasis dermatitis
Vasculitis (nodular lesions)
Xerosis

Lips

Actinic cheilitis
Allergic contact dermatitis
Angioedema
Aphthous ulcer
Fordyce's spots (upper lips)
Herpes simplex
Labial melanotic macule
Leukoplakia
Mucous cyst
Perlèche

Pyogenic granuloma
Squamous cell carcinoma
Venous lake
Wart

Neck (Side and Front)

Acanthosis nigricans
Acne
Acrochordon (skin tags)
Atopic dermatitis
Berloque dermatitis
Contact dermatitis
Epidermal cyst
Folliculitis
Poikiloderma of Civatte
Pseudofolliculitis
Pseudoxanthoma elasticum
Sycosis barbae (fungal, bacterial)
Tinea
Wart

Neck (Back)

Acne
Acne keloidalis
Cutis rhomboidalis nuchae
Epidermal cyst
Folliculitis
Furunculosis
Lichen simplex chronicus
Neurotic excoriations
Salmon patch
Tinea

Nose

Acne
Actinic keratosis
Basal cell carcinoma
Discoid lupus erythematosus
Herpes simplex
Impetigo
Nevus
Rhinophyma
Rosacea
Seborrheic dermatitis
Squamous cell carcinoma
Telangiectasias

Penis

Candidiasis (under foreskin)
Chancroid

Condyloma (warts)
Contact dermatitis (from
    condoms)
Erythroplasia of Queyrat
    (Bowen's disease)
Fixed drug eruption
Herpes simplex
Herpes zoster
Lichen planus
Lichen sclerosis et atrophicus
    (balanitis xerotica obliterans)
Molluscum contagiosum
Nevus
Pearly penile papules
Penile melanosis
Psoriasis
Scabies
Sclerosing lymphangitis (non-
    venereal)
Seborrheic keratosis
Squamous cell carcinoma
Syphilis (chancre)

Periorbital Area

Acrochordons (skin tags)
Angioedema
Atopic dermatitis
Contact dermatitis
Dermatomyositis
Milia
Molluscum contagiosum
Seborrheic dermatitis
Senile comedones
Syringoma
Xanthelasma

Scalp

Actinic keratosis
Alopecia neoplastica
    (metastases)
Basal cell carcinoma
Contact dermatitis
Folliculitis
Kerion (inflammatory tinea)
Lichen planopilaris
Lupus erythematosus (discoid)
Neurotic excoriations
Nevi
Nevus sebaceus
Pediculosis capitis

Pilar cyst (wen)
Prurigo nodularis
Psoriasis
Seborrheic dermatitis
Seborrheic keratosis
Tinea

Scrotum

Angiokeratoma of Fordyce
Condyloma
Epidermal cyst
Extramammary Paget's disease
Lichen simplex chronicus
Nevus
Scabies
Seborrheic keratosis

Thigh (Inner Surface and Inguinal Groove)

Acrochordons (skin tags)
Candidiasis
Eczema
Erythrasma
Extramammary Paget's disease
Fissures
Hidradenitis suppurativa
Intertrigo
Tinea

Trunk

Accessory nipple
Ash leaf spot
Atopic dermatitis
Capillary hemangiomas
Chickenpox
Cutaneous T-cell lymphoma
    (mycosis fungoides)
Drug eruption (maculopapular)
Epidermal cyst
Familial atypical mole syndrome
Fixed drug eruption
Folliculitis (classic and hot tub)
Granuloma annulare
    (generalized)
Halo nevus
Herpes zoster
Keloids
Lichen planus (generalized)
Lichen sclerosis et atrophicus

Lupus erythematosus (subacute cutaneous)
Miliaria
Nevus anemicus
Pediculosis (lice)
Pemphigus foliaceous
Pityriasis rosea
Pityrosporum folliculitis
Poikiloderma vasculare atrophicans
Psoriasis (guttate)
Scabies
Seborrheic dermatitis
Steatocystoma multiplex
Syphilis (secondary)

Tinea
Tinea versicolor
Transient acantholytic dermatosis (Grover's disease)
Urticaria pigmentosa
Viral exanthem
von Recklinghausen's neurofibromatosis

Vulva

Allergic contact dermatitis
Angiokeratoma of Fordyce
Candidiasis
Chancroid
Epidermal cyst

Erythrasma
Extramammary Paget's disease
Fibroepithelial polyp
Furunculosis
Hidradenitis suppurativa
Intertrigo
Leukoplakia
Lichen planus
Lichen sclerosis et atrophicus
Lichen simplex chronicus
Molluscum contagiosum
Nevus
Pediculosis
Psoriasis
Warts

C

Quantity of Cream
to Apply and Dispense

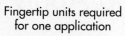

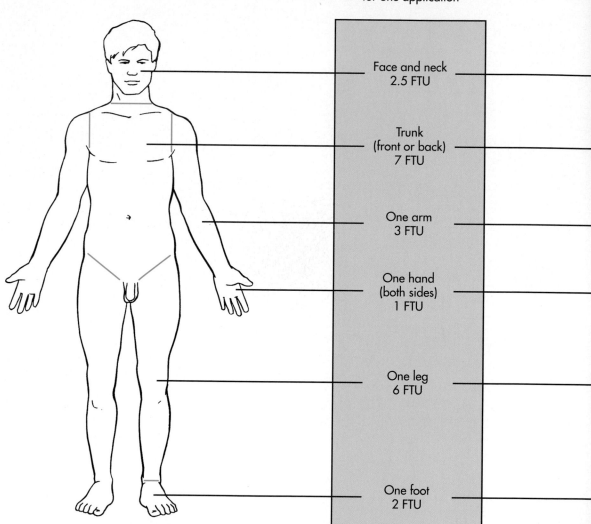

Fingertip units required
for one application

Face and neck
2.5 FTU

Trunk
(front or back)
7 FTU

One arm
3 FTU

One hand
(both sides)
1 FTU

One leg
6 FTU

One foot
2 FTU

Modified from Long CC, Finlay AY: *Clin Exp Dermatol* 16:444-447, 1991.

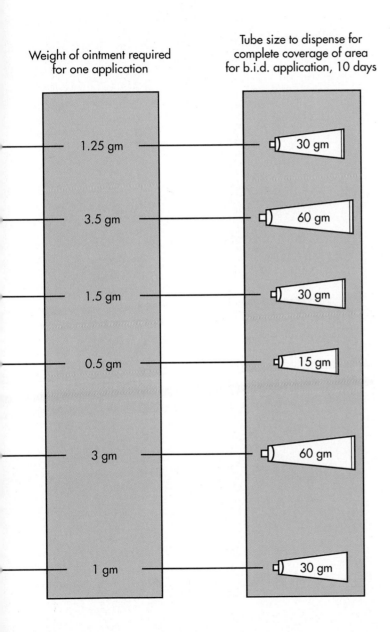

Weight of ointment required
for one application

Tube size to dispense for
complete coverage of area
for b.i.d. application, 10 days

1.25 gm — 30 gm

3.5 gm — 60 gm

1.5 gm — 30 gm

0.5 gm — 15 gm

3 gm — 60 gm

1 gm — 30 gm

Fingertip Unit (FTU)

The amount of ointment expressed
from tube applied to the fingertip.
One FTU weighs about 0.5 gm.

**Hand Unit (one side
of the hand)**

½ FTU covers 1 side of the hand
½ FTU weighs 0.25 gm

0.25 gm × Number of hand units =
Weight of cream required
for one application

Corticosteroids

■ TOPICAL

Group I: Super potency   Group II: High potency   Group III-V: Medium potency   Group VI-VII: Low potency

GROUP	BRAND NAME	%	GENERIC NAME	TUBE SIZE (GM; UNLESS NOTED)
I (super)	Cormax Scalp Appl.	0.05	Clobetasol propionate USP	25 ml, 50 ml
	Cormax cream	0.05		15 , 30 , 45
	Cormax ointment	0.05		15 g, 45
	Cordran Tape	—	Flurandrenolide	24" and 80" rolls, (12) 2" × 3" patches
	Temovate cream	0.05		15, 30, 45, 60
	Embeline E cream	0.05	Clobetasol propionate	15 , 30, 45
	Temovate ointment	0.05		15, 30, 45, 60
	Temovate gel	0.05		15, 30, 60
	Temovate emollient	0.05		15, 30, 60
	Temovate solution	0.05		25, 50 ml
	Ultravate cream	0.05	Halobetasol propionate	15, 50
	Ultravate ointment	0.05		15, 50
	Diprolene lotion	0.05	Augmented betamethasone dipropionate	30 ml, 60 ml
	Diprolene ointment	0.05		15, 45
	Diprolene gel	0.05		15, 45
	Psorcon E cream	0.05	Diflorasone diacetate	15, 30, 60
	Psorcon E ointment	0.05	Diflorasone diacetate	15, 30, 60
II (high)	Cyclocort ointment	0.1	Amcinonide	15, 30, 60
	Diprolene AF cream	0.05	Augmented betamethasone dipropionate	15, 50
	Diprosone ointment	0.05	Betamethasone dipropionate	15, 45
	Halog cream	0.1	Halcinonide	15, 30, 60, 240
	Halog ointment	0.1		15, 30, 60, 240
	Halog solution	0.1		20, 60 ml
	Halog-E cream	0.1		15, 30, 60
	Lidex cream	0.05	Fluocinonide	15, 30, 60, 120
	Lidex gel	0.05		15, 30, 60
	Lidex ointment	0.05		15, 30, 60, 120
	Lidex solution	0.05		20, 60 ml
	Lidex-E cream	0.05		15, 30, 60
	Topicort cream	0.25	Desoximetasone	15, 60
	Topicort gel	0.05		15, 60
	Topicort ointment	0.25		15, 60
III (medium)	Cutivate ointment	0.005	Fluticasone propionate	15, 30, 60
	Cyclocort lotion	0.1	Amcinonide	20, 60 ml
	Diprosone cream	0.05	Betamethasone dipropionate	15, 45
	Elocon ointment	0.1	Mometasone furoate	15, 45
	Florone cream	0.05	Diflorasone diacetate	15, 30, 60
	Florone E emollient	0.05		15, 30, 60

Continued

■ TOPICAL—cont'd

Group	Brand Name	%	Generic Name	Tube Size (gm; Unless Noted)
IV (medium)	Cordran ointment	0.05	Flurandrenolide	15, 30, 60
	Cyclocort cream	0.1	Amcinonide	15, 30, 60
	Elocon cream	0.1	Mometasone furoate	15, 45
	Elocon lotion	0.1		30, 60 ml
	Kenalog ointment	0.1	Triamcinolone acetonide	15, 60, 80, 240
	Synalar ointment	0.025	Fluocinolone acetonide	15, 60
	Westcort ointment	0.2	Hydrocortisone	15, 45, 60
V (medium)	Aristocort A	0.1	Triamcinolone acetonide	15, 60, 240
	Cordran cream	0.05	Flurandrenolide	15, 30, 60
	Cordran lotion	0.05		15, 60 ml
	Cutivate cream	0.05	Fluticasone propionate	15, 30, 60
	Dermatop cream	0.1	Prednicarbate	15, 60
	Kenalog cream	0.1	Triamcinolone acetonide	15, 80, 454
	Kenalog lotion	0.1		60 ml
	Kenalog ointment	0.025		15
	Locoid Lipocream	0.1	Hydrocortisone butyrate	15, 45
	Synalar cream	0.025	Fluocinolone acetonide	15, 60
	Valisone cream	0.1	Betamethasone valerate	15, 45
	Valisone lotion	0.1		20, 60 ml
	Westcort cream	0.2	Hydrocortisone	15, 45, 60
VI (low)	Aclovate cream	0.05	Prednicarbate	15, 60
	Aclovate ointment	0.05	Prednicarbate	15, 60
	DesOwen cream	0.05	Desonide	15, 60, 90
	DesOwen ointment			15, 60
	DesOwen lotion			2, 4 oz
	Kenalog cream	0.025	Triamcinolone acetonide	15, 60, 80
	Synalar solution	0.01		20, 60 ml

VII (low)
Topical with hydrocortisone, dexamethasone, flumethasone, prednisolone, and methylprednisolone
The potency of Luxiq (betamethasone valerate foam) has not been classified.

■ ORAL

Generic Name	Brand Name	Preparation	Equivalent Dose (mg)
Betamethasone	Celestone	0.6 mg, 0.6 mg/5 ml	0.6
Dexamethasone	Decadron	0.25, 0.5, 0.75, 1.5, 4, 6 mg	0.75
Dexamethasone	Hexadrol	0.5, 0.75, 1.5, 4 mg, 5 mg/5 ml	0.75
Methylprednisolone	Medrol	2, 4, 8, 16, 24, 32 mg	4
Prednisolone	Delta-Cortef	5 mg	5
	Prelone	15 mg/5 ml	5
Prednisone	Deltasone	1, 2.5, 5, 10, 20, 50 mg	5
	Liquid Pred	5 mg/5 ml	5
	Meticorten	1, 5 mg	5
	Orasone	1, 5, 10, 20, 50 mg	5
Triamcinolone	Aristocort	1, 2, 4, 8, 16 mg, 2 mg/5 ml	4
	Kenacort	1, 2, 4, 8 mg, 4 mg/5 ml	4

Dermatologic Formulary

■ ACNE AND ROSACEA MEDICATIONS
RETINOIDS, TRETINOIN AND RELATED COMPOUNDS WITH COMEDOLYTIC ACTIVITY

PRODUCT	BASE	CONCENTRATION	PACKAGING	
Retin-A (tretinoin)	Cream	0.025%	20 gm	45 gm
		0.05%	20 gm	45 gm
		0.1%	20 gm	45 gm
	Gel	0.01%	15 gm	45 gm
		0.025%	15 gm	45 gm
	Liquid	0.05%	28 ml	—
Retin-A Micro (tretinoin)	Gel	0.1%	20 gm	45 gm
Avita (tretinoin)	Cream	0.025%	20 gm	45 gm
	Gel	0.025%	20 gm	45 gm
Tazorac (tazarotene)	Gel	0.05%	30 gm	100 gm
		0.1%	30 gm	100 gm
Differin (adapalene)	Gel	0.1%	15 gm	45 gm
	Solution	0.1%	30 ml	—
	Pledgets	0.1%	#60	—
Azelex	Cream	20%	30 gm	50 gm

BENZOYL PEROXIDE CLEANSERS

PRODUCT	FORMULATION	PACKAGING
Benzac AC wash 2.5%	Liquid 2.5%	8 oz
Benzac AC wash 5%	Liquid 5%	8 oz
Benzac AC wash 10%	Liquid 10%	8 oz
Benzac W wash	Liquid 5%	4 oz, 8 oz
Benzac W wash	Liquid 10%	8 oz
Brevoxyl Cleansing Lotion (Rx)	Liquid 4%	10.5 oz
Brevoxyl Creamy wash	Liquid 4%	6 oz
Brevoxyl Cleansing Lotion	Liquid 8%	10.5 oz
Brevoxyl Creamy wash	Liquid 8%	6 oz
Desquam-X 5% wash	Liquid 5%	150 ml
Desquam-X 10% wash	Liquid 10%	150 ml
Desquam-X 10% bar (Rx)	Bar 10%	4-oz bar
PanOxyl 5 bar (OTC)	Bar 5%	4-oz bar
PanOxyl 10 bar (OTC)	Bar 10%	4-oz bar
Triaz cleanser 3%	Liquid 3%	6 oz, 12 oz
Triaz cleanser 6%	Liquid 6%	6 oz, 12 oz
Triaz cleanser 10%	Liquid 10%	3 oz, 6 oz, 12 oz

BENZOYL PEROXIDE GELS (2.5%)

PRODUCT	BASE	PACKAGING
Benzac AC 2.5%	Water	60, 90 gm
Clear By Design (OTC)	Water	45, 90 gm
Desquam-E 2.5	Water	1.5 oz
PanOxyl AQ 2.5	Water	60, 120 gm

BENZOYL PEROXIDE GELS (3%, 4%, 6%, 8%)

PRODUCT	BASE	PACKAGING
Brevoxyl 4%	Water	42.5, 90 gm
Brevoxyl 8%	Water	42.5, 90 gm
Triaz 3%	Glycerin	1.5 oz
Triaz 6%	Glycerin	1.5 oz

BENZOYL PEROXIDE GELS (5%)

PRODUCT	BASE	PACKAGING
Benoxyl 5 (OTC)	Water	1, 2 oz
Benzac 5	12% alcohol	60 gm
Benzac AC 5%	Water	60, 90 gm
Benzac W 5	Water	60, 90 gm
5-Benzagel	14% alcohol	42.5, 85 gm
Desquam-X 5	Water	45, 90 gm
Desquam-E 5	Water	1.5 oz
PanOxyl 5	20% alcohol	60, 120 gm
PanOxyl AQ 5	Water	60, 120 gm
Sulfoxyl Regular 5 (contains 2.5% sulfur)	Water	30 ml

BENZOYL PEROXIDE GELS (10%)

PRODUCT	BASE	PACKAGING
Benzac 10	12% alcohol	60 gm
Benzac AC 10%	Water	60, 90 gm
Benzac W 10	Water	60, 90 gm
10-Benzagel	14% alcohol	42.5, 85 gm
Desquam-X 10	Water	42.5, 85 gm
Desquam-E 10	Water	1.5 oz
PanOxyl 10	20% alcohol	60, 120 gm
PanOxyl AQ 10	Water	60, 120 gm
Sulfoxyl Strong 10 (contains 5% sulfur)	Water	2 oz
Triaz 10	Glycerin	1.5 oz

TOPICAL ANTIBIOTICS FOR ROSACEA

PRODUCT	ANTIBIOTIC	PACKAGING
MetroCream	Metronidazole 0.75%	1.5-oz tube
MetroGel	Metronidazole 0.75%	1-, 1.5-oz tube
Metrolotion	Metronidazole 0.75%	2-oz bottle
Noritate cream	Metronidazole 1.0%	1-oz tube
Sulfacet-R lotion	Sodium sulfacetamide/ sulfur	25 gm
Plexion cleanser	Sodium sulfacetamide/ sulfur	6, 12 oz

TOPICAL ANTIBIOTICS FOR ACNE

PRODUCT	ANTIBIOTICS	BASE	PACKAGING
Akne-Mycin	2% erythromycin	68% alcohol	60 ml liquid
Akne-Mycin	2% erythromycin	2% ointment	25 gm
A/T/S	2% erythromycin	66% alcohol	60 ml liquid
A/T/S	2% erythromycin	92% alcohol	30 gm gel
Benzamycin	3% erythromycin 5% benzoyl peroxide	16% alcohol	23.3 gm gel
Cleocin T	1% clindamycin	50% alcohol	30, 60 ml liquid 30, 60 ml gel
Cleocin T	1% clindamycin	Water based	60 ml lotion
Cleocin T	1% clindamycin	50% alcohol	#60 pledgets
Erycette	2% erythromycin	66% alcohol	#60 swabs
EryDerm	2% erythromycin	77% alcohol	60 ml liquid
Erygel	2% erythromycin	92% alcohol	30, 60 gm gel
Erymax	2% erythromycin	66% alcohol	2, 4 oz liquid
Staticin	1.5% erythromycin	55% alcohol	60 ml liquid
Theramycin Z	2% erythromycin	Zinc acetate	60 ml liquid
Topicycline	2% tetracycline	40% alcohol	70 ml liquid
T-Stat	2% erythromycin	71.2% alcohol	60 ml liquid
T-Stat	2% erythromycin	71.2% alcohol	#60 swabs

DRYING-KERATOLYTIC PREPARATIONS

PRODUCT	SULFUR	SODIUM SULFACETAMIDE	PACKAGING
Novacet lotion	5%	10%	30-, 60-gm tube
Sulfacet-R lotion	5%	10%	25 gm
Sulfacet-R lotion (tint free)	5%	10%	25 gm
Klaron lotion	0%	10%	2 oz

MEDICATED BAR AND LIQUID CLEANSERS FOR ACNE

PRODUCT	ACTIVE INGREDIENT	PACKAGING
Acne-Aid Cleansing Bar	6.3% surfactant	4-, 5.8-oz bars
Fostex bar	2% sulfur	Bar
Neutrogena Oil-Free Acne Wash	2% salicylic acid	6-oz pump
Seba-Nil	Oil-removing base	8-, 16-oz bottles
SalAc	2% salicylic acid	6-oz bottle

ISOTRETINOIN (ACCUTANE)

Accutane capsules   10 mg   20 mg   40 mg

Dosing Isotretinoin by Body Weight

BODY WEIGHT		TOTAL (MG/DAY)		
KILOGRAMS	POUNDS	0.5 MG/KG	1 MG/KG	2 MG/KG
40	88	20	40	80
50	110	25	50	100
60	132	30	60	120
70	154	35	70	140
80	176	40	80	160
90	198	45	90	180
100	220	50	100	200

■ ANTIBIOTICS (ORAL)

GENERIC NAME	BRAND NAME	PREPARATION*	ADULT DOSAGE (MG, UNLESS NOTED)
Cephalosporins			
First-generation			
Cephradine	Velosef	250, 500 mg	1-2 gm/24h (bid, qid)
Cephalexin	Keflex	250, 500 mg	250-1000 qid
Cefadroxil	Duricef	500, 1000 mg	1 gm/day in single (qd) or divided (bid) doses
Second-generation			
Cefaclor	Ceclor	250, 500 mg	250-500 tid
Cefuroxime	Ceftin	125, 250, 500 mg	250-500 bid
Cefprozil	Cefzil	250, 500 mg 125 mg/5 ml 250 mg/5 ml	250 bid-500 qd
Third-generation			
Cefixime	Suprax	200, 400 mg	200 bid, 400 qd
Fluoroquinolones			
Ofloxacin	Floxin	200, 300, 400 mg	200-400 mg q12hr
Ciprofloxacin	Cipro	500, 750 mg	500-750 bid
Macrolides			
Erythromycin (erythromycin ethylsuccinate)	EES	250, 400 mg	250-800 qid*
Erythromycin (enteric coated)	ERYC, Ery-Tab, E-Mycin	125, 250, 330, 500 mg	250-500 q6h*
Clarithromycin	Biaxin	250, 500 mg	250-500 mg bid
Azithromycin	Zithromax	250 mg	500 mg first day 250 qd for 3-4 days
Dynabac	Dirithromycin	250 mg	500 mg qd for 5-7 days
Penicillins			
Ampicillin	Amcill	250, 500 mg	250-500 qid
Penicillin V	Pen-Vee K, etc.	250, 500 mg	250-500 qid
Dicloxacillin	Dynapen	125, 250, 500 mg	125-500 q6h
Cloxacillin	Generic	250, 500 mg	500 mg qid
Amoxicillin	Generic	250, 500 mg	250-500 tid
Amoxicillin clavulanate	Augmentin	250, 500 mg	250-500 q8h

■ ANTIBIOTICS (ORAL)—cont'd

Generic Name	Brand Name	Preparation*	Adult Dosage (mg, unless noted)
Sulfonamides, sulfones			
Sulfamethoxazole-trimethoprim	Bactrim DS, Septra DS	800 mg/160 mg	1 tablet bid
Dapsone	Generic	25, 100 mg	50-300 mg qid
Tetracyclines			
Clindamycin	Cleocin	75, 150, 300 mg	150-300 q6hr
Demeclocycline	Declomycin	150 mg	150 mg qid or 300 mg bid
Doxycycline	Monodox, Vibramycin	50, 100 mg	100-200/24 hr (qd-bid)
Minocycline	Minocin, Dynacin	50, 75, 100 mg	100-200/24 hr (qd-bid)

*Many preparations available in liquid form.

■ ANTIBIOTICS (TOPICAL)

Topical antibiotics for acne are listed on p. 507.

Generic Name	Brand Name	Preparation*
Bacitracin	Baciguent ointment	15, 30, 120 gm
Clioquinol (iodochlorhydroxyquin)	Vioform cream, ointment	15, 30 gm
Gentamycin	Garamycin cream, ointment	15 gm
Iodoquinol and 0.5% or 1% HC	Vytone	1-oz tube
Metronidazole	MetroGel	1 oz, 45 gm
Mupirocin 2%	Bactroban cream, ointment	15, 30 gm
Neomycin	—	7.5-60 gm
Nitrofurazone	Furacin cream, ointment, solution	28 gm, 480 gm, pt, gal
Polymyxin and bacitracin	Polysporin ointment (many brands)	15, 30 gm (ointment)
	Neosporin powder	10 gm (powder)
Polymyxin, neomycin, and bacitracin	Neosporin (many brands)	15, 30 gm
Povidone-iodine	Betadine ointment	30 gm
Silver sulfadiazine	Silvadene creme	20, 50, 400, 1000 gm
Sulfacetamide sodium	Sebizon lotion	85 gm
Tetracycline HCl	Achromycin ointment	14.2, 30 gm

■ ANTIFUNGAL AGENTS (ORAL)

Brand Name	Generic Name	Packaging
Diflucan	Fluconazole	50, 100, 150, 200, mg, 10 mg/ml
Fulvicin-U/F	Griseofulvin microsize	250, 500 mg
Grifulvin V	Griseofulvin microsize	250, 500 mg; 125 mg/5 ml in 4-oz bottle
Grisactin	Griseofulvin microsize	250, 500 mg
Fulvicin-P/G	Griseofulvin ultramicrosize	125, 165, 250, 330 mg
Gris-PEG	Griseofulvin ultramicrosize	125, 250 mg
Grisactin Ultra	Griseofulvin ultramicrosize	125, 250, 330 mg
Nizoral	Ketoconazole	200 mg
Lamisil	Terbinafine	250 mg
Sporanox	Itraconazole	100 mg
Mycelex troches for oral *Candida*		10 mg troche; bottle of 70 or 140 Dissolve 5/day in mouth for 14 days

■ ANTIFUNGAL AGENTS (TOPICAL)
Topical Agents Active Against Dermatophytes and *Candida*

Brand Name	Generic Name	Packaging
Exelderm	Sulconazole	15, 30, 60 gm cream
		30 ml solution
Fungoid Crème	Miconazole	2 oz cream
Halotex	Haloprogin	15, 30 gm cream
Lamisil	Terbinafine	15, 30 gm cream
Loprox	Ciclopirox olamine	15, 30, 90 gm cream
		30, 60 ml lotion
		30, 45 gm gel
Lotrimin	Clotrimazole	15, 30, 45, 90 gm cream
		10, 30 ml lotion
Lotrisone*	Clotrimazole and betamethasone dipropionate	15, 45 gm cream
Monistat-Derm	Miconazole	15, 30, 90 gm cream
		30, 60 ml lotion
Mentax	Butenafine	15 gm, 30 gm
Naftin	Naftifine	15, 30, 60 gm cream
		20, 40, 60 gm gel
Nizoral	Ketoconazole	15, 30, 60 gm
Oxistat	Oxiconazole	15, 30, 60 gm cream
		30 ml lotion
Penlac (for onychomycosis)	Ciclopirox	3.3 ml
Spectazole	Econazole	15, 30, 85 gm cream

*A preparation containing an antifungal agent and potent topical steroid; it is useful for inflamed fungal infections. Potent topical steroids should be used only for short durations in intertriginous areas such as the groin. The physician should change to an antifungal agent once inflammation is controlled.

Topical Agents Active Against *Candida*

Brand Name	Generic Name	Packaging
Fungoid Tincture	Miconazole	2-oz bottle liquid
Mycostatin	Nystatin	15, 30 gm cream
		15, 30 gm ointment
		60 ml suspension (oral)
Mycolog II*	Nystatin and triamcinolone	15, 30, 60, 120 gm cream or ointment
Mycelex troches†	Clotrimazole	10 mg troche
		Bottle of 70 or 140

*A preparation containing an anti-*Candida* agent and topical steroid, it is useful for inflamed yeast infections. Topical steroids should be used only for short durations in intertriginous areas such as the groin. The physician should change to an anti-*Candida* agent once inflammation is controlled.
†Dissolve in mouth 5/day for 14 days.

■ ANTIHISTAMINES

GENERIC NAME	BRAND NAME	PREPARATION	ADULT DOSAGE	SEDATIVE EFFECT
First-generation*				
Alkylamines				
Brompheniramine	Dimetane	4 mg	4 mg q4-6hr	+
		8 mg, TR	q8-12hr	
		12 mg, TR	q12hr	
		2 mg/5 ml	Up to 24 mg/24 hr	
		10 mg/ml injection		
Chlorpheniramine	Chlor-Trimeton	4 mg	4-8 mg q4-12hr	+
		8 mg, TR	Up to 24 mg/day	
		12 mg, TR		
		2 mg/5 ml		
		10 mg/ml injection		
		for IV, IM, or SC		
		100 mg/ml injection		
		for IM or SC		
Dexchlorpheniramine	Polaramine	4 mg	2 mg q4-6hr	+
		4 mg, TR	4 mg q8-12hr	
			6 mg, TR	
		6 mg q8-12hr		
		2 mg/5 ml		
		1.25 mg/5 ml		
Ethanolamines				
Clemastine	Tavist-1	1.34 mg	1.34-2.68 mg q8-12hr	++
	Tavist	2.68 mg		
		0.67 mg/5 ml		
Diphenhydramine	Benadryl	25 mg	25-50 mg q6-8hr	+++
		50 mg		
			12.5 mg/tsp	
		10 mg/ml injection		
		50 mg/ml injection		
Ethylenediamine				
Tripelennamine	PBZ	25 mg	25-50 mg q4-6hr up to	++
		50 mg	600 mg/d	
		37.5 mg/5 ml		
Phenothiazine				
Promethazine	Phenergan	12.5 mg	12.5 mg q8hr	+++
		25 mg	25 mg qhs	
Piperazines				
Hydroxyzine HCl	Atarax	10, 25, 50, 100 mg	10-100 mg q4-8hr	+
Hydroxyzine pamoate	Vistaril Pamoate	10, 25, 50, 100 mg	10-100 mg q4-8hr	+
Piperidines				
Azatadine	Optimine	1 mg	1-2 mg q12hr	++
Cyproheptadine	Periactin	4 mg	4-8 mg q8hr up to	+
			32 mg/day	
		2 mg/5 ml		

*Bind nonselectively to central and peripheral H1 receptors and can result in central nervous system stimulation or depression.

TR, Timed release.

■ ANTIHISTAMINES—cont'd

Generic Name	Brand Name	Preparation	Adult Dosage	Sedative Effect
First-generation*—cont'd				
H1 and H2 blockers				
Doxepin	Adapin	10 mg 25 mg	10-25 mg q6-8hr	+++
Doxepin	Zonalon	30-gm tubes: cream	qid	+
Second-generation†				
Citirizine	Zyrtec	5 mg, 10 mg	5-10 mg qd	−+
Fexofenadine	Allegra	60, 180 mg	60 mg bid 180 mg qd	
Loratadine	Claritin	10 mg	10 mg qd	−+

†Selective for peripheral H1 receptors and are less sedating.

■ ANTINEOPLASTIC AGENTS (TOPICAL)

Product	Fluorouracil	Packaging
Efudex	2% fluorouracil	10 ml liquid
	5% fluorouracil	10 ml liquid
	5% fluorouracil	25 gm cream
Fluoroplex	1% fluorouracil	30 ml solution
	1% fluorouracil	30 gm cream

■ ANTIPERSPIRANTS

Brand Name	Active Ingredient	Packaging
Certain-dri (OTC)	Aluminum chloride (hexahydrate)	1-, 2-oz roll-on Pump spray nonaerosol
Drysol (Rx)	20% aluminum chloride (hexahydrate) in 93% anhydrous ethyl alcohol 35-ml bottle with Dab-O-Matic applicator	37.5-ml bottle
Xerac AC (Rx)	6.25% aluminum chloride (hexahydrate) in 96% anhydrous ethyl alcohol	35-, 60-ml bottles with Dab-O-Matic applicator

■ ANTIPRURITIC LOTIONS AND CREAMS

Brand Name	Active Ingredient	Packaging
Itch-X	1% pramoxine	35.4 gm gel; 60 ml spray
PrameGel	1% pramoxine, 0.5% menthol	118 gm gel
Prax	1% pramoxine	15, 120, 240 ml lotion; 113.4 gm, 1 pound cream
Sarna	0.5% each of camphor and menthol	7.5-oz bottle
Zonalon (Rx)	5% doxepin hydrochloride	30, 45 gm cream

■ ANTIVIRAL AGENTS

Famvir (famciclovir)	125-, 250-, 500-mg tablets
Valtrex (valacyclovir)	500-mg, 1-gm capsules
Zovirax (acyclovir)	200-, 400-, 800-mg capsules
Zovirax ointment 5%	3- and 15-gm tubes
Denavir (penciclovir) ointment	2-gm tube

TOPICAL THERAPY FOR POSTHERPETIC NEURALGIA

Zostrix (capsaicin, 0.025% cream)	1.5 oz, 3 oz tubes (OTC)

■ DEPIGMENTING AND COSMETIC COVERING AGENTS
SKIN BLEACHES AND DEPIGMENTING AGENTS

BRAND NAME	ACTIVE INGREDIENT	SUN PROTECTANT	PACKAGING
Benoquin cream (Rx)*	20% monobenzone	None	114-oz tube
Eldopaque Forte 4% cream (Rx)†	4% hydroquinone	Sunblock	1-oz tube
Eldoquin Forte 4% cream (Rx)	4% hydroquinone	None	1-oz tube
Lustra	4% hydroquinone	None	1-, 2-oz jar
Lustra-AF	4% hydroquinone	Sunscreen	1-, 2-oz jar
Melanex topical solution‡	3% hydroquinone	None	1-oz bottle
Solaquin Forte 4% cream (Rx)	4% hydroquinone	Sunscreen	1-oz tube
Solaquin Forte 4% gel (Rx)	4% hydroquinone	Sunscreen	1-oz tube
Ultraquin	Hydroquinone crystals for compounding		

*Indicated for extensive vitiligo to depigment entire body.
†Flesh-tinted cream base.
‡Packaged with a narrow plastic, broad-tipped sponge applicator

MASKING AGENTS (COSMETIC COVERING AGENTS)

BRAND NAME	BASE	PACKAGING	SHADES
Covermark* (www.covermark.com)	Cream Stick Crayon	Many products	15 different shades
Dermablend cover cream* (www.sheen.com)	Cream	Many products	15 different shades
Dy-O-Derm† (www.delasco.com)	Liquid	4 oz	
Vitadye† (http://icncanda.com)	Liquid	15 ml	

*Waterproof concealing makeup.
†A solution for masking vitiligo; transmits most UVA radiation, so it can be used with psoralens in vitiligo therapy.

■ HAIR-RESTORATION PRODUCTS

Rogaine	Minoxidil solution	2%, 5%	60-ml bottle
Propecia	Finasteride	1 mg	

■ LUBRICATING AGENTS
EMOLLIENTS

Emollients are complex mixtures containing many ingredients. They are listed under their primary ingredient.

Emollients Containing Urea

Urea promotes hydration and removal of excess keratin.

PRODUCT	ACTIVE INGREDIENTS	PACKAGING
Carmol 10 lotion	10% urea	6 oz
Carmol 20 cream	20% urea	3 oz
Carmol 40 cream (Rx)	40% urea	1, 3 oz
Nutraplus		
Cream	10% urea	90 gm, 1 lb
Lotion	10% urea	8, 16 oz
U-Lactin	10% urea, lactic acid	2, 4 oz
Ultra Mide lotion	25% urea	8 oz
Ureacin-10 lotion	10% urea, 3% lactic acid	8 oz
Ureacin-20 cream	20% urea, 3% lactic acid	2.5 oz

Emollients Containing Lactic Acid

Lactic acid promotes hydration and removal of excess keratin.

PRODUCT	ACTIVE INGREDIENTS	PACKAGING
Epilyt lotion	5%	4 oz
Lac-Hydrin cream (Rx)	12%	225-gm tube
Lac-Hydrin cream (Rx)	12%	400-gm bottles
Lacticare lotion	5%	8-, 12-oz bottles
Lactinol lotion	10%	12 oz
Lactinol-E cream	10%	4 oz
U-Lactin lotion	—	8 oz

Emollients Containing Glycolic Acid

Glycolic acid promotes hydration and may reserve mild photoaging changes.

PRODUCT	ACTIVE INGREDIENTS	PACKAGING
Aqua Glycolic face cream	10%	2 oz
Aqua Glycolic facial cleanser	—	8, 12 oz
Aqua Glycolic hand/body lotion	14%	4-, 8-oz bottles
Aqua Glycolic shampoo	14%	8 oz
Aqua Glyde astringent	11%	8 oz
Aqua Glyde shave and aftershave	—	4 oz

GEL THAT REMOVES EXCESS KERATIN

Hydrisalic gel, 6% salicylic acid and propylene glycol	1 oz
Keralyt gel, 6% salicylic acid and propylene glycol	1 oz

Emollients Containing Glycerin

Corn Huskers Lotion
Curel Skin Lotion
Keri Light
Nutraderm 30 lotion
Neutrogena Norwegian Formula emulsion (scented and unscented)
Neutrogena Norwegian Formula emulsion hand cream (scented and unscented)
Shepard's Dry Skin Care
Wibi Lotion

Emollients Containing Mineral Oil

Lotions
Cetaphil
Dermassage
Formula 405
Jeri-Lotion
Keri
Lubriderm
Nivea moisturizing
Nivea skin oil
Nutraderm, Nutraderm 30

Creams
Cetaphil
DML Forté
Eucerin
Formula 405
Keri
Lubriderm
Nivea moisturizing
Nutraderm

OINTMENTS

Ointments containing petrolatum
  Aquaphor
  Dermasil lotion, cream
  DML Forté
  Eucerin

Greaseless ointments
  Acid Mantle
  Unibase

BATH OILS

Alpha-Keri therapeutic
Aveeno Bath
Lubath

■ POWDERS, PROTECTING LOTIONS, AND PROTECTING BARRIER CREAMS

POWDERS

Brand Name	Ingredient	Size	Use
Pedi-Dri Topical Powder	Nystatin	2 oz	—
	Talcum		Drying, mildly absorptive
Zeasorb	Talcum, cellulose, acrylic	75, 240 gm	Drying, absorptive
Zeasorb-AF	Talcum, cellulose, acrylic		—
	Miconazole nitrate 2%		—

PROTECTING LOTIONS

Brand Name	Generic Name	Size	Use
Calamine	Zinc oxide, ferric oxide	—	Cooling, drying shake
	Zinc oxide, 12.5% lotion	30, 60 ml	Protecting, lubricating

PROTECTING BARRIER CREAMS

BRAND/GENERIC NAME	SIZE	USE
Chimal skin shield	3, 8 oz	(www.asurefit.com/Chimal_Skin_Shield/index.htm)
Dermaguard	2, 12 oz	Industrial (protects against acids)
Desitin ointment	30, 60, 120, 240, 480 gm	Protective ointment
Ivy Shield	1.25, 4, 16 oz	Helps prevent poison ivy and oak dermatitis
Kerodex 51	120, 480 gm	Protective cream for dry, oily work
Kerodex 71	120, 480 gm	Protective cream (water repellent)
pH-Stabil	60, 240 gm	Protective cream
Zinc oxide		
20% ointment	60 gm	Protective ointment
25% paste	30, 60, 480 gm	Protective paste

■ PSORIASIS AND SEBORRHEIC DERMATITIS SHAMPOOS
ANTIMICROBIAL ANTISEBORRHEIC SHAMPOOS (PYRITHIONE ZINC AND OTHERS)

BRAND NAME	ACTIVE INGREDIENT	PACKAGING
Betadine	7.5% povidone-iodine	118 ml
Capitrol (Rx)	2% chloroxine	85 gm
Danex	1% pyrithione zinc	120 ml
DHS Zinc	2% pyrithione zinc	6, 12 oz
FS Shampoo (Rx)	0.01% fluocinolone acetonide	120 ml
Head & Shoulders	2% pyrithione zinc	51, 75, 120, 210 gm cream
		120, 210, 330, 450 ml lotion
Nizoral	1% (OTC), 2% (Rx) ketoconazole	4 oz
Zincon Dandruff Shampoo	1% pyrithione zinc	120, 240 ml
ZNP Bar	2% pyrithione zinc	4.2-oz bar

ANTISEBORRHEIC PREPARATIONS

BRAND NAME	ACTIVE INGREDIENT	PACKAGING
Nizoral cream	1% (OTC), 2% (Rx) ketoconazole	15, 30, 60 gm
Sebizon	10% Sulfacetamide sodium	85 gm

CORTICOSTEROID, TAR, AND OTHER MEDICATED SCALP PREPARATIONS

BRAND NAME	ACTIVE INGREDIENT	BASE	PACKAGING
Derma-Smoothe/FS (Rx)	Fluocinolone acetonide 0.01%	Peanut oil	120 ml
10% liquor carbonis detergens in nivea oil*	Liquor carbonis detergens, 8, 16 oz	Nivea oil	Prescribe
Neutrogena tar gel solution	2% coal tar, 2% salicylic acid	Alcohol free	2 oz

*Pharmacist compounded.

SELENIUM SULFIDE SHAMPOOS

BRAND NAME	CONCENTRATION	PACKAGING
Exsel	2.5%	120 ml
Head & Shoulders (Intensive Treatment)	1%	15.2 oz
Selsun	2.5%	120 ml
Selsun Blue	1%	120, 210, 330 ml

SULFUR AND SALICYLIC ACID SHAMPOOS

PRODUCT	SULFUR	SALICYLIC ACID	PACKAGING
Ionil Plus	—	2%	240 ml
Meted	5%	3%	120 ml
Sebulex	2 %	2%	120 ml
			120, 240 ml
Sulfoam	2%	—	4, 8, 16 oz
Tiseb	—	2%	8 oz
Vanseb	2%	1%	90 gm cream
			120 ml lotion
Xseb	—	4%	4, 8 oz
P & S	—	2%	4, 8 oz

TAR AND TAR-COMBINATION SHAMPOOS

BRAND NAME	CONCENTRATION	PACKAGING
Denorex	2% coal tar gel	60, 120 ml
	2% coal tar lotion	120, 240 ml
DHS Tar	0.5% coal tar USP	4, 8, 16 oz
DHS Tar gel	0.5% coal tar USP	8 oz
Ionil-T Plus	2% crude coal tar	240 ml
Liquor carbonis detergens	10%-15% coal tar	Any amount in Green soap*
MG 217	5% coal tar, 2% salicylic acid	120, 240 ml
Neutrogena T/gel	2% Neutar	4.4, 8.5, 16 oz
Neutrogena T/gel extra strength	4% Neutar (1% coal tar)	6 oz
Neutrogena T/sal	3% salicylic acid	4.5 oz
Packer's pine tar	0.82% pine tar	180 ml
Pentrax tar	4.3% crude coal tar	120, 240 ml
Pentrax Gold	4% solubilized coal tar	168 ml
Polytar	1% mixture of tars	180, 360 ml
Sebutone	0.5% coal tar, 2% salicylic acid, 2% sulfur	120, 240 gm lotion
Tarsum shampoo	10% LCD	4, 8 oz
Tegrin Medicated	5% coal tar extract	60, 132 ml cream
		112.5, 198 ml lotion
Theraplex T shampoo	1% coal tar	8 oz
Tiseb-T	0.5% coal tar product	—
Vanseb-T	5% coal tar	120 ml lotion
Xseb-T	2% crude coal tar	4, 8 oz
Zetar	1% whole coal tar	180 ml

*Pharmacist compounded.

■ PSORIASIS MEDICATIONS (ORAL)
SORIATANE (ACITRETIN)

Capsules   10, 25 mg

METHOTREXATE

Tablets	2.5 mg	—
Injection	25 mg/ml	2-, 10-ml vials
Preservative-free injection	20 mg	20 mg/vial
Powder for injection	20, 50, 100, 250 mg	20-ml vials or single-use vials

NEORAL (CYCLOSPORINE)

Capsules	25 mg,
Oral solution	100 mg/ml

■ PSORIASIS MEDICATIONS (TOPICAL)
ANTHRALIN (DITHRANOL)

BRAND NAME	CONCENTRATION	BASE	PACKAGING
Anthra-Derm	0.1%, 0.25%, 0.5, 1%	Ointment	42.5-gm tubes
Drithocreme	0.1%, 0.25%, 0.5%	Cream	50-gm tube
Drithocreme HP 1%	1%	Cream	50-gm tube
Dritho-Scalp	0.25%, 0.5%	Cream	50-gm tube*
Micanol	1%	Ointment	50-gm tube

*With special applicator.

TOPICAL VITAMIN D₃ ANALOG

BRAND NAME	ACTIVE INGREDIENT	PACKAGING
Dovonex ointment	Calcipotriene 0.005	30-, 60-, 100-gm tubes
Dovonex cream	Calcipotriene 0.005	30-, 60-, 100-gm tubes
Dovonex solution	Calcipotriene 0.005	60 ml

TOPICAL RETINOIDS

BRAND NAME	ACTIVE INGREDIENT	PACKAGING
Tazorac topical gel 0.05%	Tazarotene	30-, 100-gm tube
Tazorac topical gel 0.1%	Tazarotene	30-, 100-gm tube

TAR-CONTAINING BATH OILS

BRAND NAME	SIZE	PACKAGING
Balnetar	2.5% coal tar	225 ml
Doak Oil	2% tar distillate	237 ml
Cutar Bath	7.5 coal tar	180 ml
Polytar Bath	25% polytar	240 ml
Zetar emulsion (Rx)	30% whole coal tar	177 ml

TAR CREAMS AND SOLUTION

BRAND NAME	CONCENTRATION	OTHER INGREDIENTS	BASE	PACKAGING
Aqua Tar	2.5% coal tar extract	—	Gel (water base)	90 gm
Doak Tar Lotion	5% tar distillate	—	Lotion	4 oz
Estar	5% coal tar	13.8% alcohol	Gel	90 gm
Fototar	2% coal tar, USP	—	Cream	85-gm, 1-lb jar
Ichthyol	10% ichthammol	—	Ointment	30 gm
Liquor carbonis detergens*	20% coal tar solution	—	Solution	4 oz, pt, gal
M G217	5% coal tar, 2% salicylic acid	—	Lotion	120 ml
Oxipor VHC	48.5% coal tar solution	1% salicylic acid	Lotion	2 oz
P & S Plus	8% coal tar solution	2% salicylic acid	Gel	105 gm
Packer's	5.87% pine tar	—	Soap	—
PolyTar Soap	Blend of tars	—	Soap	Bar
Pragmatar	4% coal tar distillate	3% salicylic acid, 3% sulfur	Ointment	—
PsoriGel	7.5% coal tar solution	1% alcohol	Gel	4 oz
T/Derm	5% coal tar extract	Alcohol free	Oil	4 oz
Tegrin Medicated	5% crude coal tar extract	—	Lotion	6 oz
			Cream	60, 132 gm
Unguentum Bossi	5% tar distillate	5% ammoniated Hg	Ointment	60, 480 gm

*Used by the pharmacist for compounding in Unibase and other ointment bases.

GELS THAT REMOVE EXCESS KERATIN

Hydrisalic gel, 6% salicylic acid and propylene glycol   1 oz
Keralyt gel, 6% salicylic acid and propylene glycol   1 oz

■ SCABICIDES AND PEDICULICIDES
SCABICIDES

BRAND NAME	GENERIC NAME	PACKAGING
Elimite	Permethrin	5% cream: 60 gm
Acticin	Permethrin	5% cream: 60 gm
Eurax*	Crotamiton	10% cream: 60 gm
		10% lotion: 2 oz, 1 pt
Kwell	Lindane	1% cream: 1 oz, 2 oz, 16 oz, 1 gal
		1% lotion: 2 oz, 16 oz
Kwell shampoo	Lindane	1% lotion: 1 ox, 2 oz, 16 oz 1 gal
	Sulfur	5%-10% precipitated sulfur in petrolatum†
	Ivermectin	6-mg tablets

*Eurax has been reported to be less effective than lindane.
†Pharmacist compounded.

PEDICULOCIDES

BRAND NAME	GENERIC NAME	PACKAGING
Clear Total Lice Elimination system	0.33% pyrethrins	In kit containing shampoo, lice egg remover, and nit comb
End Lice	0.33% pyrethrins	177 ml
A-200 shampoo (OTC)	0.17% pyrethrins	2-, 4-oz shampoo
NIX cream rinse	Permethrin	2 oz with comb
Ovide	0.5% malathion	2-oz lotion
R & C shampoo (OTC)	0.3% pyrethrins	2-, 4-oz shampoo
RID shampoo (OTC)	0.3% pyrethrins	2, 4, 8 oz
Step 2*	8% formic acid	Cream rinse
	Lindane	Bulk

*For removal of lice eggs (nits); does not kill lice.

■ SHAMPOO: FRAGRANCE FREE, DYE FREE

DHS Clear   8, 16 oz

■ SOAP-FREE CLEANSERS

Often used in the management of atopic dermatitis.

Aquanil lotion	8, 16 oz
Aveeno Cleansing	Bar
Cetaphil lotion	4, 8, 16 oz
Lowila cake	Bar
Neutrogena: nondrying	5.5 oz
SFC lotion	8, 16 oz

■ SOAPS: BAR (MILD, NONIRRITATING)

Alpha-Keri	Dove	Oilatum
Basis glycerin	Neutrogena dry skin	Purpose
Basis superfatted	Nivea Creme	Cetaphil

■ WART MEDICATIONS
KERATOLYTIC COMBINATIONS FOR TREATING WARTS AND MOLLUSCUM CONTAGIOSUM

BRAND NAME	SALICYLIC ACID	LACTIC ACID	PODOPHYLLIN	CANTHARIDIN	PACKAGING
Cantharone Plus	30%	—	5%	1%	7.5 ml
Duofilm	16.7%	16.7%	—	—	15 ml
Verrex	30%	—	10%	—	7.5 ml
Verrusol	30%	—	5%	1%	7.5 ml
Viranol solution	16.7%	16.7%	—	—	10 ml

CANTHARIDIN

BRAND NAME	CANTHARIDIN	PACKAGING
Cantharone	0.7% in film-forming vehicle	7.5 ml
Verr-Canth	0.7% in film-forming vehicle	7.5 ml

SALICYLIC ACID PREPARATIONS FOR TREATING WARTS, CALLUSES, AND HYPERKERATOTIC SKIN (ALL OTC)

BRAND NAME	SALICYLIC ACID	PACKAGING
Compound W Liquid	17%	9.3 ml liquid
Duofilm	17%	15 gm gel
Keralyt	6%	30 gm gel
Mediplast	40%	2" (3" patches
Occlusal-HP	17%	10 ml liquid
Salacid	40%	Plaster
Sal-Acid Plaster	40%	14 pkg
Sal-Plant	17%	14 gm gel
Trans-Ver-Sal PediaPatch	15%	Cartons of 6-mm (20 pads), securing tapes
Trans-Ver-Sal PlantarPatch	15%	Cartons of 20-mm (20 pads), securing tapes, and emery file
Trans-Ver-Sal AdultPatch	15%	Cartons of 6, or 12, (1r 40 pads), securing tapes, and emery file

PODOPHYLLIN/PODOFILOX/IMIQUIMOD

BRAND NAME	PODOPHYLLIN	PACKAGING
Condylox	0.5% podofilox (podophyllotoxin)	3.5 ml gel, solution
Pod-Ben-25	25% in tincture of benzoin	30 ml
Podocon	25% in tincture of benzoin	15 ml
Podofin	25% in tincture of benzoin	7.5 ml
—	Podophyllin in tincture of benzoin or alcohol	Compounded
Aldara	5% imiquimod	250-mg single-use packets

■ WET DRESSINGS

GENERIC/BRAND NAME	ACTIVE INGREDIENT
Acetic acid	Vinegar in 5% acetic acid
Buro-Sol powder	Aluminum acetate
Burow's solution (Domeboro, Bluboro Pedi-Boro, Buro-Sol)	Aluminum acetate
Domeboro otic solution	2% acetic acid (60 ml)
Domeboro powder, Bluboro, Pedi-Boro	Aluminum sulfate, calcium acetate (boxes of 12, 100 packets)
Domeboro tablets, Bluboro, Pedi-Boro	Aluminum sulfate, calcium acetate (boxes of 2, 100 tablets)
Potassium permanganate	0.025%-0.1%, stains skin purple (prepared by pharmacist)
Silver nitrate	0.1%-0.5%, stains skin black (prepared by pharmacist)

Index

M

P

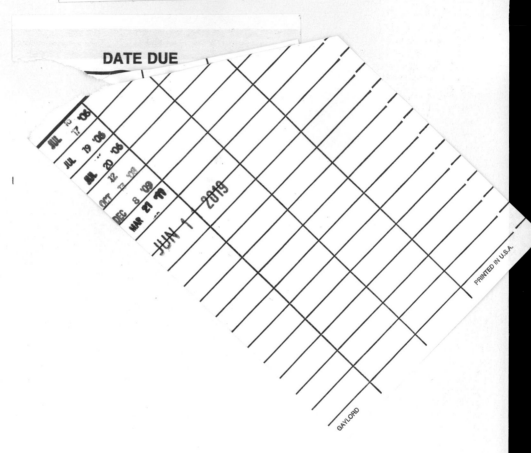

DATE DUE